Motivations Associated with Food Choices and Eating Practices

Motivations Associated with Food Choices and Eating Practices

Editor

Raquel P. F. Guiné

MDPI • Basel • Beijing • Wuhan • Barcelona • Belgrade • Manchester • Tokyo • Cluj • Tianjin

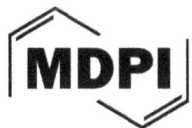

Editor
Raquel P. F. Guiné
CERNAS Research Centre and
Department of Food Industry
Polytechnic Institute of Viseu
Viseu
Portugal

Editorial Office
MDPI
St. Alban-Anlage 66
4052 Basel, Switzerland

This is a reprint of articles from the Special Issue published online in the open access journal *Foods* (ISSN 2304-8158) (available at: www.mdpi.com/journal/foods/special_issues/Motivations_Food_Choices).

For citation purposes, cite each article independently as indicated on the article page online and as indicated below:

LastName, A.A.; LastName, B.B.; LastName, C.C. Article Title. *Journal Name* **Year**, *Volume Number*, Page Range.

ISBN 978-3-0365-1414-7 (Hbk)
ISBN 978-3-0365-1413-0 (PDF)

© 2021 by the authors. Articles in this book are Open Access and distributed under the Creative Commons Attribution (CC BY) license, which allows users to download, copy and build upon published articles, as long as the author and publisher are properly credited, which ensures maximum dissemination and a wider impact of our publications.

The book as a whole is distributed by MDPI under the terms and conditions of the Creative Commons license CC BY-NC-ND.

Contents

About the Editor vii

Preface to "Motivations Associated with Food Choices and Eating Practices" ix

Raquel P. F. Guiné
Motivations Associated with Food Choices and Eating Practices
Reprinted from: *Foods* **2021**, *10*, 834, doi:10.3390/foods10040834 1

Vítor João Pereira Domingues Martinho
Food Marketing as a Special Ingredient in Consumer Choices: The Main Insights from Existing Literature
Reprinted from: *Foods* **2020**, *9*, 1651, doi:10.3390/foods9111651 5

Raquel P. F. Guiné, Sofia G. Florença, Maria João Barroca and Ofélia Anjos
The Link between the Consumer and the Innovations in Food Product Development
Reprinted from: *Foods* **2020**, *9*, 1317, doi:10.3390/foods9091317 27

Raquel P. F. Guiné, Elena Bartkiene, Viktória Szűcs, Monica Tarcea, Marija Ljubičić, Maša Černelič-Bizjak, Kathy Isoldi, Ayman EL-Kenawy, Vanessa Ferreira, Evita Straumite, Małgorzata Korzeniowska, Elena Vittadini, Marcela Leal, Lucia Frez-Muñoz, Maria Papageorgiou, Ilija Djekić, Manuela Ferreira, Paula Correia, Ana Paula Cardoso and João Duarte
Study about Food Choice Determinants According to Six Types of Conditioning Motivations in a Sample of 11,960 Participants
Reprinted from: *Foods* **2020**, *9*, 888, doi:10.3390/foods9070888 49

João P. M. Lima, Sofia A. Costa, Teresa R. S. Brandão and Ada Rocha
Food Consumption Determinants and Barriers for Healthy Eating at the Workplace—A University Setting
Reprinted from: *Foods* **2021**, *10*, 695, doi:10.3390/foods10040695 67

Anca Bacârea, Vladimir Constantin Bacârea, Cristina Cînpeanu, Claudiu Teodorescu, Ana Gabriela Seni, Raquel P. F. Guiné and Monica Tarcea
Demographic, Anthropometric and Food Behavior Data towards Healthy Eating in Romania
Reprinted from: *Foods* **2021**, *10*, 487, doi:10.3390/foods10030487 81

Rungsaran Wongprawmas, Cristina Mora, Nicoletta Pellegrini, Raquel P. F. Guiné, Eleonora Carini, Giovanni Sogari and Elena Vittadini
Food Choice Determinants and Perceptions of a Healthy Diet among Italian Consumers
Reprinted from: *Foods* **2021**, *10*, 318, doi:10.3390/foods10020318 97

Katia Laura Sidali, Roberta Capitello and Akhsa Joanne Taridaasi Manurung
Development and Validation of the Perceived Authenticity Scale for Cheese Specialties with Protected Designation of Origin
Reprinted from: *Foods* **2021**, *10*, 248, doi:10.3390/foods10020248 121

Raquel P. F. Guiné, Sofia G. Florença, Solange Carpes and Ofélia Anjos
Study of the Influence of Sociodemographic and Lifestyle Factors on Consumption of Dairy Products: Preliminary Study in Portugal and Brazil
Reprinted from: *Foods* **2020**, *9*, 1775, doi:10.3390/foods9121775 139

Egle Zokaityte, Vita Lele, Vytaute Starkute, Paulina Zavistanaviciute, Darius Cernauskas, Dovile Klupsaite, Modestas Ruzauskas, Juste Alisauskaite, Alma Baltrusaitytė, Mantvydas Dapsas, Karolina Siriakovaite, Simonas Trunce, Raquel P. F. Guiné, Pranas Viskelis, Vesta Steibliene and Elena Bartkiene
Antimicrobial, Antioxidant, Sensory Properties, and Emotions Induced for the Consumers of Nutraceutical Beverages Developed from Technological Functionalised Food Industry By-Products
Reprinted from: *Foods* **2020**, *9*, 1620, doi:10.3390/foods9111620 . . . . **167**

Ágoston Temesi, Dawn Birch, Brigitta Plasek, Burak Atilla Eren and Zoltán Lakner
Perceived Risk of Fish Consumption in a Low Fish Consumption Country
Reprinted from: *Foods* **2020**, *9*, 1284, doi:10.3390/foods9091284 . . . . **197**

Ana Paula Cardoso, Vanessa Ferreira, Marcela Leal, Manuela Ferreira, Sofia Campos and Raquel P. F. Guiné
Perceptions about Healthy Eating and Emotional Factors Conditioning Eating Behaviour: A Study Involving Portugal, Brazil and Argentina
Reprinted from: *Foods* **2020**, *9*, 1236, doi:10.3390/foods9091236 . . . . **211**

Nikola Tomic, Ilija Djekic, Gerard Hofland, Nada Smigic, Bozidar Udovicki and Andreja Rajkovic
Comparison of Supercritical CO_2-Drying, Freeze-Drying and Frying on Sensory Properties of Beetroot
Reprinted from: *Foods* **2020**, *9*, 1201, doi:10.3390/foods9091201 . . . . **225**

Raquel P. F. Guiné, Sofia G. Florença, Keylor Villalobos Moya and Ofélia Anjos
Edible Flowers, Old Tradition or New Gastronomic Trend: A First Look at Consumption in Portugal versus Costa Rica
Reprinted from: *Foods* **2020**, *9*, 977, doi:10.3390/foods9080977 . . . . **239**

About the Editor

Raquel P. F. Guiné

Raquel Guiné is Director of Research Centre and Full Professor in Food Industry Department. License degree in Chemical Engineering, Master in Engineering Science and PhD in Chemical Engineering, all at University of Coimbra, and Habilitation in Food Science at University of Algarve, Portugal. She is a University Teacher at Polytechnic Institute of Viseu (Portugal), has been President of Scientific Board; President of Assembly of Representatives; Director of Bachelor and Master Courses. Authored: 20 books, 68 chapters, 270 research papers, 292 conference proceedings; presented 28 keynotes, 180 oral communications, and 144 posters. Research interest in Food Engineering, Food Science and Nutrition. Global leader of a team of 69 researchers working for the International Project "EISuFood"involving 18 countries: Brazil, Cape Verde, Colombia, Croatia, Greece, Latvia, Lebanon, Lithuania, Mexico, Morocco, Nigeria, Poland, Portugal, Romania, Serbia, Slovenia, Spain, Turkey.

Preface to "Motivations Associated with Food Choices and Eating Practices"

This book is generally focused on food choice, and which factors are associated with the decisions that define people's eating behaviour. These reasons are highly variable and include influences from the surrounding environment, as well as the individual characteristics of each person. The chapters that compose the book address these issues from different points of view. Some explore the psychology of food choices or the cultural aspects and tradition, as well as the influence of surrounding contexts. Others focus on the role of lifestyle on eating practices and health motivations, but also the food marketing and the sensory aspects of food, as a way to incentive consumption. Finally, sustainability concerns and environmental impacts can also shape and help change people's food choices.

The book was derived from the international project "EATMOT - Psycho-social motivations associated with food choices and eating practices" developed in various countries simultaneously, to study the different psychic and social motivations that determine people's food choices or eating habits. The project addressed, in particular, some key topics: health motivations, economic factors, emotional aspects, cultural influences, marketing and commercials, and environmental concerns. For this reason, the book contains a set of chapters about the outcomes from the project, and authored by its team members. Additionally, some other chapters were authored by scientists external to the project but working on related topics, which enhance the final quality of the book and expand its contents.

Within the chapters gathered on this book you will find key topics that apply to everyday food choices or that can help target food consumption goals towards better health, more sustainable food chains and happier lifestyles.

The Editor would like to thank MDPI publishing for supporting the publication of the book and CI&DETS and CERNAS research centres at Polytechnic Institute of Viseu for approval and financial support to the project EATMOT (references: PROJ/CI&DETS/2016/0008 & PROJ/CI&DETS/CGD/0012).

Raquel P. F. Guiné
Editor

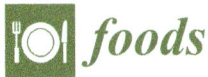

Editorial

Motivations Associated with Food Choices and Eating Practices

Raquel P. F. Guiné

CERNAS Research Centre, Department of Food Industry, Polytechnic Institute of Viseu, 3504-510 Viseu, Portugal; raquelguine@esav.ipv.pt

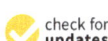

Citation: Guiné, R.P.F. Motivations Associated with Food Choices and Eating Practices. *Foods* **2021**, *10*, 834. https://doi.org/10.3390/foods10040834

Received: 2 April 2021
Accepted: 8 April 2021
Published: 12 April 2021

Publisher's Note: MDPI stays neutral with regard to jurisdictional claims in published maps and institutional affiliations.

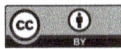

Copyright: © 2021 by the author. Licensee MDPI, Basel, Switzerland. This article is an open access article distributed under the terms and conditions of the Creative Commons Attribution (CC BY) license (https://creativecommons.org/licenses/by/4.0/).

The principal reason that influences people's eating characteristics is to satisfy basic body stimuli, like feeling hunger and the need for satiety. Nevertheless, people's food choices are not determined solely by physiological needs or nutritional demands. Actually, in addition to the central factors that lay behind the act of eating, it is possible to enumerate an extensive diversity of other factors which also condition the food choices. The human behaviors regarding foods are associated with a number of reasons, some of sociological nature and others of psychological essence. Hence, it is important to better understand the different psychic and social motivations that determine people's eating patterns, either in relation to their food choices or to their eating habits. The possible different types of motivations that shape food consumption can include areas such as, but not exclusively, health motivations, economic factors, emotional aspects, cultural influences, marketing and commercials or environmental concerns.

Presently, the close relation between eating habits and the prevention of a large number of pathologies is well-established. Unhealthy diets comprise minimal fruit and vegetable intake and excessive consumption of processed convenience foods high in salt, fat and sugar. However, an excess of fats, sugars or salt has been associated with many chronic diseases [1,2]. It has been demonstrated that eating inappropriate amounts of fats, and particularly saturated and trans fats, constitutes an increased risk of heart diseases such as stroke, atherosclerotic vascular diseases and, in particular, coronary heart disease, cardiac dysfunction (indirect and direct cardiac effects, including inflammation, hypertrophy, fibrosis and contractile dysfunction) or increased LDL (Low Density Lipoproteins) cholesterol and triglycerides. Salt has also been recognized as a major contributor to cardiovascular diseases, as it progressively raises blood pressure levels with age. On the other hand, the presence of added sugars in the diet is associated with an increased risk of obesity and other obesity-related chronic diseases, including type 2 diabetes. Additionally, an excess of weight has been identified as a major risk factor for a range of preventable chronic diseases, including cardiovascular disease, cancer, osteoarthritis or diabetes. On the other hand, the insufficient ingestion of fruits and vegetables, as a result of modern trends towards the consumption of high levels of processed convenience foods, results in deficiencies in vitamins, dietary minerals, dietary fibers and bioactive substances such as, for example, antioxidants, among other extremely important food constituents.

It is unquestionable that food is essential to provide the human body with the energy it needs to function, as well as macro and micro components and bioactive components with major roles in maintaining health. However, food is also recognized as an inseparable part of traditions and culture, as well as social environments, and hence, eating has a strong emotional component. Some people may have had certain eating habits for so long that they do not even realize they are unhealthy. On the other hand, for many people, even if a need to change their eating habits is identified, it might be very hard to do it for a number of reasons: the present habits have become part of their daily life, so they do not think much about them; they want to change but familiar or friends' influences may overcome their intentions; the role of publicity and marketing must also be accounted for; or simply they have become addicted to bad foods and it is difficult to overcome this addiction.

One's emotional status influences all features of human life, and naturally also eating behavior. People tend to establish regular dietary patterns or make different food choices adaptable to their emotional status or temporary moods. Emotional eating is associated with a trend to overeat as a compensation for negative emotions, like, for example, depression, anxiety or irritability. Conversely, for other individuals, feelings of sadness, loneliness or depression can block their appetite, preventing them from ingesting appropriate amounts of the nutrients essential for the correct body functioning. Therefore, emotions assume an incredibly relevant role in people's eating behavior [3,4].

Economic factors have also been demonstrated to have a modulatory effect on eating patterns, evidencing differences, for example, at the level of low household income families when compared to those societies with a higher average income and characterized by a higher level of industrialization [5]. However, other factors, besides price, also contribute to define consumer trends, such as availability or cultural aspects. In the present global markets, food products are commercialized amongst many different countries and across cultures, and the role of tradition is also relevant, especially when it comes to protected regional foods. The willingness to consume traditional food products is directly related to the concept of authenticity and how this is perceived by consumers [6–8].

The sustainability across the food supply chain is also driving modern consumers towards sustainable or green consumer behavior, which relates to food choices that aim at preserving the environment and ecosystems' biodiversity. Sustainable consumers refuse to buy and consume foods that bring detrimental effects to the environment, and instead look for products which cause a minimal impact on the planet, or even that are beneficial for global sustainability. Hence, nowadays a great deal of importance is given to the development of nutritionally improved foods, with good acceptability and which at the same time bear additional environmental impacts. This is the case with the utilization of food industry by-products, that otherwise would have to be discarded, being incorporated into new foods [9].

Funding: FCT—Foundation for Science and Technology, I.P., project Ref^a UIDB/00681/2020.

Acknowledgments: As Guest Editor of the Special Issue "Motivations Associated with Food Choices and Eating Practices", I would like to express my deep appreciation to all authors whose valuable work was published under this issue and thus contributed to the success of this edition. I also would like to leave a word of hope to all other authors who submitted works that were not accepted at this stage, and encourage them to pursue excellence and wish them future triumph.

Conflicts of Interest: The author declares no conflict of interest.

References

1. Wongprawmas, R.; Mora, C.; Pellegrini, N.; Guiné, R.P.F.; Carini, E.; Sogari, G.; Vittadini, E. Food Choice Determinants and Perceptions of a Healthy Diet among Italian Consumers. *Foods* **2021**, *10*, 318. [CrossRef] [PubMed]
2. Bacârea, A.; Bacârea, V.C.; Cînpeanu, C.; Teodorescu, C.; Seni, A.G.; Guiné, R.P.F.; Tarcea, M. Demographic, Anthropometric and Food Behavior Data towards Healthy Eating in Romania. *Foods* **2021**, *10*, 487. [CrossRef] [PubMed]
3. Guiné, R.P.F.; Bartkiene, E.; Szűcs, V.; Tarcea, M.; Ljubičić, M.; Černelič-Bizjak, M.; Isoldi, K.; EL-Kenawy, A.; Ferreira, V.; Straumite, E.; et al. Study about Food Choice Determinants According to Six Types of Conditioning Motivations in a Sample of 11,960 Participants. *Foods* **2020**, *9*, 888. [CrossRef] [PubMed]
4. Lima, J.P.M.; Costa, S.A.; Brandão, T.R.S.; Rocha, A. Food Consumption Determinants and Barriers for Healthy Eating at the Workplace—A University Setting. *Foods* **2021**, *10*, 695. [CrossRef] [PubMed]
5. Cardoso, A.P.; Ferreira, V.; Leal, M.; Ferreira, M.; Campos, S.; Guiné, R.P.F. Perceptions about Healthy Eating and Emotional Factors Conditioning Eating Behaviour: A Study Involving Portugal, Brazil and Argentina. *Foods* **2020**, *9*, 1236. [CrossRef] [PubMed]
6. Guiné, R.P.F.; Florença, S.G.; Barroca, M.J.; Anjos, O. The Link between the Consumer and the Innovations in Food Product Development. *Foods* **2020**, *9*, 1317. [CrossRef] [PubMed]
7. Martinho, V.J.P.D. Food Marketing as a Special Ingredient in Consumer Choices: The Main Insights from Existing Literature. *Foods* **2020**, *9*, 1651. [CrossRef] [PubMed]

8. Sidali, K.L.; Capitello, R.; Manurung, A.J.T. Development and Validation of the Perceived Authenticity Scale for Cheese Specialties with Protected Designation of Origin. *Foods* **2021**, *10*, 248. [CrossRef] [PubMed]
9. Zokaityte, E.; Lele, V.; Starkute, V.; Zavistanaviciute, P.; Cernauskas, D.; Klupsaite, D.; Ruzauskas, M.; Alisauskaite, J.; Baltrusaitė, A.; Dapsas, M.; et al. Antimicrobial, Antioxidant, Sensory Properties, and Emotions Induced for the Consumers of Nutraceutical Beverages Developed from Technological Functionalised Food Industry By-Products. *Foods* **2020**, *9*, 1620. [CrossRef] [PubMed]

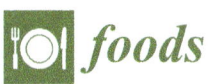

Review

Food Marketing as a Special Ingredient in Consumer Choices: The Main Insights from Existing Literature

Vítor João Pereira Domingues Martinho

Agricultural School (ESAV) and CERNAS-IPV Research Centre, Polytechnic Institute of Viseu (IPV), 3504-510 Viseu, Portugal; vdmartinho@esav.ipv.pt

Received: 26 October 2020; Accepted: 10 November 2020; Published: 12 November 2020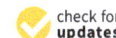

Abstract: The choices and preferences of food consumers are influenced by several factors, from those related to the socioeconomic, cultural, and health dimensions to marketing strategies. In fact, marketing is a determinant ingredient in the choices related to food consumption. Nonetheless, for an effective implementation of any marketing approach, the brands play a crucial role. Creating new brands in the food sector is not always easy, considering the relevant amount of these goods produced within the agricultural sector and in small food industries. The small dimension of the production units in these sectors hinders both brand creation and respective branding. In this context, it would seem important to analyse the relationships between food marketing and consumer choice, highlighting the role of brands in these frameworks. For this purpose, a literature review was carried out considering 147 documents from Scopus database for the topics of search "food marketing" and "choices" (search performed on 16 October 2020). As main insights, it is worth highlighting that the main issues addressed by the literature, concerning food marketing and consumer choices, are the following: economic theory; label and packaging; marketing strategies; agriculture and food industry; market segments; social dimensions; brand and branding. In turn, food marketing heavily conditions consumer choices; however, these related instruments are better manipulated by larger companies. In addition, this review highlights that bigger companies have dominant positions in these markets which are not always beneficial to the consumers' objectives.

Keywords: literature survey; Scopus; brands; consumer preferences

1. Introduction

The food choices by consumers are influenced by several factors, where the prices traditionally have great importance, as highlighted by the economic theory. However, there are new tendencies, and some segments currently privilege healthy [1] and sustainable characteristics [2]. Food consumption has several dimensions, including that of a social and cultural magnitude, and this sometimes compromises policies to change unadjusted behaviours [3] and influence food perceptions [4]. The sociodemographic and behavioural factors also have their implications [5] on consumer behaviour. On the other hand, labelling and packaging have a significant impact on consumer choices and preferences [6].

In these contexts, marketing strategies are useful and powerful approaches in order to create and maintain a market in any economic sector and, specifically, in the food industry [7]. However, in the food market, it is important to distinguish two production sectors, agriculture and industry. These two distinct sectors with different dynamics have implications on the respective markets. This is important to highlight, because this makes the food sector different from other economic sectors.

Agriculture has several particularities that constrain the design of effective marketing plans. In fact, the structural context of farms, often, in small dimensions, in great numbers and the producing commodities are limited in the ability to create a custom positioning, a crucial ingredient for any marketing approach. The main problem of this atomised structure is associated with the reduced individual level of production, focused on parts of the year that prove difficult to maintain a regular presence in the market and the respective branding. These weaknesses of the sector limit the market choices of farmers [8]. Of course, the brand and the agricultural sector are only a part of the food marketing framework.

In turn, the food industry is often conditioned to be more competitive and to generate value added through the creation of brands. In fact, this is a sector with the dynamics and the competitiveness predicted by the economic theory for the industry, i.e., as having activities with increasing returns to scale. The performance in terms of productivity and efficiency allows for another presence in the markets and possibilities to further develop marketing plans and strategies for a more sustainable development [9].

Considering that marketing approaches influence consumer food choices, the literature survey highlights the relevance of a systematic review concerning two dimensions: food marketing and consumer choices, taking into account the specificities of the two sectors related to food production.

From this perspective, the research carried out intends to highlight the main insights from the scientific literature into the relationships between food marketing and the choices of consumption performed by consumers. To achieve this objective, 147 documents (only articles and reviews) from the Scopus database [10] were obtained, considering as topics for searches carried out on 16 October 2020 "food marketing" and "choices". These documents were analysed through a literature survey. To better perform the literature analysis, a previous bibliographic analysis and literature survey were considered, and this approach allowed for organisation of the literature review with the following structure: economic theory; label and packaging; marketing strategies; agriculture and food industry; market segments; social dimensions; brand and branding. This approach was complemented using the PRISMA (Preferred Reporting Items for Systematic Reviews and Meta-Analyses) methodology [11]. For the PRISMA approach, 137 documents (only articles and reviews) were also considered from the Web of Science Core Collection [12] for the same topics. When the documents from Scopus and Web of Science were considered together, through the Zotero software [13], a great majority were duplicated (around 100). From this perspective, considering the relevant number of documents duplicated across the two scientific databases and the Scopus platform having more documents, the decision was made to opt only for the documents from this database. The topics of search "food marketing" and "choices" were selected to find documents in the scientific databases related to the interrelationships between food marketing and consumer choices. The search topics "food", "marketing", and "choices" could be considered, for instance, but this search option would greatly increase the number of documents found, taking the level to an infeasible amount for a literature review; furthermore, the studies obtained were outside the intended scope ("food marketing").

2. Bibliographic Sample Characterisation

The information presented in this section is relative to a sample obtained from the Scopus database for a search carried out with the following topics/keywords: "food marketing" and "choices". In addition, it is important to highlight that the identification of the sample and its analysis considered other scientific contributions concerning systematic reviews [14–17].

The number of documents related to the topics considered has increased from 1970 until today, with relevant breaks in 2013 and 2016, with a total of 16 documents in 2020 (Figure 1). This context shows that there are opportunities to increase the number of documents published with regard to these fields, considering the annual average number of studies published and the relevance of the topics.

A large part of the documents focused on subject areas such as the following (Figure 2): medicine; nursing; agricultural and biological sciences; business, management and accounting; psychology; social sciences; economic, econometrics, and finance; and environmental science. This framework reveals the multidisciplinary dimension of the issues related with the topics addressed here.

The majority of the studies were carried out by authors affiliated to institutions from the United States, Australia, the United Kingdom, Canada, Italy, New Zealand, Belgium, China, and Germany

(Figure 3). The several dimensions associated with these topics are relevant to several countries around the world. In this way and considering the values presented in Figure 3, there are opportunities to be further explored regarding these topics by affiliated authors in institutions from important countries, such as, China, India, Brazil, and the European Union member-states.

Source titles having two or more documents are those presented in Figure 4. The following journals were noted: Appetite (13); Public Health Nutrition (8); Food Quality and Preference (5); Nutrients (5); British Food Journal (4); Childhood Obesity (3); Journal of the Academy of Nutrition and Dietetics (3); Obesity Reviews (3).

Figure 5 was obtained using VOSviewer software [18,19] with the 147 documents obtained from the Scopus database. This figure was obtained using bibliographic data for co-occurrence links and all keyword items. In this figure, the circle/label size represents the number of keyword occurrences, and relatedness (proximity of circles/labels) is determined on the basis of the number of documents in which the keywords occur together [19]. Figure 5 highlights the relevance of keywords, for example, obesity, child, advertising, review, interview, adolescents, market, policy, labelling, perception, willingness to pay, health, choice experiment, index method, case study, apps, and television. These keywords reveal some relevant dimensions related to food and marketing and consumer choices (obesity, health, children and youths, labelling, perceptions, taste, willingness to pay, policies, and media) and some methodological approaches (review, interview, choice experiment, index method, and case study). On the other hand, there is a great amount of relatedness (number of documents in which the keywords occur together) between food marketing and human obesity, especially in men and children.

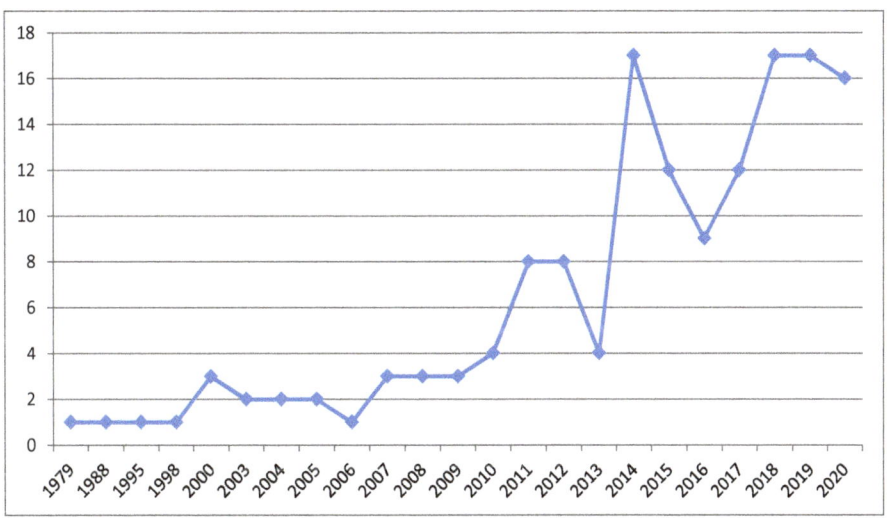

Figure 1. Distribution of the documents across years.

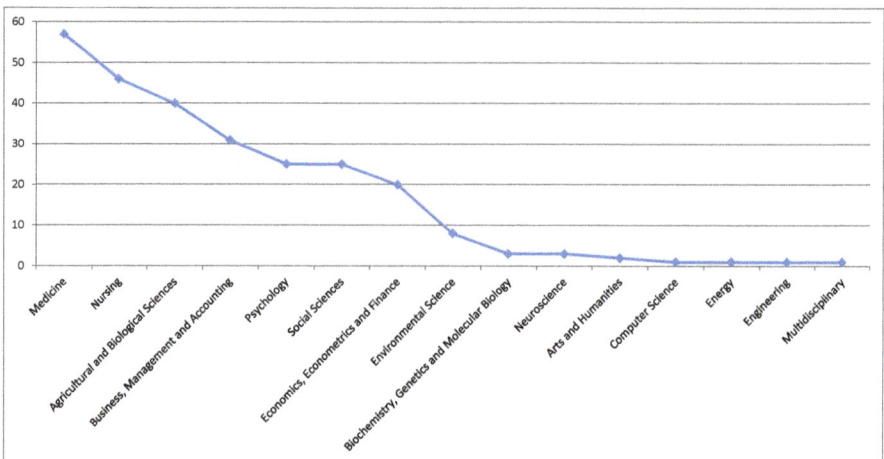

Figure 2. Distribution of the documents across subject areas.

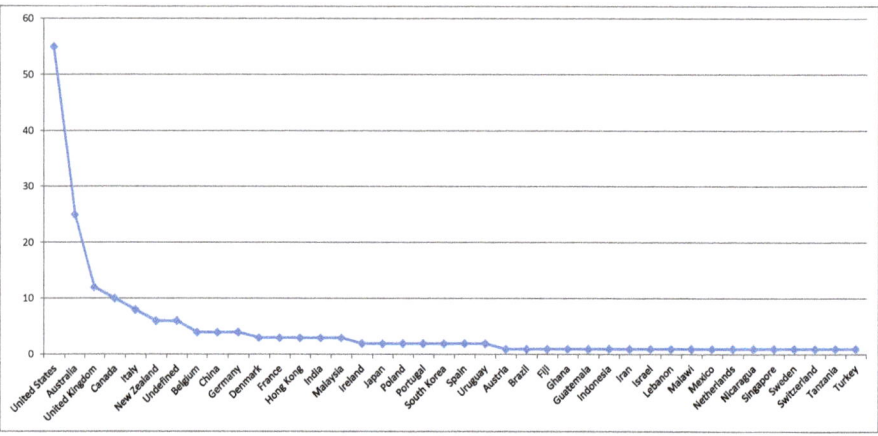

Figure 3. Distribution of the documents across countries.

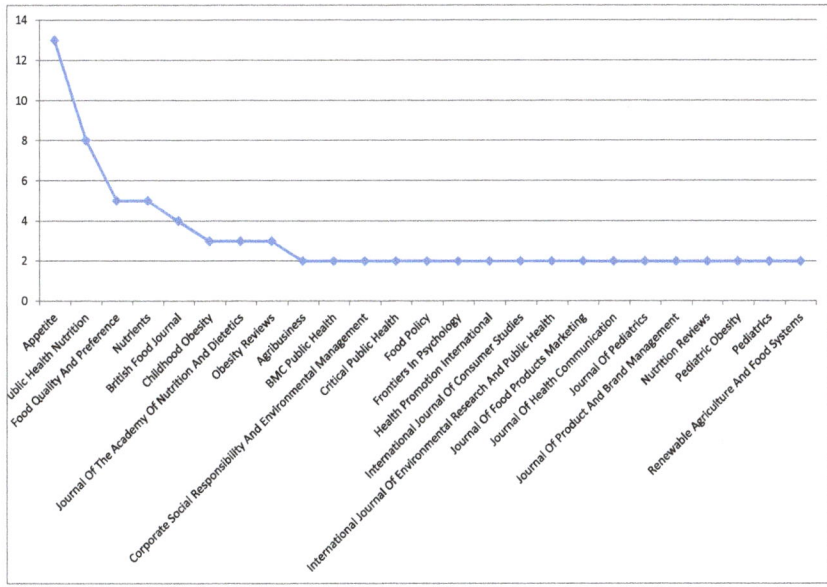

Figure 4. Source titles with two or more documents.

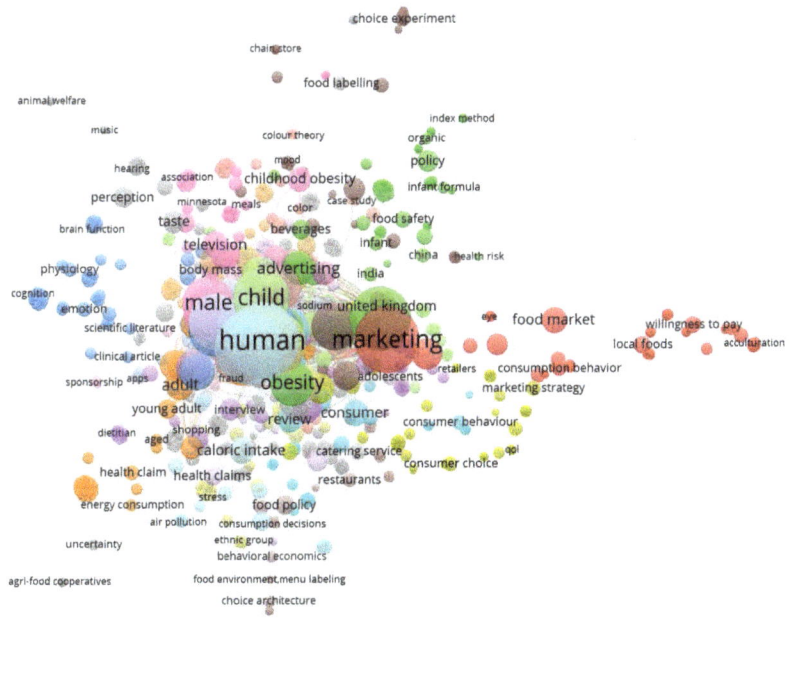

Figure 5. Co-occurrences of all keywords (one as a minimum number of occurrences of a keyword).

3. Literature Survey

Considering the bibliographic analysis and a preliminary literature survey, this section is divided into the following subsections: economic theory; labelling and packaging; marketing strategies; agriculture and food industry; market segments; social dimensions; brand and branding.

3.1. Economic Theory

As predicted by the theory of demand, the consumption of goods and services by consumers to satisfy their daily needs is dependent on market prices. In addition, the theory of utility explains that, when consumers intend to satisfy their needs, they also expect to maximise utility, depending on their income. This is true in every market, including in the food markets from low-income countries [20]. Consumer demand is dependent on several factors, but the prices (own product, substitute product, and complementary product prices) are amongst the most important variables. Of course, other variables, such as product quality and the economic conjuncture of each country, have their influences on consumption. In these frameworks, consumers combine quantities of goods and services so as to obtain the maximum satisfaction from their consumption. The level of satisfaction achieved is dependent on the available revenue to consume. The economic theory assumes that the economic agents are rational, and this means that consumers want to consume more when prices are lower with the exception of luxury products or goods and services of basic needs [21]. The marketing plans, in general, bear these contexts in mind, because the consideration of these fields is determinant for a successful strategy in the food sector.

On the other hand, some dimensions are multidisciplinary and networked, such as those, for example, related to welfare [22]. Welfare is, in fact, the focus of research for several disciplines such as biology, economy, psychology, and sociology. This transversal perspective could prove interesting as a means for cross-approaches, including insights from economic theory, to promote more adjusted patterns of food consumption, mainly those more compatible with health requirements [23]. The impact on health from food consumption is a concern for several stakeholders; however, it is not an easy challenge to mitigate these implications, due to the market power of certain stronger brands.

Economic options and the respective economic dynamics, with consequences on prices and on consumer incomes, have direct and indirect impacts on food choices and, consequently, on the health of the respective population [24]. In turn, the economic theory may provide interesting insights for more effective health policies and programmes that incentivise, in a greater way, food choices which are more compatible with a balanced human life environment [25]. The economic theory may also be a relevant ally towards supporting better knowledge about company frameworks for a more effective market and marketing approaches [26].

The price elasticities, for example, may provide relevant support in these strategies and enable us to predict future patterns of food consumption [27]. The prices do indeed have a determinant impact on food markets [28], despite their particular price and income elasticities. In general, the food markets, specifically, those more linked with the production sector (agriculture), have lower, inelastic price elasticities. This means that the consumers are not sensitive in their consumption to price changes, mainly due to the fact that food products are often essential goods and services of basic needs and where the prices are lower. The same happens for income elasticities, meaning that, when consumers have more revenue, they have a tendency to increase their consumption of products other than food goods. In other words, when consumer income increases, they are willing to increase industrial and service consumption rather than consume more food [21]. This is a great task for the food industry, where the brand and respective branding are called upon here to play their contribution, whilst sometimes having implications on consumer health.

3.2. Label and Packaging

Food labelling and packaging are used to inform consumers about the product's characteristics, in accordance with legislation, and for marketing purposes [29], but they may also provide support for healthier choices [30]. The legislation regulates the information which may be considered for labelling, and this can sometimes be too bureaucratic and may bring about additional difficulties to market strategies. For example, in some food/beverage sectors, prior to any change in the label, there needs to be previous approval from the competent institutions, and this limits the strategic tasks of the respective companies, mainly when the intention is to provide something more personalised for the consumers.

Despite this regulation, the objectives of labelling to protect human health are, sometimes, compromised. The labelling text and design condition the perceptions of the consumers about food goods and services and influence their choices [31], especially when questions related to health are implicit [32]. The influence of the label design also has relevance in the perceptions and choices among children [33], where cartoon characters and nutritional statements have their importance [34].

The regional and Mediterranean labels are, in general, designed to promote marketing strategies and highlight product attributes [35]. The regional brands and respective labels are ways to highlight local food characteristics and to create value added in endogenous resources. In fact, the big challenge in some food sectors is to create value added for stakeholders, and these regional brands support the objectives to bring more value added to several operators. In general, these regional brands are umbrella products that promote other endogenous goods and services.

The type of packaging has an influence on consumer perceptions about the healthfulness of the respective food. For example, milk in glass packaging is perceived as being healthier than milk packaged in a carton [36]. Packaging influences children and adults in different ways. For example, for adults, the package size and shape are important attributes, more than the information present on the labels [37]. Different generations have distinct patterns of consumption, and millennials, having a different educational environment, where social media has a great impact, have other preferences and vulnerabilities.

Nonetheless, the labelling and packaging are, in some cases, more useful in aiding consumers to identify healthier food rather than trying to influence them to buy these products [38]. In addition, the presence of cartoons on packages positively influences children to choose fruit and vegetables, but this is unfortunately used more for choices of energy-dense and poor nutritional foods [39]. Cartoon characters on packaging do in fact have a great impact on children's food choices [40]. The taste perceptions are determinant for children's choices, and the packaging design influences these assessments. Children identify the product name, prices, and images as being the most relevant packaging characteristics for their choices [41]. The information that stimulates human sensations, such as images and songs, is powerful in influencing consumers.

Sometimes, some information on the packaging may mislead consumers about the real properties of the food chosen [42] or does not conveniently inform consumers about the nutritional characteristics [43]. This is particularly disturbing in some nutritional and health claims [44]. The messages on the packaging must be clear [45] and appropriate for what the products really are [46].

In general, researchers seem to agree on the need for some control by legislation of the information present on packaging [47], primarily that which promotes unhealthy food choices [48] in children [49]. These concerns are transversal around the world, including, for example, studies carried out in Brazil [50], Australia [51–53], United States (US) [54,55], since the 1970s [56], India [57,58], Philippines [59], Malaysia [60], and Ireland [61]. In any case, the decisions related to regulation towards preventing health issues should bear in mind the international commitments and consequent constraints [62].

From another perspective, health standards are sometimes not uniform across organizations and countries [63]. This may create additional difficulties for the producers and retailers who operate in international markets. It could be important, for example, in the context of the World Trade

Organization or the World Health Organization, to find transversal standards for the domains relative to healthy food attributes.

3.3. Marketing Strategies

Food marketing is an important tool [64] to build and maintain markets through the creation of ties of confidence and loyalty between the producers/sellers and the consumers. Food marketing is dependent on several different dimensions, especially those related to the particularities of the sectors associated with food goods and services; in this way, the marketing plans are no easy task [65].

In any circumstance, the marketing of food as an external factor which influences consumer choices [66] is a powerful instrument that may be used to promote public campaigns, such as those related to healthy eating [67] across the several points of food sale, including restaurant kids' menus [68] and supermarkets [69]. However, for companies, the trade-off between health and profit is not easy to solve and this is visible in many of the strategies adopted.

For example, supermarket checkout areas are especially strategic for marketing plans and deserve special attention in terms of their impact upon human health [70]. From another perspective, the tie-in offers in fast food menus for children could be restricted to healthy promotions [71]. The same concern could be present when sport celebrities are associated with the marketing plans [72] for children and parents [73] or in the criteria used to choose sport sponsors [74]. In turn, in the definition of marketing approaches, the message for healthy food promotions should be clear, well designed, and well oriented [75] to avoid misunderstandings [76], principally by children [77], as well as to obtain the intended objectives [78].

The media is a determinant way to communicate with consumers [79], which calls for adjusted advertising when it comes to promoting healthy consumption. However, often times, the consumers, especially youths, are not prepared to deal with these aggressive forms of publicity [80] and are not able to decide on the most important information [81], explicitly that which is related to nutritional characteristics [82]. In fact, the youth and children who are more engaged with, for example, social media are more vulnerable to being influenced into buying unhealthy food [83].

The marketing strategies designed by food operators are very persuasive, and this implies that the consumers who are exposed to food marketing campaigns seem to be more prone to agreeing with their strategies, including those for unhealthy food choices [84]. The television and internet seem to be the most powerful ways to influence exposed consumers [85], specifically through neuromarketing approaches which encourage children to favour taste when making food choices [86]. Television cooking shows are particularly influential on the consumption patterns of children and the youth [87]. The same happens on children's websites [88] and social media [89]. The taste is, indeed, a decisive ingredient in food marketing strategies [90] and, usually, food marketing uses contexts related to this attribute to design its plans and influence customers.

Neuromarketing is an emergent technique that applies approaches to measure spontaneous reactions [91], with relevant impacts on the consumers' choices [92], especially on young people [93]. The songs, image sequence, and colour are tools usually considered to support neuromarketing policies [94]. The evolution of these approaches allows for current expressions such as "musical flavour" to be normal and accepted by the several stakeholders [95]. Usually, consumers are influenced in their consumption without any perception of this factor. The stimuli for human senses have a strong impact on the consumers' perceptions, and these tools are used to intentionally encourage consumers by marketing professionals in a subconscious way.

Magazines, as well as television and the internet, are powerful ways to advertise to consumers [96], sometimes in a more persuasive way [97]. This is because, in some cases, the control approaches are more focused on television and the internet, whilst the written forms of advertisement are forgotten about although they do have similar tools to influence consumers.

The several strategies related to food marketing have an impact on dietary choices, consumption preferences, and cultural values [98]. These changes in the pattern of consumption, as a consequence of food marketing, are particularly visible in countries that became more vulnerable to external advertisements, due to political, social, or a conjuncture of changes. In any event, a familiar environment and parents' behaviour have a determinant impact on the several food choices [99].

An emerging area in the marketing of food is the guilt-free approach [100]; however, this a multidisciplinary field where several disciplines are called upon to add their contributions. It is important to find food marketing strategies that combine the profit aims of the companies with the health of consumers [101].

3.4. Agriculture and Food Industry

The food industry is interlinked with the agricultural sector, making this sector and its marketing strategy dependent on the options made by the farmers [102], specifically, in terms of farming practices compatible with the environment and animal welfare [103], as well as with the safety of the products themselves [104]. For example, organic farming products may have for the food markets a set of virtues and advantages, relative to conventional agriculture, but may also bring about a set of barriers and difficulties (because of the higher prices, for example) [105]. In any case, farming practices which are compatible with the environment will be the future in many countries around the world, especially in the European Union member-states. In fact, the several measures of the Common Agricultural Policy (CAP), mainly since 1992, have gone in this very direction. Due to structural and environmental problems, the CAP since 1992 has become more directed towards promoting sustainable development in an integrated rural approach, where the agri-environmental (organic farming, integrated production, etc.) measures have gained more relevance. The recent instruments created in the CAP framework, such as Greening, are examples of an agricultural policy which is more concerned about the environment within the European context [106,107].

Nonetheless, the food industry is an interesting way to bring about value added to agriculture, because, in farms, due to their characteristics, marketing strategies have, in certain circumstances, less importance in the market than other factors [108]. Agriculture as a sector of food commodities has additional difficulties in order to be presented into the market in a differentiated way, and this compromises marketing strategies.

The Protected Designation of Origin (PDO) products and the associated producers' organizations are examples that may support some market differentiation and provide more structured and effective marketing strategies [109]. These PDO and the respective certification brands allow for the protection of local and regional food attributes and are interesting tools to create marketing strategies common to the respective stakeholders. Of course, the PDO brands are not the same as individual trademarks, but may bring interesting contributions, primarily for smaller farmers, for example, with more budgetary difficulties to implement strategies complementary to production techniques, to create value added in the markets, and to increase their income.

The broad diversity of farms, in terms of size, characteristics, and organization, makes the agricultural sector specific, with particular dynamics that influence the strategies adopted for food marketing [110]. The different programmes and policies designed for the agricultural sector have relevant impacts on the agriculture industry's dynamics [111] and implicitly on the respective markets [112]. This has been a concern for the several policymakers and policy design in the European Union context bearing in mind these agricultural market characteristics, but it continues to require some further adjustments for some local particularities.

Local markets appear, in general, as great opportunities for farmers who have achieved consumer preference or loyalty, principally in terms of quality [113]. These local markets are relevant ways to shorten the agricultural chain. In certain circumstances, consumers are willing to pay more for local food [114]. Usually, the greater margin of value added in agricultural markets remains with the intermediaries and the retailers. Local markets and short agri-food chains (farm events, farm tourism, farm shops, etc.) may support farmers to maintain a large part of the total amount of value added generated in the markets. Nonetheless, the channels used in the markets depend, in some cases, on their structural characteristics, mainly those linked with their experience in the sector [115].

In the agricultural food industry market, questions sometimes appear such as those related to patriotism, where dimensions associated with food safety may contribute to adjusted marketing strategies that provide support to overcome these aspects [116]. Consumers are concerned with the health impacts of food consumption and, in this way, are sensitive to claims associated with food safety.

For an effective marketing plan in the agricultural sector, considering their specificities, the associations and cooperatives are fundamental, when well managed and organised. However, sometimes, the management structure of these organizations is not the best adjusted, and this has consequences on the sector's performance [117]. The associations and cooperatives are crucial for technical support to the farmers and to concentrate the agricultural supply of the farmers who have worse conditions and dimensions in terms of storing production. On the other hand, the output concentration allows further capacity to negotiate contracts and prices with retailers.

The new technologies of information and communication may be useful tools to support marketing strategies in farms, and some farmers are indeed willing to pay for electronic platforms [118]. Social media is one of the cheaper and easier ways to promote food products, and this may be used without relevant difficulties by the several stakeholders. Some years ago, publicity and advertising were expensive and restricted to the traditional means of communication, such as television, radio, newspapers, and magazines.

3.5. Market Segments

Food markets are characterised by heterogeneous segments of consumers [119], involving a great diversity of realities [120], some more sensitized to health statements and others more influenced by nutritional information [121]. These contexts bring about interesting challenges for the marketing professional and for researchers, due to the great number of brands that operate in these markets. This diversity implies that food markets could be segmented considering food features, sales structure, and consumer characteristics [122].

Insufficient nutritional information seems to be one of the main factors that, in some segments, hinders the prevention of unhealthy food consumption [123]. This is particularly alarming in countries with a lower income [124]. Children and low-income consumers are vulnerable segments to persuasive and targeted marketing campaigns: children because of their lower skills to deal with marketing strategies to sell more and low-income consumers because of their vulnerability to lower-priced products.

As a result of these frameworks, the terms used to describe the nutritional dimensions, targeted at specific segments, need proper regulation, since the personal perceptions of consumers concerning the real definition of these expressions are not consensual [125] and this, therefore, opens up an element of free will for the marketing designers/strategists.

In some segments, the perceptions about food safety are more important for consumer choices than their socioeconomic characteristics [126]. In a similar pattern, consumers are, in some cases, prepared to pay more for beneficial health claims than for nutritional claims [127]. Nonetheless, the consumer's choices of food with heath claims are, in general, interrelated with several factors, such as those related with the socioeconomic domains [128]. Depending on the segments considered, the food choices may be influenced by personality, health, sensory attributes, price, and convenience [129], as well as, by environmental, ethnic, and cultural contexts [130].

More adjusted regulations may support the promotion of more healthy advertising to more vulnerable segments [131]. However, there are areas that need to be worked on, across several segments, concerning regulations, recommendations, and policies. Some of these dimensions that deserve special attention are the accuracy [132] and the perception [133] of consumers relative to these fields associated with healthier food. The main fields to be considered by regulations to promote a healthier choice by children are the usual persuasive techniques such as promotional offers, nutrition and health claims, and appeals towards taste and fun [134].

Tourism is an important market segment that may bring significant contributions to food marketing strategies, considering the several interrelationships between the associated sectors in these interlinkages [135]. The relationships between food and tourism are well known and strong, and they should be considered in joint strategies to promote the two sectors in an integrated way. Nonetheless, the externalities that may be created in this common strategy could also spread positive effects to other sectors (transport, support services, etc.).

3.6. Social Dimensions

The interlinkages between the social responsibility of firms and the market response to the respective consumers are positive [136]; however, the traditional consumer determinants, such as the price, continue to be relevant [137]. The strong impacts from the level of prices on consumer choices are particularly problematic in lower-income countries and consumer segments [138]. Knowledge about price relevance in consumer choice may be further considered so as to promote heathy strategies and be complemented with nutritional education [139]. Adjusted educational campaigns are fundamental for a healthier food choice [140] and lifestyles [141], mainly for young people [142] to obtain critical skills [143] in making more informed decisions [144]. Educational campaigns to inform and create skills in consumers to deal with the abundance in daily advertisements are crucial in preventing health problems related to ill-informed consumption, mostly those related to obesity and diabetes. Another question concerns lifestyles that need to be adjusted in order to be healthier and prevent other diseases associated with an unbalanced diet. Cancers and cardiovascular diseases are examples of civilizational diseases related to population lifestyles and social contexts. The media could better support these healthier campaigns [145], considering its influence on adolescents [146], for example, in terms of food choices [147].

On the other hand, it is important to increase the social conscientiousness of the companies which support self-regulatory approaches. Public health policies may play an important role here to influence companies to voluntarily improve their social responsibility concerning the negative implications of marketing practices that promote the consumption of unhealthy foods [148]. Sugar and salt are among the main nefarious ingredients in unhealthy products [149], having several impacts on society's dynamics, and they are sometimes presented on packaging along with other information in a misleading way [150]. The design of adjusted healthy food policies needs multidisciplinary approaches [151] that consider the several human dimensions [152], in which, of course, health professionals should be included [153]. Scientific research may also bring about significant insight and support here [154]. Children's health, changing industry practices, intervention from public institutions, and consumer support are all consensual dimensions for the several stakeholders to promote healthier food production and choice [155].

Social condition has a great impact on food choices [156]. Indeed, the social and economic contexts have direct implications on the amount of income available to consume and on the level of prices afforded. However, in some cases, retailers are not clearly informed about the impacts of the price changes on their sales [157]. Food may also be used as an expression of social identity and a way to make a difference from the mainstream [158].

In general, food choice patterns followed by consumers are similar to those considered in other decisions of their lives [159]. In fact, consumers concerned with sustainability tend to consume foods of a higher quality and are less vulnerable to promotional advertisements [160]. The consumption patterns of these more sustainable consumers may be considered by, for example, policymakers as benchmarks and practices to be spread over other social segments. It is important to know the several dimensions related to food choices and consumption in order to promote more balanced lifestyles. For example, Chinese teenagers are influenced, in their food choices, by personal, family, peer, and retailer frameworks and the following features were highlighted as influencing their options:

nutrition, safety, taste, image, price, convenience, and fun [161]. The social dimensions around the world are very different, and any adjusted approach needs to consider and be aware of the local particularities.

3.7. Brand and Branding

Brands and branding are fundamental instruments for an effective marketing plan in each step of the food chain [162]. From production to retailers' markets, brands are crucial to create value added and to differentiate products from their competition. Only with brands is it possible to carry out a marketing strategy across all dimensions.

Commercial brands are more important for the brand-schematic consumers than for brand-aschematic consumers. The brand-aschematic consumers, in wine markets, for example, give greater importance to the Protected Designation of Origin label and the associated categories [163]. The wine market is a very complex context, due to its great number of individual and certified brands. Markets with a great diversity of brands may confuse consumers when they want to make a choice. In these cases, the main challenge is to have a brand that may be easily identified, amongst many others, and be positioned in the mind of the customers. Consumers, in general, maintain two brands by category in their minds, and the great task is to be included as one of these two brands. Here, positioning approaches are crucial for an efficient branding [164].

Credence features are decisive for the marketing of food, and the brand itself is among these characteristics jointly with organic foods, health, and ingredients [165]. The branding processes usually create ties of confidence and loyalty with consumers to maintain the market and the respective sales. These dimensions distinguish the concerns and objectives of sales technicians from marketing professionals. In addition, the scientific literature highlights that consumer satisfaction is interrelated with their behaviour and loyalty [166], showing that consumer loyalty is, indeed, a central dimension in marketing strategies and that brands are crucial in creating ties of confidence [167]. However, loyalty and satisfaction of consumers are, also, influenced by their lifestyle and personality [168].

Iconic and old brands, such as Coca-Cola, are examples of market drivers [169] and may bring important contributions for strategic plans to lead consumers towards a more adjusted and healthy consumption, principally among children and youths. On the other hand, the display of brand characters has an important impact on consumer choice, and this deserves special attention from the several stakeholders for healthier food consumption [170].

4. Discussion and Conclusions

The study presented here aimed to highlight the main contributions from the literature concerning the dimensions related to the interrelationships between food marketing and consumer choice. For this purpose, 147 documents from the Scopus database were considered in a search carried out on 16 October 2020 for the topics "food marketing" and "choices". These documents were first analysed through bibliographic characterisation and after surveyed by literature review.

The bibliographic data reveals that there are opportunities to explore regarding these topics, considering the annual average number of documents published, the subject areas addressed, and the countries of the authors' affiliation. On the other hand, there is great relatedness between food marketing and human obesity, especially in young people. In fact, the literature review highlighted that there is a great concern from several stakeholders about the impact of marketing strategies on the health of children and adolescents.

The literature review may be summarised in a SWOT (strengths, weaknesses, opportunities, and threats) analysis approach, to better highlight the main insights, principally considering food marketing and consumer choice when building the matrix (see Figure 6).

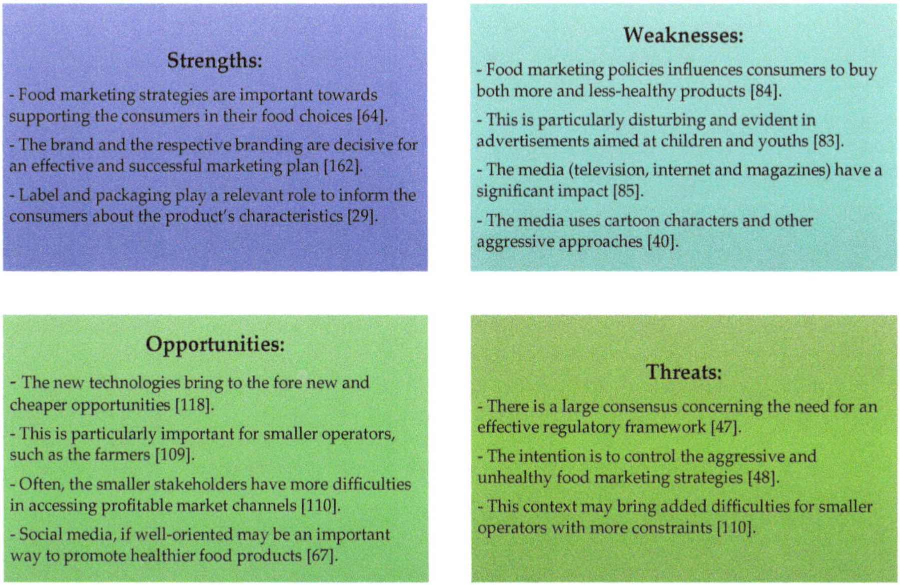

Strengths:
- Food marketing strategies are important towards supporting the consumers in their food choices [64].
- The brand and the respective branding are decisive for an effective and successful marketing plan [162].
- Label and packaging play a relevant role to inform the consumers about the product's characteristics [29].

Weaknesses:
- Food marketing policies influences consumers to buy both more and less-healthy products [84].
- This is particularly disturbing and evident in advertisements aimed at children and youths [83].
- The media (television, internet and magazines) have a significant impact [85].
- The media uses cartoon characters and other aggressive approaches [40].

Opportunities:
- The new technologies bring to the fore new and cheaper opportunities [118].
- This is particularly important for smaller operators, such as the farmers [109].
- Often, the smaller stakeholders have more difficulties in accessing profitable market channels [110].
- Social media, if well-oriented may be an important way to promote healthier food products [67].

Threats:
- There is a large consensus concerning the need for an effective regulatory framework [47].
- The intention is to control the aggressive and unhealthy food marketing strategies [48].
- This context may bring added difficulties for smaller operators with more constraints [110].

Figure 6. SWOT (strengths, weaknesses, opportunities, and threats) analysis to summarise the literature review.

Figure 6 shows that adjusted food image and name approaches, interrelated with the label, packaging, and brand, are crucial for a successful marketing strategy [6]. However, these powerful marketing instruments are often used by companies, through the media, to promote unhealthy food, especially for children and adolescents [49]. In parallel, new technologies and social media offer new and attractive opportunities for smaller operators, opening up new channels for them to communicate with consumers [118]. Nonetheless, these smaller stakeholders may be those most affected by restrictive policies to mitigate negative food marketing impacts on consumer health [47].

Traditionally, prices are amongst the most influential factors that condition consumption, including food choices, and the economic theory confirms this influence. Nonetheless, there are specific segments and new tendencies where quality, healthy attributes, and sustainability aspects are emergent dimensions. The sociodemographic, cultural, and behavioural domains also play their part in food consumption and preferences. This explains, in part, the emerging importance of neurosciences in marketing plans. In the universe of food marketing and consumer choice, it is important to highlight the relevance of the agricultural sector and its particularities, in the production of commodities, which condition the definition of effective marketing plans for the entire sector.

In terms of practical implications, it seems to be consensual that food marketing strategies have relevant implications on human health, and this framework deserves special attention from several stakeholders, particularly in the design of more adjusted policies in a standard way across countries, through World Trade Organization and World Health Organization negotiations. However, these regulations should be designed in order to have the right desired effect and avoid worsening the fragile context of smaller producers.

For future studies, it would be advisable to survey several stakeholders with regard to suggestions for designing new and efficient policies and regulations, so as to obtain a more adjusted regulatory framework and increase the operators' compliance.

Funding: This work is funded by National Funds through the FCT—Foundation for Science and Technology, I.P., within the scope of the project Ref^a UIDB/00681/2020.

Acknowledgments: We would like to thank the CERNAS Research Centre and the Polytechnic Institute of Viseu for their support.

Conflicts of Interest: The author declares no conflict of interest.

References

1. Arroyo, P.E.; Linan, J.; Vera Martinez, J. Who really values healthy food? *Br. Food J.* **2020**. [CrossRef]
2. Proserpio, C.; Fia, G.; Bucalossi, G.; Zanoni, B.; Spinelli, S.; Dinnella, C.; Monteleone, E.; Pagliarini, E. Winemaking Byproducts as Source of Antioxidant Components: Consumers' Acceptance and Expectations of Phenol-Enriched Plant-Based Food. *Antioxidants* **2020**, *9*, 661. [CrossRef] [PubMed]
3. Daly, J. A social practice perspective on meat reduction in Australian households: Rethinking intervention strategies. *Geogr. Res.* **2020**, *58*, 240–251. [CrossRef]
4. De Dominicis, S.; Bonaiuto, F.; Fornara, F.; Cancellieri, U.G.; Petruccelli, I.; Crano, W.D.; Ma, J.; Bonaiuto, M. Food Reputation and Food Preferences: Application of the Food Reputation Map (FRM) in Italy, USA, and China. *Front. Psychol.* **2020**, *11*, 1499. [CrossRef] [PubMed]
5. Szolnoki, G.; Hauck, K. Analysis of German wine consumers' preferences for organic and non-organic wines. *Br. Food J.* **2020**, *122*, 2077–2087. [CrossRef]
6. Li, S.; Zeng, Y.; Zhou, S. The congruence effect of food shape and name typeface on consumers' food preferences. *Food. Qual. Prefer.* **2020**, *86*, 104017. [CrossRef]
7. Martinho, V.J.P.D. The Behaviour of External Markets for the Portuguese Wine: Its Implications in the Sustainability of the Sector. In *Proceedings of the 4th International Conference on Energy & Environment (icee 2019): Bringing Together Engineering and Economics*; Ferreira, P., Soares, I., Eds.; Univ Minho: Guimaraes, Portugal, 2019; pp. 406–411, ISBN 978-989-97050-9-8.
8. Martinho, V.J.P.D. The evolution of the milk sector in Portugal: Implications from the Common Agricultural Policy. *Open Agric.* **2020**, *5*, 582–592. [CrossRef]
9. Martinho, V.J.P.D. The Competitiveness of the Portuguese Wine Sector: An Important Indicator for a Sustainable Development. In *Proceedings of the 4th International Conference on Energy & Environment (icee 2019): Bringing Together Engineering and Economics*; Ferreira, P., Soares, I., Eds.; Univ Minho: Guimaraes, Portugal, 2019; pp. 372–377, ISBN 978-989-97050-9-8.
10. Scopus Scopus (Article Title, Abstract, Keywords). Available online: https://www.scopus.com/search/form.uri?display=basic (accessed on 16 October 2020).
11. Liberati, A.; Altman, D.G.; Tetzlaff, J.; Mulrow, C.; Gøtzsche, P.C.; Ioannidis, J.P.A.; Clarke, M.; Devereaux, P.J.; Kleijnen, J.; Moher, D. The PRISMA Statement for Reporting Systematic Reviews and Meta-Analyses of Studies That Evaluate Health Care Interventions: Explanation and Elaboration. *PLoS Med.* **2009**, *6*. [CrossRef]
12. Web of Science Web of Science (Core Collection). Available online: https://apps.webofknowledge.com/WOS_GeneralSearch_input.do?product=WOS&search_mode=GeneralSearch&SID=D52GU5AnotDfa7ZAPDL&preferencesSaved=. (accessed on 2 November 2020).
13. Zotero Zotero Software. Available online: https://www.zotero.org/ (accessed on 2 November 2020).
14. Baumeister, R.F.; Leary, M.R. Writing Narrative Literature Reviews. *Rev. Gen. Psychol.* **1997**, *1*, 311–320. [CrossRef]
15. Campbell, M.; Thomson, H.; Katikireddi, S.V.; Sowden, A. Reporting of narrative synthesis in systematic reviews of public health interventions: A methodological assessment. *Lancet* **2016**, *388*, S34. [CrossRef]
16. Jahan, N.; Naveed, S.; Zeshan, M.; Tahir, M.A. How to Conduct a Systematic Review: A Narrative Literature Review. *Cureus* **2016**, *8*, e864. [CrossRef] [PubMed]
17. Lagorio, A.; Pinto, R. Food and grocery retail logistics issues: A systematic literature review. *Res. Transp. Econ.* **2020**, 100841. [CrossRef]
18. VOSviewer VOSviewer—Visualizing Scientific Landscapes. Available online: https://www.vosviewer.com// (accessed on 21 October 2020).
19. Van Eck, N.J.; Waltman, L. VOSviewer Manual. Available online: https://www.vosviewer.com/documentation/Manual_VOSviewer_1.6.15.pdf (accessed on 21 October 2020).

20. Agnew, J.; Henson, S.; Cao, Y. Are Low-Income Consumers Willing to Pay for Fortification of a Commercially Produced Yogurt in Bangladesh. *Food Nutr. Bull.* **2020**, *41*, 102–120. [CrossRef] [PubMed]
21. Samuelson, P.; Nordhaus, W. *Economics*, 19th ed.; McGraw-Hill Education: Boston, MA, USA, 2009; ISBN 978-0-07-351129-0.
22. Watson, F.; Ekici, A. Well-being in Alternative Economies: The Role of Shared Commitments in the Context of a Spatially-Extended Alternative Food Network. *J. Macromark.* **2017**, *37*, 206–216. [CrossRef]
23. McMahon, A.-T.; Williams, P.; Tapsell, L. Reviewing the meanings of wellness and well-being and their implications for food choice. *Perspect. Public Health* **2010**, *130*, 282–286. [CrossRef] [PubMed]
24. Phillips, T.; Ravuvu, A.; McMichael, C.; Thow, A.M.; Browne, J.; Waqa, G.; Tutuo, J.; Gleeson, D. Nutrition policy-making in Fiji: Working in and around neoliberalisation in the Global South. *Crit. Pub. Health* **2019**. [CrossRef]
25. Roberto, C.A. How psychological insights can inform food policies to address unhealthy eating habits. *Am. Psychol.* **2020**, *75*, 265–273. [CrossRef]
26. Rogers, R.T.; Caswell, J.A. Strategic management and the internal organization of food marketing firms. *Agribusiness* **1988**, *4*, 3–10. [CrossRef]
27. Thompson, G.D. Consumer demand for organic foods: What we know and what we need to know. *Am. J. Agric. Econ.* **1998**, *80*, 1113–1118. [CrossRef]
28. Wu, L.; Gong, X.; Chen, X.; Hu, W. Compromise Effect in Food Consumer Choices in China: An Analysis on Pork Products. *Front. Psychol.* **2020**, *11*. [CrossRef]
29. Pulker, C.E.; Li, D.C.C.; Scott, J.A.; Pollard, C.M. The impact of voluntary policies on parents' ability to select healthy foods in supermarkets: A qualitative study of australian parental views. *Int. J. Environ. Res. Public Health* **2019**, *16*, 3377. [CrossRef]
30. Scrinis, G.; Parker, C. Front-of-Pack Food Labeling and the Politics of Nutritional Nudges. *Law Policy* **2016**, *38*, 234–249. [CrossRef]
31. Grabenhorst, F.; Schulte, F.P.; Maderwald, S.; Brand, M. Food labels promote healthy choices by a decision bias in the amygdala. *NeuroImage* **2013**, *74*, 152–163. [CrossRef]
32. Amos, C.; Pentina, I.; Hawkins, T.G.; Davis, N. "Natural" labeling and consumers' sentimental pastoral notion. *J. Prod. Brand Manag.* **2014**, *23*, 268–281. [CrossRef]
33. Arrúa, A.; Curutchet, M.R.; Rey, N.; Barreto, P.; Golovchenko, N.; Sellanes, A.; Velazco, G.; Winokur, M.; Giménez, A.; Ares, G. Impact of front-of-pack nutrition information and label design on children's choice of two snack foods: Comparison of warnings and the traffic-light system. *Appetite* **2017**, *116*, 139–146. [CrossRef]
34. Ares, G.; Arrúa, A.; Antúnez, L.; Vidal, L.; Machín, L.; Martínez, J.; Curutchet, M.R.; Giménez, A. Influence of label design on children's perception of two snack foods: Comparison of rating and choice-based conjoint analysis. *Food Qual. Prefer.* **2016**, *53*, 1–8. [CrossRef]
35. Cannon, J. Notions of region and the Mediterranean diet in food advertising: Quality marks or subjective criteria? *Br. Food J.* **2005**, *107*, 74–83. [CrossRef]
36. Elliott, C. Milk in a glass, milk in a carton: The influence of packaging on children's perceptions of the healthfulness of milk. *Int. J. Health Promot. Edu.* **2018**, *56*, 155–164. [CrossRef]
37. Hallez, L.; Qutteina, Y.; Raedschelders, M.; Boen, F.; Smits, T. That's my cue to eat: A systematic review of the persuasiveness of front-of-pack cues on food packages for children vs. adults. *Nutrients* **2020**, *12*, 1062. [CrossRef]
38. Ikonen, I.; Sotgiu, F.; Aydinli, A.; Verlegh, P.W.J. Consumer effects of front-of-package nutrition labeling: An interdisciplinary meta-analysis. *J. Acad. Mark. Sci.* **2020**, *48*, 360–383. [CrossRef]
39. Kraak, V.I.; Story, M. Influence of food companies' brand mascots and entertainment companies' cartoon media characters on children's diet and health: A systematic review and research needs. *Obes. Rev.* **2015**, *16*, 107–126. [CrossRef] [PubMed]
40. Ogle, A.D.; Graham, D.J.; Lucas-Thompson, R.G.; Roberto, C.A. Influence of Cartoon Media Characters on Children's Attention to and Preference for Food and Beverage Products. *J. Acad. Nutri. Diet.* **2017**, *117*, 265–270.e2. [CrossRef] [PubMed]
41. Letona, P.; Chacon, V.; Roberto, C.; Barnoya, J. A qualitative study of children's snack food packaging perceptions and preferences. *BMC Public Health* **2014**, *14*. [CrossRef] [PubMed]

42. Lwin, M.O.; Vijaykumar, S.; Chao, J. "Natural" and "Fresh": An Analysis of Food Label Claims in Internationally Packaged Foods in Singapore. *J. Food Prod. Mark.* **2015**, *21*, 588–607. [CrossRef]
43. Monro, J.A. Evidence-based food choice: The need for new measures of food effects. *Trends Food Sci. Technol.* **2000**, *11*, 136–144. [CrossRef]
44. Sussman, R.L.; McMahon, A.T.; Neale, E.P. An audit of the nutrition and health claims on breakfast cereals in supermarkets in the illawarra region of Australia. *Nutrients* **2019**, *11*, 1604. [CrossRef]
45. Nelson, A. They are what they eat? Ensuring our children get the right nutrients. *J. Fam. Health Care* **2013**, *23*, 14–16.
46. Pulker, C.E.; Scott, J.A.; Pollard, C.M. Ultra-processed family foods in Australia: Nutrition claims, health claims and marketing techniques. *Public Health Nutr.* **2018**, *21*, 38–48. [CrossRef]
47. Roberto, C.A.; Baik, J.; Harris, J.L.; Brownell, K.D. Influence of licensed characters on children's taste and snack preferences. *Pediatrics* **2010**, *126*, 88–93. [CrossRef]
48. Roberto, C.A.; Pomeranz, J.L.; Fisher, J.O. The need for public policies to promote healthier food consumption: A comment on Wansink and Chandon (2014). *J. Consum. Psychol.* **2014**, *24*, 438–445. [CrossRef]
49. Rodrigues, A.S.; Carmo, I.D.; Breda, J.; Rito, A.I. Association between marketing of high energy food and drinks and childhood obesity. *Rev. Port. Saude Publica* **2011**, *29*, 180–187. [CrossRef]
50. Santana, M.O.; Guimarães, J.S.; Leite, F.H.M.; Mais, L.A.; Horta, P.M.; Bortoletto Martins, A.P.; Claro, R.M. Analysing persuasive marketing of ultra-processed foods on Brazilian television. *Int. J. Public Health* **2020**, *65*, 1067–1077. [CrossRef] [PubMed]
51. Scully, M.; Wakefield, M.; Niven, P.; Chapman, K.; Crawford, D.; Pratt, I.S.; Baur, L.A.; Flood, V.; Morley, B. Association between food marketing exposure and adolescents' food choices and eating behaviors. *Appetite* **2012**, *58*, 1–5. [CrossRef]
52. Smith, J. The contribution of infant food marketing to the obesogenic environment in Australia. *Breastfeed Rev.* **2007**, *15*, 23–35. [PubMed]
53. Smith, R.; Kelly, B.; Yeatman, H.; Moore, C.; Baur, L.; King, L.; Boyland, E.; Chapman, K.; Hughes, C.; Bauman, A. Advertising Placement in Digital Game Design Influences Children's Choices of Advertised Snacks: A Randomized Trial. *J. Acad. Nutri. Diet.* **2020**, *120*, 404–413. [CrossRef] [PubMed]
54. Seiders, K.; Petty, R.D. Obesity and the role of food marketing: A policy analysis of issues and remedies. *J. Public Policy Mark.* **2004**, *23*, 153–169. [CrossRef]
55. Zimmerman, F.J. Using Marketing Muscle to Sell Fat: The Rise of Obesity in the Modern Economy. *Annu. Rev. Public Health* **2011**, *32*, 285–306. [CrossRef]
56. TYEBJEE, T.T. Affirmative Disclosure of Nutrition Information and Consumers' Food Preferences: A Review. *J. Consum. Aff.* **1979**, *13*, 206–223. [CrossRef]
57. Srivastava, B. Fast-food marketing and children's fast-food consumption: A trigger to childhood obesity. *Indian J. Public Health Res. Dev.* **2019**, *10*, 173–177. [CrossRef]
58. Vecchio, M.G.; Ghidina, M.; Gulati, A.; Berchialla, P.; Paramesh, E.C.; Gregori, D. Measuring Brand Awareness as a Component of Eating Habits in Indian Children: The Development of the IBAI Questionnaire. *Indian J. Pediatrics* **2014**, *81*, 23–29. [CrossRef]
59. Stewart, J.F.; Guilkey, D.K. Estimating the health impact of industry infant food marketing practices in the Philippines. *J. Dev. Stud.* **2000**, *36*, 50–77. [CrossRef]
60. Tan, L.; Ng, S.H.; Omar, A.; Karupaiah, T. What's on YouTube? A Case Study on Food and Beverage Advertising in Videos Targeted at Children on Social Media. *Child. Obes.* **2018**, *14*, 280–290. [CrossRef]
61. Tatlow-Golden, M.; Hennessy, E.; Dean, M.; Hollywood, L. Young children's food brand knowledge. Early development and associations with television viewing and parent's diet. *Appetite* **2014**, *80*, 197–203. [CrossRef]
62. Von Tigerstrom, B. How Do International Trade Obligations Affect Policy Options for Obesity Prevention? Lessons from Recent Developments in Trade and Tobacco Control. *Can. J. Diabetes* **2013**, *37*, 182–188. [CrossRef]
63. Wootan, M.G.; Almy, J.; Ugalde, M.; Kaminski, M. How do nutrition guidelines compare for industry to market food and beverage products to children? World Health Organization nutrient profile standards versus the US children's food and beverage advertising initiative. *Child. Obes.* **2019**, *15*, 194–199. [CrossRef]
64. Vecchio, R.; Cavallo, C. Increasing healthy food choices through nudges: A systematic review. *Food Qual. Prefer.* **2019**, *78*. [CrossRef]

65. Manfredo, M.R.; Sanders, D.R. Contract design: A note on cash settled futures. *J. Agric. Food Ind. Organ.* **2003**, *1*. [CrossRef]
66. Bruce, A.S.; Lim, S.-L.; Smith, T.R.; Cherry, J.B.C.; Black, W.R.; Davis, A.M.; Bruce, J.M. Apples or candy? Internal and external influences on children's food choices. *Appetite* **2015**, *93*, 31–34. [CrossRef]
67. Aschemann-Witzel, J.; Perez-Cueto, F.J.; Niedzwiedzka, B.; Verbeke, W.; Bech-Larsen, T. Lessons for public health campaigns from analysing commercial food marketing success factors: A case study. *BMC Public Health* **2012**, *12*. [CrossRef]
68. Ayala, G.X.; Castro, I.A.; Pickrel, J.L.; Lin, S.-F.; Williams, C.B.; Madanat, H.; Jun, H.-J.; Zive, M. A cluster randomized trial to promote healthy menu items for children: The kids' choice restaurant program. *Int. J. Environ. Res. Public Health* **2017**, *14*, 1494. [CrossRef]
69. Charlton, E.L.; Kähkönen, L.A.; Sacks, G.; Cameron, A.J. Supermarkets and unhealthy food marketing: An international comparison of the content of supermarket catalogues/circulars. *Prev. Med.* **2015**, *81*, 168–173. [CrossRef] [PubMed]
70. Lam, C.C.V.; Ejlerskov, K.T.; White, M.; Adams, J. Voluntary policies on checkout foods and healthfulness of foods displayed at, or near, supermarket checkout areas: A cross-sectional survey. *Public Health Nutr.* **2018**, *21*, 3462–3468. [CrossRef] [PubMed]
71. Dixon, H.; Niven, P.; Scully, M.; Wakefield, M. Food marketing with movie character toys: Effects on young children's preferences for unhealthy and healthier fast food meals. *Appetite* **2017**, *117*, 342–350. [CrossRef]
72. Dixon, H.; Scully, M.; Niven, P.; Kelly, B.; Chapman, K.; Donovan, R.; Martin, J.; Baur, L.A.; Crawford, D.; Wakefield, M. Effects of nutrient content claims, sports celebrity endorsements and premium offers on pre-adolescent children's food preferences: Experimental research. *Pediatric Obes.* **2014**, *9*, e47–e57. [CrossRef]
73. Dixon, H.; Scully, M.; Wakefield, M.; Kelly, B.; Chapman, K.; Donovan, R. Parent's responses to nutrient claims and sports celebrity endorsements on energy-dense and nutrient-poor foods: An experimental study. *Public Health Nutr.* **2010**, *14*, 1071–1079. [CrossRef]
74. Dixon, H.; Scully, M.; Wakefield, M.; Kelly, B.; Pettigrew, S. Community junior sport sponsorship: An online experiment assessing children's responses to unhealthy food v. pro-health sponsorship options. *Public Health Nutr.* **2018**, *21*, 1176–1185. [CrossRef]
75. Dixon, H.; Scully, M.; Kelly, B.; Donovan, R.; Chapman, K.; Wakefield, M. Counter-Advertising May Reduce Parent's Susceptibility to Front-of-Package Promotions on Unhealthy Foods. *J. Nutr. Educ. Behav.* **2014**, *46*, 467–474. [CrossRef]
76. Dixon, H.; Scully, M.; Kelly, B.; Chapman, K.; Wakefield, M. Can counter-advertising reduce pre-adolescent children's susceptibility to front-of-package promotions on unhealthy foods?: Experimental research. *Soc. Sci. Med.* **2014**, *116*, 211–219. [CrossRef]
77. García, A.L.; Morillo-Santander, G.; Parrett, A.; Mutoro, A.N. Confused health and nutrition claims in food marketing to children could adversely affect food choice and increase risk of obesity. *Arch. Dis. Child.* **2019**, *104*, 541–546. [CrossRef]
78. Elliott, C. Marketing foods to children: Are we asking the right questions? *Child. Obes.* **2012**, *8*, 191–194. [CrossRef]
79. Bernhardt, A.M.; Wilking, C.; Gilbert-Diamond, D.; Emond, J.A.; Sargent, J.D. Children's recall of fast food television advertising-testing the adequacy of food marketing regulation. *PLoS ONE* **2015**, *10*. [CrossRef] [PubMed]
80. Batada, A.; Wootan, M.G. Nickelodeon Markets Nutrition-Poor Foods to Children. *Am. J. Prev. Med.* **2007**, *33*, 48–50. [CrossRef]
81. Austin, E.W.; Austin, B.W.; French, B.F.; Cohen, M.A. The Effects of a Nutrition Media Literacy Intervention on Parents' and Youths' Communication about Food. *J. Health Commun.* **2018**, *23*, 190–199. [CrossRef] [PubMed]
82. Austin, E.W.; Austin, B.W.; Kaiser, C.K. Effects of Family-Centered Media Literacy Training on Family Nutrition Outcomes. *Prev. Sci.* **2020**, *21*, 308–318. [CrossRef] [PubMed]
83. Baldwin, H.J.; Freeman, B.; Kelly, B. Like and share: Associations between social media engagement and dietary choices in children. *Public Health Nutr.* **2018**, *21*, 3210–3215. [CrossRef] [PubMed]
84. Avianty, S.; Khusun, H.; Bardosono, S.; Februhartanty, J.; Worsley, A. Exposure and approval of food marketing strategies: A mixed methods study among household food providers in Jakarta. *Malays. J. Nutr.* **2019**, *25*, S47–S62.

85. Boyland, E.J.; Whalen, R. Food advertising to children and its effects on diet: Review of recent prevalence and impact data. *Pediatric Diabetes* **2015**, *16*, 331–337. [CrossRef]
86. Bruce, A.S.; Pruitt, S.W.; Ha, O.-R.; Cherry, J.B.C.; Smith, T.R.; Bruce, J.M.; Lim, S.-L. The Influence of Televised Food Commercials on Children's Food Choices: Evidence from Ventromedial Prefrontal Cortex Activations. *J. Pediatr.* **2016**, *177*, 27–32.e1. [CrossRef]
87. Neyens, E.; Smits, T. Seeing is doing. The implicit effect of TV cooking shows on children's use of ingredients. *Appetite* **2017**, *116*, 559–567. [CrossRef]
88. Ustjanauskas, A.E.; Harris, J.L.; Schwartz, M.B. Food and beverage advertising on children's web sites. *Pediatr. Obes.* **2014**, *9*, 362–372. [CrossRef]
89. Vassallo, A.J.; Kelly, B.; Zhang, L.; Wang, Z.; Young, S.; Freeman, B. Junk food marketing on instagram: Content analysis. *J. Med. Internet Res.* **2018**, *20*. [CrossRef]
90. Choi, H.; Springston, J.K. How to use health and nutrition-related claims correctly on food advertising: Comparison of benefit-seeking, risk-avoidance, and taste appeals on different food categories. *J. Health Commun.* **2014**, *19*, 1047–1063. [CrossRef] [PubMed]
91. Stasi, A.; Songa, G.; Mauri, M.; Ciceri, A.; Diotallevi, F.; Nardone, G.; Russo, V. Neuromarketing empirical approaches and food choice: A systematic review. *Food Res. Int.* **2018**, *108*, 650–664. [CrossRef] [PubMed]
92. Lowe, M.; Ringler, C.; Haws, K. An overture to overeating: The cross-modal effects of acoustic pitch on food preferences and serving behavior. *Appetite* **2018**, *123*, 128–134. [CrossRef] [PubMed]
93. Musicus, A.; Tal, A.; Wansink, B. Eyes in the Aisles: Why Is Cap'n Crunch Looking Down at My Child? *Environ. Behav.* **2015**, *47*, 715–733. [CrossRef]
94. Nyilasy, G.; Lei, J.; Nagpal, A.; Tan, J. Colour correct: The interactive effects of food label nutrition colouring schemes and food category healthiness on health perceptions. *Public Health Nutr.* **2016**, *19*, 2122–2127. [CrossRef]
95. Ziv, N. Musical flavor: The effect of background music and presentation order on taste. *Eur. J. Mark.* **2018**, *52*, 1485–1504. [CrossRef]
96. Jones, S.C.; Kervin, L. An experimental study on the effects of exposure to magazine advertising on children's food choices. *Public Health Nutr.* **2011**, *14*, 1337–1344. [CrossRef]
97. King, L.; Hill, A.J. Magazine adverts for healthy and less healthy foods: Effects on recall but not hunger or food choice by pre-adolescent children. *Appetite* **2008**, *51*, 194–197. [CrossRef]
98. Cairns, G. A critical review of evidence on the sociocultural impacts of food marketing and policy implications. *Appetite* **2019**, *136*, 193–207. [CrossRef]
99. Campbell, K.J.; Crawford, D.A.; Hesketh, K.D. Australian parents' views on their 5-6-year-old children's food choices. *Health Promot. Int.* **2007**, *22*, 11–18. [CrossRef] [PubMed]
100. Haynes, P.; Podobsky, S. Guilt-free food consumption: One of your five ideologies a day. *J. Consum. Mark.* **2016**, *33*, 202–212. [CrossRef]
101. Just, D.R.; Payne, C.R. Obesity: Can behavioral economics help? *Ann. Behav. Med.* **2009**, *38*, S47–S55. [CrossRef] [PubMed]
102. Baah Annor, P. Smallholder farmers' compliance with GlobalGAP standard: The case of Ghana. *Emerald Emerg. Mark. Case Stud.* **2018**, *8*. [CrossRef]
103. Cao, Y.J.; Cranfield, J.; Chen, C.; Widowski, T. Heterogeneous informational and attitudinal impacts on consumer preferences for eggs from welfare enhanced cage systems. *Food Policy* **2020**. [CrossRef]
104. Cheng, L.; Yin, C.; Chien, H. Demand for milk quantity and safety in urban China: Evidence from Beijing and Harbin. *Aust. J. Agric. Resour. Econ.* **2015**, *59*, 275–287. [CrossRef]
105. Bryła, P. Organic food consumption in Poland: Motives and barriers. *Appetite* **2016**, *105*, 737–746. [CrossRef]
106. Martinho, V.J.P.D. Output Impacts of the Single Payment Scheme in Portugal: A Regression with Spatial Effects. *Outlook Agric.* **2015**, *44*, 109–118. [CrossRef]
107. Martinho, V.J.P.D. Insights from over 30 years of common agricultural policy in Portugal. *Outlook Agric.* **2017**, *46*, 223–229. [CrossRef]
108. Bauman, A.; Thilmany, D.; Jablonski, B.B.R. Evaluating scale and technical efficiency among farms and ranches with a local market orientation. *Renew. Agric. Food Syst.* **2019**, *34*, 198–206. [CrossRef]
109. Bonetti, E.; Mattiacci, A.; Simoni, M. Communication patterns to address the consumption of PDO products. *Br. Food J.* **2019**, *122*, 390–403. [CrossRef]

110. Kangile, R.J.; Mgeni, C.P.; Mpenda, Z.T.; Sieber, S. The determinants of farmers' choice of markets for staple food commodities in Dodoma and Morogoro, Tanzania. *Agriculture* **2020**, *10*, 142. [CrossRef]
111. Morgan, E.H.; Severs, M.M.; Hanson, K.L.; McGuirt, J.; Becot, F.; Wang, W.; Kolodinsky, J.; Sitaker, M.; Pitts, S.B.J.; Ammerman, A.; et al. Gaining and maintaining a competitive edge: Evidence from CSA members and farmers on local food marketing strategies. *Sustainability* **2018**, *10*, 2177. [CrossRef]
112. Neill, C.L.; Holcomb, R.B.; Lusk, J.L. Estimating potential beggar-thy-neighbor effects of state labeling programs. *Agribusiness* **2020**, *36*, 3–19. [CrossRef]
113. Murphy, A.J. Farmers' markets as retail spaces. *Int. J. Retail Disrtib. Manag.* **2011**, *39*, 582–597. [CrossRef]
114. Remar, D.; Campbell, J.; DiPietro, R.B. The impact of local food marketing on purchase decision and willingness to pay in a foodservice setting. *J. Foodserv. Bus. Res.* **2016**, *19*, 89–108. [CrossRef]
115. Plakias, Z.T.; Demko, I.; Katchova, A.L. Direct marketing channel choices among US farmers: Evidence from the Local Food Marketing Practices Survey. *Renew. Agric. Food Syst.* **2020**, *35*, 475–489. [CrossRef]
116. Ortega, D.L.; Chen, M.; Wang, H.H.; Shimokawa, S. Emerging markets for U.S. Pork in China: Experimental evidence from mainland and Hong Kong consumers. *J. Agric. Resour. Econ.* **2017**, *42*, 275–290.
117. Sánchez-Navarro, J.L.; Arcas-Lario, N.; Hernández-Espallardo, M. Antecedents of opportunism in agri-food cooperatives. *CIRIEC Esp. Rev. Econ. Publica Soc. Coop.* **2019**, 111–136. [CrossRef]
118. Vassalos, M.; Lim, K.H. Farmers' willingness to pay for various features of electronic food marketing platforms. *Int. Food Agribus. Manag. Rev.* **2016**, *19*, 131–149.
119. Guilkey, D.K.; Stewart, J.F. Infant feeding patterns and the marketing of infant foods in the Philippines. *Econ. Dev. Cult. Chang.* **1995**, *43*, 369–399. [CrossRef]
120. Hasnah Hassan, S. Consumption of functional food model for Malay Muslims in Malaysia. *J. Islam. Mark.* **2011**, *2*, 104–124. [CrossRef]
121. Ballco, P.; De Magistris, T. Spanish consumer purchase behaviour and stated preferences for yoghurts with nutritional and health claims. *Nutrients* **2019**, *11*, 2742. [CrossRef]
122. Hawkes, C. Sales promotions and food consumptionnure. *Nutr. Rev.* **2009**, *67*, 333–342. [CrossRef] [PubMed]
123. Bibeau, W.S.; Saksvig, B.I.; Gittelsohn, J.; Williams, S.; Jones, L.; Young, D.R. Perceptions of the food marketing environment among African American teen girls and adults. *Appetite* **2012**, *58*, 396–399. [CrossRef] [PubMed]
124. Bragg, M.A.; Eby, M.; Arshonsky, J.; Bragg, A.; Ogedegbe, G. Comparison of online marketing techniques on food and beverage companies' websites in six countries. *Glob. Health* **2017**, *13*. [CrossRef]
125. Bucher, T.; Hartmann, C.; Rollo, M.E.; Collins, C.E. What is nutritious snack food? A comparison of expert and layperson assessments. *Nutrients* **2017**, *9*, 874. [CrossRef]
126. Chalak, A.; Abiad, M. How effective is information provision in shaping food safety related purchasing decisions? Evidence from a choice experiment in Lebanon. *Food Qual. Prefer.* **2012**, *26*, 81–92. [CrossRef]
127. Viscecchia, R.; Nocella, G.; De Devitiis, B.; Bimbo, F.; Carlucci, D.; Seccia, A.; Nardone, G. Consumers' trade-off between nutrition and health claims under regulation 1924/2006: Insights from a choice experiment analysis. *Nutrients* **2019**, *11*, 2881. [CrossRef]
128. Contini, C.; Casini, L.; Stefan, V.; Romano, C.; Juhl, H.J.; Lähteenmäki, L.; Scozzafava, G.; Grunert, K.G. Some like it healthy: Can socio-demographic characteristics serve as predictors for a healthy food choice? *Food Qual. Prefer.* **2015**, *46*, 103–112. [CrossRef]
129. Gama, A.P.; Adhikari, K.; Hoisington, D.A. Factors influencing food choices of Malawian consumers: A food choice questionnaire approach. *J. Sens. Stud.* **2018**, *33*. [CrossRef]
130. Kumanyika, S.K. Environmental influences on childhood obesity: Ethnic and cultural influences in context. *Physiol. Behav.* **2008**, *94*, 61–70. [CrossRef] [PubMed]
131. Chapman, K.; Nicholas, P.; Banovic, D.; Supramaniam, R. The extent and nature of food promotion directed to children in Australian supermarkets. *Health Promot. Int.* **2006**, *21*, 331–339. [CrossRef] [PubMed]
132. Huang, Y.; Pomeranz, J.L.; Cash, S.B. Effective National Menu Labeling Requires Accuracy and Enforcement. *J. Acad. Nutri. Diet.* **2018**, *118*, 989–993. [CrossRef]
133. Elliott, C. Parents' choice: Examining parent perspectives on regulation and child-targeted supermarket foods. *Food Cult. Soc.* **2013**, *16*, 437–455. [CrossRef]
134. Jenkin, G.; Madhvani, N.; Signal, L.; Bowers, S. A systematic review of persuasive marketing techniques to promote food to children on television. *Obes. Rev.* **2014**, *15*, 281–293. [CrossRef]
135. Seo, S.; Yun, N.; Kim, O.Y. Destination food image and intention to eat destination foods: A view from Korea. *Curr. Issues Tour.* **2017**, *20*, 135–156. [CrossRef]

136. Boccia, F.; Malgeri Manzo, R.; Covino, D. Consumer behavior and corporate social responsibility: An evaluation by a choice experiment. *Corp. Soc. Responsib. Environ. Manag.* **2019**, *26*, 97–105. [CrossRef]
137. Boccia, F.; Sarnacchiaro, P. Chi-squared automatic interaction detector analysis on a choice experiment: An evaluation of responsible initiatives on consumers' purchasing behavior. *Corp. Soc. Responsib. Environ. Manag.* **2020**, *27*, 1143–1151. [CrossRef]
138. Chandon, P.; Wansink, B. Does food marketing need to make us fat? A review and solutions. *Nutr. Rev.* **2012**, *70*, 571–593. [CrossRef]
139. Disantis, K.I.; Grier, S.A.; Oakes, J.M.; Kumanyika, S.K. Food prices and food shopping decisions of black women. *Appetite* **2014**, *77*, 104–112. [CrossRef] [PubMed]
140. Kim, R.B. Consumer Attitude of Risk and Benefits toward Genetically Modified (GM) Foods in South Korea: Implications for Food Policy. *Eng. Econ.* **2012**, *23*, 189–199. [CrossRef]
141. Kline, S. Countering children's sedentary lifestyles an evaluative study of a media-risk education approach. *Childhood* **2005**, *12*, 239–258. [CrossRef]
142. Lai Yeung, W.-L.T. Combating deceptive advertisements and labelling on food products—An exploratory study on the perceptions of teachers. *Int. J. Consum. Stud.* **2003**, *27*, 235. [CrossRef]
143. Lai Yeung Wai-ling, T. Combating deceptive advertisements and labelling on food products—An exploratory study on the perceptions of teachers. *Int. J. Consum. Stud.* **2004**, *28*, 117–126. [CrossRef]
144. Truman, E.; Elliott, C. Health-promoting skills for children: Evaluating the influence of a media literacy and food marketing intervention. *Health Educ. J.* **2020**, *79*, 431–445. [CrossRef]
145. Putnam, M.M.; Cotto, C.E.; Calvert, S.L. Character Apps for Children's Snacks: Effects of Character Awareness on Snack Selection and Consumption Patterns. *Games Health J.* **2018**, *7*, 116–120. [CrossRef]
146. Qutteina, Y.; Hallez, L.; Mennes, N.; De Backer, C.; Smits, T. What Do Adolescents See on Social Media? A Diary Study of Food Marketing Images on Social Media. *Front. Psychol.* **2019**, *10*. [CrossRef]
147. Sivathanu, B. Food marketing and its impact on adolescents' food choices. *Ind. J. Mark.* **2017**, *47*, 46–60. [CrossRef]
148. Harris, J.L.; LoDolce, M.E.; Schwartz, M.B. Encouraging big food to do the right thing for children's health: A case study on using research to improve marketing of sugary cereals. *Crit. Pub. Health* **2015**, *25*, 320–332. [CrossRef]
149. Harris, J.L.; Schwartz, M.B.; Ustjanauskas, A.; Ohri-Vachaspati, P.; Brownell, K.D. Effects of serving high-sugar cereals on children's breakfast-eating behavior. *Pediatrics* **2011**, *127*, 71–76. [CrossRef] [PubMed]
150. Harris, J.L.; Thompson, J.M.; Schwartz, M.B.; Brownell, K.D. Nutrition-related claims on children's cereals: What do they mean to parents and do they influence willingness to buy? *Public Health Nutr.* **2011**, *14*, 2207–2212. [CrossRef] [PubMed]
151. Liu, P.J.; Wisdom, J.; Roberto, C.A.; Liu, L.J.; Ubel, P.A. Using behavioral economics to design more effective food policies to address obesity. *Appl. Econ. Perspect. Policy* **2014**, *36*, 6–24. [CrossRef]
152. Mandlik, M.; Oetzel, J.G.; Kadirov, D. Obesity and health care interventions: Substantiating a multi-modal challenge through the lens of grounded theory. *Health Promot. J. Aust.* **2020**. [CrossRef] [PubMed]
153. Ravasco, P.; Ferreira, C.; Camilo, M.E. Food for health: Primary-care prevention and public health relevance of the medical role. *Acta Med. Port.* **2011**, *24*, 783–790.
154. Maziak, W.; Ward, K.D.; Stockton, M.B. Childhood obesity: Are we missing the big picture? *Obes. Rev.* **2008**, *9*, 35–42. [CrossRef]
155. Kraak, V.I.; Swinburn, B.; Lawrence, M.; Harrison, P. A Q methodology study of stakeholders' views about accountability for promoting healthy food environments in England through the Responsibility Deal Food Network. *Food Policy* **2014**, *49*, 207–218. [CrossRef]
156. Jiang, H.; Yang, Z.; Sun, P.; Xu, M. When does social exclusion increase or decrease food self-regulation? The moderating role of time orientation. *J. Consum. Behav.* **2018**, *17*, 34–46. [CrossRef]
157. Díaz, E.R.; Ivanic, A.S.; Durazo-Watanabe, E. A study of food retailing: How does consumer price sensitivity vary across food categories and retailer types in Mexico? *Contad. Adm.* **2020**, *65*. [CrossRef]
158. Cronin, J.M.; McCarthy, M.B.; Collins, A.M. Covert distinction: How hipsters practice food-based resistance strategies in the production of identity. *Consum. Mark. Cult.* **2014**, *17*, 2–28. [CrossRef]
159. Kumcu, A.; Woolverton, A.E. Feeding Fido: Changing Consumer Food Preferences Bring Pets to the Table. *J. Food Prod. Mark.* **2015**, *21*, 213–230. [CrossRef]

160. Von Meyer-Höfer, M.; von der Wense, V.; Spiller, A. Characterising convinced sustainable food consumers. *Br. Food J.* **2015**, *117*, 1082–1104. [CrossRef]
161. Veeck, A.; Yu, F.G.; Yu, H.; Veeck, G.; Gentry, J.W. Influences on food choices of urban chinese teenagers. *Young Consum.* **2014**, *15*, 296–311. [CrossRef]
162. Hamlin, R.P.; Lindsay, S.; Insch, A. Retailer branding of consumer sales promotions. A major development in food marketing? *Appetite* **2012**, *58*, 256–264. [CrossRef]
163. Carsana, L.; Jolibert, A. The effects of expertise and brand schematicity on the perceived importance of choice criteria: A Bordeaux wine investigation. *J. Prod. Brand Manag.* **2017**, *26*, 80–90. [CrossRef]
164. Ries, A.; Ries, L. *The 22 Immutable Laws of Branding*, 1st ed.; Harper Business: New York, NY, USA, 2002; ISBN 978-0-06-000773-7.
165. Fernqvist, F.; Ekelund, L. Credence and the effect on consumer liking of food—A review. *Food Qual. Prefer.* **2014**, *32*, 340–353. [CrossRef]
166. Foscht, T.; Maloles, C.; Schloffer, J.; Swoboda, B.; Chia, S.-L. Exploring the impact of customer satisfaction on food retailers' evolution: Managerial lessons from Austria. *J. Int. Food Agribus. Mark.* **2009**, *21*, 67–82. [CrossRef]
167. Morganosky, M.A.; Cude, B.J. Large format retailing in the US: A consumer experience perspective. *J. Retail. Consum. Serv.* **2000**, *7*, 215–222. [CrossRef]
168. Sheikhesmaeili, S.; Hazbavi, S. Model construction of engagement and outcomes in consumers food life: Evidence from chain stores customer. *Br. Food J.* **2019**, *121*, 218–239. [CrossRef]
169. Lonier, T. Alchemy in Eden: Entrepreneurialism, branding, and food marketing in the United States, 1880-1920. *Enterp. Soc.* **2010**, *11*, 695–708. [CrossRef]
170. McGale, L.S.; Halford, J.C.G.; Harrold, J.A.; Boyland, E.J. The Influence of Brand Equity Characters on Children's Food Preferences and Choices. *J. Pediatrics* **2016**, *177*, 33–38. [CrossRef] [PubMed]

Publisher's Note: MDPI stays neutral with regard to jurisdictional claims in published maps and institutional affiliations.

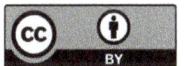 © 2020 by the author. Licensee MDPI, Basel, Switzerland. This article is an open access article distributed under the terms and conditions of the Creative Commons Attribution (CC BY) license (http://creativecommons.org/licenses/by/4.0/).

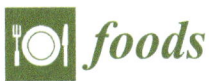

Review

The Link between the Consumer and the Innovations in Food Product Development

Raquel P. F. Guiné [1], Sofia G. Florença [2], Maria João Barroca [3,4,*] and Ofélia Anjos [5,6,7]

1. Research Centre for Natural Resources, Environment and Society (CERNAS), Polytechnic Institute of Viseu, 3504-510 Viseu, Portugal; raquelguine@esav.ipv.pt
2. Faculty of Nutrition and Food Sciences (FCNAUP), University of Porto, 4150-180 Porto, Portugal; sofiaguine@gmail.com
3. Polytechnic Institute of Coimbra, Coimbra College of Agriculture, Bencanta, 3045-601 Coimbra, Portugal
4. Department Chemistry, Molecular Physical-Chemistry R&D Unit, University of Coimbra, 3004-535 Coimbra, Portugal
5. Polytechnic Institute of Castelo Branco, 6000-084 Castelo Branco, Portugal; ofelia@ipcb.pt
6. CEF, Forest Research Centre, School of Agriculture, University of Lisbon, 1349-017 Lisbon, Portugal
7. CBP-BI, Plant Biotechnology Centre of Beira Interior, 6001-909 Castelo Branco, Portugal
* Correspondence: mjbarroca@gmail.com

Received: 7 August 2020; Accepted: 15 September 2020; Published: 18 September 2020

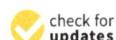

Abstract: New lifestyles, higher incomes and better consumer awareness are increasing the demand for a year-round supply of innovative food products. In past decades, important developments have been achieved in areas related to food and the food industry. This review shows that factors influencing performance in new product development (NPD) are dynamic and continuously guiding project development. The data obtained by direct involvement of consumers can impact positively successful product development and enhance the company's financial performance. The study of consumer behaviour and attitudes towards new foods encompasses multiple aspects, such as preference, choice, desire to eat certain foods, buying intentions and frequency of consumption. Additionally, both the consumers' willingness to purchase and the willingness to pay a premium are important in NPD, launching and success.

Keywords: buying intention; consumer acceptance; marketing innovation; price

1. Introduction

Today's manufacturing companies rely much on the success of new products, and this has become critical for a healthy business performance, having in mind the present competitive and fast shifting markets [1,2].

Developing appropriate strategies for achieving successful new product development (NPD) has required increasing consideration. Attention has been given to exposing the drivers of successful new product performance while at the same time highlighting the importance of measuring that performance ensuring viable product life-cycle (PLC). Still, it has been observed that the majority (50–75%) of consumer-packaged goods do not achieve desired levels of success, in general, and this is also a reality in the case of the food industry, for which contributes some degree of food neophobia [1,2].

Presently, the food sector is considered one of the most important in the current global economy. Nevertheless, food industry or food service companies still face many challenges in managing their products and competing in the market. In fact, the food manufacturing industry has been recognized as an area with high degrees of new product failure [1,3–5].

Products aim to fulfil certain needs, which are not constant because of differences among users, constraints, usage scenarios and social values, among others. Hence, in order to meet these differences, manufacturers rely on variety as a way to target different needs and preferences (Figure 1). In this sense, it is important to clarify some concepts: Variety or assortment is defined as a number or collection of different items of a particular class of the same general kind, while variant is an instance of a class that exhibits usually slight differences from the common type. Product variety is beneficial in a way that offers potential to expand markets, with economic benefits by increasing sales' volume and revenues. This market expansion can have two dimensions: on one hand, to reach entirely new customer segments, while on the other, being able to sell to existing customer segments more customized products repositioned as premium options. Nevertheless, this positive result is not automatic, and therefore, it must be evaluated. Variety is not necessarily always good, and more product variants may not be the best for customers when making purchase choices. It has been shown that when consumers have to choose among items in a wide assortment, frequently, they become too confused and cannot really perceive the differences between product variants and product quality. Besides, offering additional products with improved characteristics can bring increased costs from product design to production, inventory, marketing and service. Therefore, a deep evaluation must be done before making decisions about diversification of the present offer [6–8].

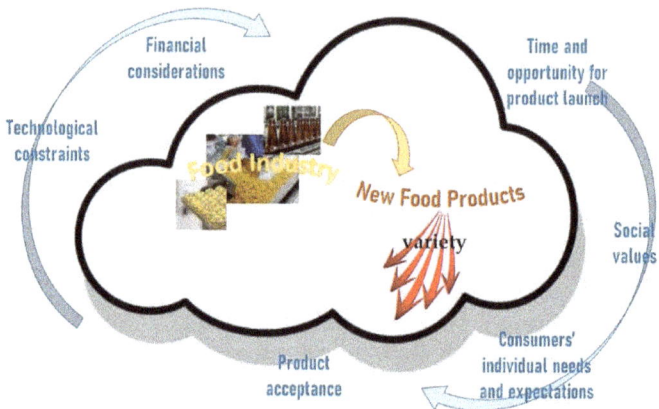

Figure 1. Industrial food development strategy (author's own work).

Historically, three main research perspectives in new food product development can be pointed out: (1) a technological perspective, according to which technological progress was the main driver of research and innovation in early times. Examples include technologies such as freezing or pasteurization or more recently extrusion, all technologies that were quite innovative in their own time. (2) A market-oriented perspective, according to which, back in the mid-60s, the establishment of marketing and appearance of supermarkets allied to new packaging and increased competition led to innovations in manufacture and marketing of distinguishable foods. (3) A consumer-led product development, which has more recently attracted attention to increase new products' success [1,9].

These approaches appear relatively independent, with technological aspects and product performance traditionally studied by food scientists and consumer researchers, whereas marketing and promotion of new food products would be in the field of economics, management and marketing. Nevertheless, at present, it is demonstrated that there is a need to integrate marketing, consumer research, food design and food technology to improve new food product performance [1,9]. Attempts have been made to establish an integrated approach to food product development, combining the different subjects that altogether contribute for the positive appreciation of the product by the final consumers (ex., technology, design, marketing, product benefits, consumer research). These go way back to the early stages of development until the final launch of the product in the market and evaluation [1,9].

The factors influencing NPD performance are dynamic and continuously influence the project of development, so that changes in those factors must be somewhat anticipated and measured multiple times throughout a product's life [1]. For a new product to be entirely successful, it must achieve excellence in three different areas: (a) reduced NPD cycle time, (b) high level of innovation and (c) reuse of company knowledge resources. To be successful in these three complementary areas, companies must pay attention to the factors that drive innovation: people, knowledge and systems. Product Lifecycle Management (PLM) focuses on the later (systems) and can constitute a key role for innovation and success [3,9].

2. Objective and Methodology

The objective of this review was to explore some aspects related to the role of consumer in the development of new foods, the factors that determine consumers' acceptance, the innovation in traditional products, the increasing market of novel healthy foods and willingness-to-pay for innovations in food product development.

The methodology that was followed in the elaboration of this review included on a first step the selection of the topics to be addressed. For this, the specific needs of industrials and developers were taken in consideration in view of the difficulty to find information gathered about these specific issues, thus giving place to the structure of this review:

- The role of consumer;
- New foods acceptance;
- Innovation in traditional foods;
- The market of innovative functional foods;
- Willingness to pay for innovation in new product development.

Industrials and developers want to make sure that their investment in new products will pay off by revenues in sales but will depend naturally on consumer acceptance. In the second step, after establishing the studied subjects, a search was conducted on the following scientific databases: science direct, B-on, SciELO, Science Citation Index and Mendeley. For each of the topics addressed, i.e., for each of the sections in this review, appropriate keywords were used to search for relevant works. Although this was not a systematic review, some inclusion criteria were established for each of the read articles based on the relevance for the particular aspects focused in our review and the publication date as recent as possible.

3. The Role of Consumer

To assess the ideal fitting of the new product with the needs of the target consumers, there are different methods available for the food industries to rely on, such as collecting data about consumers' needs and preferences [10,11]. A more traditional strategy includes a wide variety of tests designed to gather information about consumers' response to new ideas and concepts of possible food products as well as concrete developed products. These allow a more directly assessment of the level of acceptance by consumers regarding those new products, so important for successful launch [11]. Other types of approach make use of indirect data, which can also be used to determine the optimal degree of fit of the new product with the expectation of consumers (Figure 2). Examples of these include data on current food trends or aggregated data on environmental factors that affect consumers' needs and preferences, such as demographics, economical aspects, social and cultural factors or technological developments [11,12]. While the first, focusing on consumer involvement data collection and corresponding methodologies, have been more studied, the second group, namely study of consumer trends and socio-environmental factors, have been less analysed [10]. Ultimately, data obtained through direct involvement of consumers in NPD, like for example a consumer co-creation, constitute a rich source of product ideas and can have a positive impact on the successful product development and consequently improve the company's financial performance [13,14]. Nevertheless, food firms that use food trend and socio-environmental data, which point to future changes in consumers' needs and preferences, can more effectively develop products with longer PLC and in that way make their NPD more profitable [11,15].

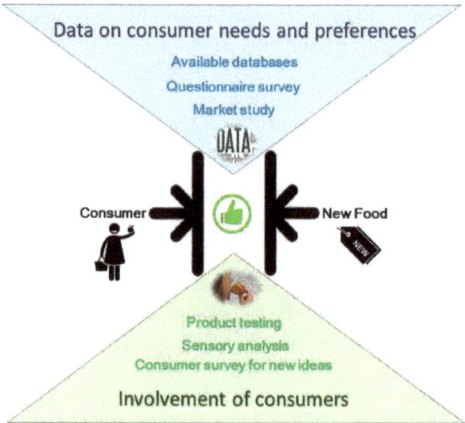

Figure 2. Fitting of the new food product with target consumers (author's own work).

Many studies have focused on consumer involvement data obtained and used only up to the launch of the new products. However, consumers' needs and tastes change over time. Hence, the fitting of the new product with the consumer is dynamic and sometimes obliges food industries to redesign and reformulate their products, even after they had already been launched to be marketed. Even in this case, a successful redesign or reformulation must be based on knowledge regarding what consumers like, or dislike, about the existing product. Hence, it is also important to understand whether food firms obtain and employ consumer data and analyse the fitness of the new product after its launch and also during the PLC [11].

4. New Foods Acceptance

The study of consumer food behaviour has been based on two types of variables, i.e., some related with behavioural aspects and others linked to attitudes. While the first include measures like preference, choice, purchase or consumption, the attitudes include affective measures of the desire to select or eat foods, purchase intent or desired frequency of consumption [16,17].

Research and development (R&D) activities in the food sector should be supported by a program of research on sensory analysis and consumer acceptance of foods, and that should be well established in the company for quite some time. The NPD is supported by intrinsic as well as extrinsic factors that impact consumer acceptance, regardless of being towards conventional or novel foods. These include the role of sensorial perceptions, cognitive evaluations and situational variables [18,19].

Although the measurements of food preference and acceptance attained through attitudinal judgments can become poor predictors of consumption, owing to their degree of motivational willingness, still these types of measures continue to be used to predict consumer behaviours toward new foods, regardless of being at industrial or academic levels. This is mostly due to the easiness in assessing these measurements, in a rapid and relatively simple way, with a controlled participation of the subjects. Although with an affective nature, these evaluations in response to a tasted food have become fundamental for studying consumer behaviour towards new foods and therefore are used to orient new product development or product improvement while ensuring quality in the food industry [16].

At present, innovation practices in the food industry rely very strongly on the voice of the consumer, recognized as vital for success. Hence, strategies to develop a successful new product include an appropriate sensory evaluation allied to an understanding of the consumers' acceptance criteria, which should be as detailed as possible [20]. When food scientists design tests intended to truthfully predict consumer behaviour at the point of purchase, they must not forget to include a proper number of variables related to marketing in their experimental design specifications, in order to guarantee that the right consumers will respond suitably to the new products [21,22]. However, for the assessment of a correct prediction of consumer behaviour, a high number of assessors is needed to evaluate food preferences regarding a specific product, which could represent a constraint.

The role of the sensory analysis for success when launching a new food product is complemented with defining the target consumers. In truth, for success on the market, it is crucial to direct, eventually, the product to the right people, leading to target segmentation. Hence, food products should be market oriented according to consumers' needs and expectations. To target a market segment, different criteria can be adopted (Figure 3): geographic variations; demographic characteristics (like sex or age); psychographic factors (including healthy or sportive lifestyles) or, lastly, behavioural criteria, like consumer's habits and types of purchase [23].

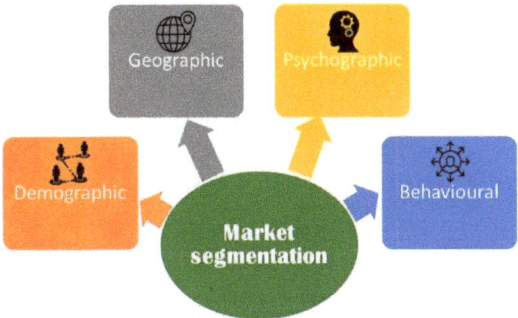

Figure 3. Marketing segmentation (author's own work).

When it comes to innovation, the food sector faces higher challenges when compared to other business areas, because people are more protective towards what they eat since, contrarily to other products, foods will enter their bodies and go all the way through the gastrointestinal tract, ending up absorbing many of their components. The concept of food neophobia, which consists in the fear of new foods, shows how this can be problematic. Although this phenomenon has been reported to have particular incidence in children, the truth is that there are people whose food neophobia persists into adulthood and truly determines their decisions when it comes to choosing between new unknown or old fully recognizable foods [17].

Consumer research and marketing dedicate attention to those segments of market interested in new products, and at the same time, the neophobic consumers shall not be neglected during the new product development process and marketing studies, because, depending on the specific product, they may represent an important share of the target market [24,25]. Some areas in which this is of particular importance include for example irradiation technology or gene mutation biotechnology, much owing to the fear of risks that these may bring for health [26–29].

The assessment of consumers' perceptions towards foods is of vital importance in the development and marketing of new foods [30]. Therefore, understanding how consumers respond to tests helps develop effective food marketing and communication strategies. Although communication and information do not really change the characteristics of the products, they can shape the attitudes of consumers and influence their choices and behaviours [31].

5. Innovation in Traditional Foods

Traditional food products (TFP) have been playing an important role in European culture, heritage and identity. The growth of this segment in the European food market has been providing a higher variety of food choices for consumers [32]. Moreover, traditional food may be viewed as an opportunity to rethink rural development and sustainability patterns in many countries and to add value to the market [33,34]. There are different definitions of traditional foods in the literature that intend to capture the various dimensions of this food concept [35–39]. Different conceptions to define traditional food contribute to explaining consumers' motivations to purchase traditional foods but may also cause low consumer awareness of TFPs [40]. From the general definitions, it follows that TFPs are characterized by historical, geographical and sociological dimensions. One possible definition of "traditional" related to foods was given by the European Commission as "traditional means proven usage in the community market for a time period showing transmission between generations; this time period should be the one generally ascribed as one human generation, at least 25 years" [41]. In 2007, the EuroFIR FP6 Network of Excellence developed an elaborative definition, which includes statements about traditional ingredients, traditional type of production and/or processing and composition [42,43]. Guerrero et al. [32] introduced in 2009 the perspective of consumers' point of view in traditional food product definition based on a study across six European countries that analysed the data using an ordinary semantic and textual statistical on four main dimensions (habit and natural, origin and locality, processing and elaboration and sensory properties). A traditional food product, from the consumers' perspective, was defined as "a product frequently consumed or associated with specific celebrations and/or seasons, normally transmitted from one generation to another, made accurately in a specific way according to the gastronomic heritage, with little or no processing/manipulation, distinguished and known because of its sensory properties and associated with a certain local area, region or country". Later, in 2010, Guerrero et al. [44] added the dimensions of health, heritage and variety to the definition of traditional foods. Furthermore, the study also notes that Central and Nordic regions tend to associate the term "traditional" primarily with practical issues such as usefulness, convenience and health whereas Southern regions tend to focus on broader concepts such as culture, heritage or history.

Although there are different definitions of TFP available in the literature, the concepts related to these food products are regulated by a European regulatory framework established in 1992 and updated in 2012 [45]. Furthermore, as part of its policy on food safety and quality and to boost competitiveness and profitability, the European Union (EU) has promoted a set of criteria for the registration and recognition of TFPs, namely, PDO (Protected Designation of Origin), PGI (Protected Geographical Indication) and TSG (Traditional Speciality Guaranteed), produced under predefined quality standards (Table 1).

Table 1. European Union labels for protected traditional products [46].

Protection Scheme	Symbol	Products	Specifications	Label
Protected designation of origin (PDO)		Food, agricultural products and wines.	Every part of the production, processing and preparation process must take place in the specific region. For wines, the grapes have to come exclusively from the geographical area where the wine is made.	Mandatory for food and agricultural products. Optional for wine.
Protected geographical indication (PGI)		Food, agricultural products and wines.	For most products, at least one of the stages of production, processing or preparation takes place in the region. In the case of wine, this means that at least 85% of the grapes used have to come exclusively from the geographical area where the wine is actually made.	Mandatory for food and agricultural products. Optional for wine.

Table 1. Cont.

Protection Scheme	Symbol	Products	Specifications	Label
Geographical indication of spirit drinks and aromatised wines (GI)		Spirit drinks and aromatised wines.	For most products, at least one of the stages of distillation or preparation takes place in the region. However, raw products do not need to come from the region.	Optional for all products.
Traditional speciality guaranteed (TSG)		Food and agricultural products.	It highlights the traditional aspects such as the way the product is made or its composition, without being linked to a specific geographical area.	Mandatory for all products.

Despite the controversial concept of innovation in the context of traditional foods, innovation can become an important tool to maintain and expand the market share of TFP through the improvement in convenience, safety or healthy products. Innovations in the traditional food sector have also the potential to strengthen and augment the market for traditional food products in accordance with the emerging difficulties, such as poor imitations and changing preferences and eating patterns towards more processed and convenience foods [43,47]. Other challenges such as the effective communication in the labels, legal protection of collective brands and quality assurance can contribute for the growth of traditional food market [35]. In fact, some TFPs in the EU are protected with designation quality schemes to protect producers and consumers from copycat goods. However, due to the low awareness of consumers and producers about the labels and poor understanding of the differences between them, these labels have little impact on the consumption of these traditional products. In this market, privately owned brand names are often more important quality signals to consumers than designation labels [48,49].

Innovations in traditional food are mainly introduced in the product characteristics or in packaging, which preserve the sensory quality and improve the shelf life (e.g., resealable packaging), but also in size, form and composition or in new ways of using the product but preserving the sensory quality. Given the impact of process on the authentic identity of the product, the innovation in production processes is less common and mainly refers to new technical solutions to improve quality assurance and traceability along the chain network. The organisational and market innovation can be valuable, but it is not yet recognized by all chain members of the traditional food sector and is limited to joint product development and formation of research organisations or networks [50].

For the successful introduction of innovations in traditional food products, it is also important to have a good understanding of consumers' perceptions and attitudes towards traditional food products and of consumers' needs and preferences when applying even small innovations to the traditional food products [51,52]. In this sense, consumers' acceptance and improvements of traditional foods are related with product quality, innovations oriented to safer and healthier products that do not compromise their sensory properties, labels with the guarantee of origin and more product variety and convenience-oriented innovations [50]. Innovation in the traditional food sector also aims to further guarantee quality by introducing full traceability along the chain, reinforcing the message of authenticity [36]. The integration of chain partners in the innovation increases the ability to innovate while at the same time diminishes the risks involved in their implementation [53,54].

Globally, any innovation related with TFPs has to be evaluated taking into account the specifications of the product, whose market success largely depends on how consumers perceive the innovation [55].

6. The Market of Innovative Functional Foods

Both functional foods and nutraceuticals are food products that bear some additional health benefits beyond just nutrition. Food innovation is, among other factors, also driven by the aim to improve health or prevent disease (the scope of functional foods) or even contribute to prevent or treat certain disorders or diseases (the ambit of nutraceuticals). Although without globally accepted or legally established definitions, functional foods are recognized as providing additional benefits besides the most general functions of satisfying hunger or desire to eat and of nutrient intake [56,57].

Although there are some food categories in which more intensive development of functional foods has been made, there has been functional food development in all food categories (foods and beverages of different nature), by fortification, modification of characteristics, etc. To cite some categories in which a higher diversity and number of functional foods have been developed, one could mention the dairy sector, confectionery, soft-drinks, bakery and baby-foods [58]. Table 2 presents some relevant literature to expand the knowledge about innovations in some selected domains of functional foods.

Table 2. Some relevant literature focusing on innovations in the domain of functional foods.

Category	Product	Scope	Reference
Dairy	Fermented dairy products	Scientific evidence about consumption of fermented dairy products and their health benefits	[59]
	Yogurt	Development of functional yogurts enriched with antioxidants extracted from wine	[60]
	Yogurt	Adding apple pomace as a functional ingredient to yogurt and yogurt drinks has the potential to increase the level of dietary fibre and phytochemicals, enhancing their health effects	[61]
	Dairy products	The effect of ohmic heating on probiotic metabolism and the application of this technology for the development of functional products	[62]
	Dairy products	Goat milk as a raw material for the production of functional dairy products due to the presence of functional prebiotics and probiotic bacteria	[63]
	Yogurt	Enrichment of yogurts in conjugated linolenic acid by the utilization of pomegranate and jacaranda seeds as functional components	[64]
	Yogurt	Development of yogurt formulations containing strawberries and chia seeds as health enhancing components	[65]
	Fermented dairy product	Study the feasibility for production of a functional fermented dairy-based product rich in menaquinone-7 by using iron oxide hydroxide (FeOOH) nanoparticles	[66]
Confectionary and bakery	Biscuits and breads	Use of an olive oil by-product as a functional ingredient in bakery products	[67]
	Bakery products	The use of by-products from the food industry as functional ingredients added in bakery products	[68]
	Bakery products	The use of functional ingredients in bakery products originating from marine foods	[69]
	Bakery products	The application of fibre concentrate from mango fruit as a functional ingredient with antioxidant activity in bakery products	[70]
	Biscuits and breads	Fortification of breads and biscuits with millet, oilseeds and herbs	[71]
	Bread	Fortification of bread with wheat bran protein concentrate	[72]
	Bread	Development of high-fibre wheat bread using microfluidized corn bran	[73]
Soft drinks	Plant-based dairy alternatives	Impact of the EU regulatory framework on innovation in the industry and consumers of vegetable drinks alternative to dairy products	[74]
	Fermented fruit drink	Use of coconut water and inulin as a source of soluble fibre for the development of a symbiotic fermented functional drink	[75]
	Fruit drink	The development of a functional non-alcoholic drink based on prekese fruits	[76]
	Fruit drink	Development of a functional beverage by microencapsulation of lyophilised wild pomegranate flavedo phenolics	[77]

From a product point of view, functional foods can be classified into [78,79]:

- Food fortified with additional nutrients (labelled fortified products)—example: fruit juices fortified with vitamins or dietary minerals;
- Food with additional new nutrients or components not usually present in a particular food (labelled enriched products)—example: probiotics or prebiotics;

- Food from which a harmful component has been removed, reduced or replaced by another with beneficial effects (labelled altered products)—example: use of fibres as fat releasers in high fat content foods;
- Food in which one of the components has been naturally enhanced (labelled enhanced commodities)—example: eggs with increased omega-3 content.

From the functional point of view, i.e., having in mind the objectives of the functional foods, another classification is used [80]:

- Functional foods that add benefits to life or improve children's life—example: prebiotics and probiotics;
- Functional foods that reduce an existing health risk problem—example: foods that decrease high cholesterol or high blood pressure;
- Functional foods which make life easier—example: lactose-free or gluten-free products, for people with food allergies or intolerances.

The development of novel functional foods and nutraceuticals has been increasing largely because, on one hand, the market is demanding these products, and on the other hand, the chemistry and biochemistry of natural products as well as food technology and biotechnology have allowed important advancements. Moreover, countless studies undertaken to confirm the health claims of this type of product or their bioactive components have contributed for a great development of this market [57,81–86].

In Europe, claims of health benefits for marketing of food products are subject to Regulation (EC) No 1924/2006: Nutrition and Health Claims Made on Foods [87], which determines that any health benefits of foods announced must be scientifically proven. This regulation intends to protect consumers from deceptive or false benefits, as well as to harmonise the markets within the countries of the European Union (EU). Additionally, this regulation also aims to stimulate reliable food innovation and development. The Regulation 1924/2006 defines a health claim as any voluntary statement that refers to the relationship between food and health and establishes three classes of health claims: (1) general function claims, which can be based on generally accepted (Art. 13.1) or newly developed scientific evidence (Art. 13.5), (2) reduction of disease risk claims (Art. 14.1a) and (3) claims referring to children's development and health (Art. 14.1b) [56,87].

Complementary health approaches include natural products and mind and body practices, as recognized by the National Centre for Complementary and Integrative Health of the USA [88]. Natural products are also considered as dietary supplements, complementary medicines, alternative medicines or traditional medicines, and are recognized by the World Health Organization as playing an important role in health promotion all over the world [89,90]. In the United States of America (USA), The Dietary Supplement Health and Education Act (DSHEA) system was introduced in 1994 to regulate supplements with health benefits [91].

In Japan, a country with a long history of utilization of foods with health benefits and the place of birth of functional foods, a functional food regulation called "foods for specified health uses" (FOSHU) was introduced in 1991. After its introduction, countless clinically proven FOSHU products with health benefits have been developed and launched in the market. Most of these products claim to be beneficial for the gastro-intestinal health, by using probiotics, prebiotics and synbiotics. Other targeted health functions with claims include lowering triglycerides level, blood pressure, LDL (low-density lipoprotein)-cholesterol and blood glucose. After 2007, in Japan, the market for FOSHU products was nearly saturated. Nevertheless, a new functional regulatory system called "Foods with Function Claims" (or New Functional Foods) was introduced in 2015, and allowed the development of many New Functional Foods due to two main reasons: higher flexibility regarding health claims as compared to FOSHU and no need for governmental approval [92,93].

Because nowadays the boundaries between the food and pharmaceutical industries are somewhat blurred, the perceptions of the consumers towards these health-related borderline products need to be investigated. The success of these products is influenced by consumers' perception of their safety, efficacy, appearance and the placement of the product into one of those categories: food or pharmaceutical. In a survey conducted by Khedkar et al. [94] in Germany, it was found that consumers, and particularly young and highly educated women, were not convinced of the health effects of these borderline products with alleged health benefits. Although they perceived these products as GRAS (Generally Recognized as Safe), they did not consider their consumption as an easy way to stay healthy.

The attractiveness of functional foods and intention to try and eventually purchase such foods vary according to the type of product. Foods that are perceived by the consumer as healthier are judged more positively, and therefore, consumer acceptance is higher. It is important to evaluate the general principles that influence consumer responses to the health-related aspects of functional foods, including the claims, much beyond the product's characteristics alone. One of the first aspects to consider is how believable the claims are to the consumer, since in principle, consumers frequently show some scepticism towards health or nutritional claims like those found on food labels. The construct of believability is not necessarily a strong cause for purchase intent. Still, it is supposed to interact with a number of other variables. While for some foods, the purchase intention has been influenced by low levels of scepticism towards the information provided on the product label, this is not entirely true for other foods, for which purchase intentions persist high even if the product is not fully perceived to entirely fulfil the advertised claims. Some causes that may explain this include the consumers' familiarity with the claim and/or associated ingredients, the way in which the claim is phrased and framed, and finally the familiarity with the product itself and the extent to which the claim is consistent with the nature of the product. Another factor that influences the consumer acceptance and behaviour is the source of the claim, i.e., whether the information refers to a claim that was approved by some regulatory authority or if it is a hedonic claim made by the product manufacturer. While in many countries or regions there are strict regulations about this matter, in some others it is admissible by manufacturers to make the claims without supporting scientific evidence [95–98].

Other factors are related with the consumers' intentions to try or purchase new foods, functional foods included, such as age, gender, education level, nutrition knowledge, dietary pattern, taste preferences or marketing and advertising. The market segmentation according to these categories, so as to consider the individual differences, has been used for long in food-related consumer research, including also the market for functional foods [98–100].

Lifestyle corresponds to a social concept shared by a group of people with similar attitudes towards certain variables and is strongly affected by their simultaneous needs for integration (sense of belonging) and differentiation (sense of individuality). Lifestyles of people sharing a common culture or social class and having similar professional activities are not necessarily equal. Hence, lifestyle cannot be solely attributed to demographic parameters like gender, age, education, or income but can also relate to integration or individual self-expression [98–100].

Consumers' behaviours and attitudes concerning foods with health claims are also partially influenced by their own general state of health or some particular diseases, as well as the perception of how relevant the health claim might be. Additionally, the attributes that shape the perception of a food being or not helpful for a certain health/disease condition differ between groups of people [98,99,101,102].

Regarding the development of new functional foods aimed at specific markets, like older people, there are important challenges to be considered. In this ambit, care must be devoted to the sensory properties of the products, and the consumers have to be seen as particular because they show inconstant behaviours, including many of the times negative attitudes towards innovative foods or beverages [103,104]. Nevertheless, in general, it could be expected that older consumers would eventually be open to new functional foods, because these are formulated in such a way that they provide additional nutritional and health benefits, and older people tend to be more interested in maintaining health and preventing chronic diseases, when they come to a certain age where those are more probable to appear. Henceforth, to achieve success when developing new functional foods and beverages, the communication of the health benefits associated with the products must be effective to the targeted consumers [103,105,106].

Alicia et al. [107] conducted a study to understand the factors that affect consumer choice regarding foods that contain functional ingredients, by recurring to Multicriteria Decision Methods (MCDM) that are valuable to help in the decision process when designing the products in the stage of product development. The study was done with Venezuelan consumers of yoghurt, who rated with highest utility value the yogurt containing pieces of fruit, with a firm texture, which regulates intestinal function, low in fat, with sweetener (Splenda) and at an intermediate price [107].

Functional foods which increase satiety are frequently used to control appetite and help in weight loss. In order to understand the consumers' perceptions towards this type of products, Hunter el al. [99] evaluated the influence of claims of appetite control in trustworthiness and purchasing intentions, in a sample of Australian individuals trying to lose or maintain weight. Their results showed that believability of product concept statements was highly variable, depending on the type of product. Furthermore, it was shown that consumers actively trying to lose weight demonstrated higher purchase intent as compared to consumers that were only trying to maintain their current weight, even though these two types of consumers tended to have similar levels of trust in the product concept. Variables such as age, gender or sceptical attitude towards functional foods were not found to greatly determine the purchase intent or trust regarding these functional food products [99].

7. Willingness to Pay for Innovation in NPD

It has been observed that people around the world spend a considerable amount on natural products, for example, as reported in Asia, Canada or Australia. In the USA, these natural products are bought in the form of dietary supplements, a domain in which there has been an increase in expenditure, with costs going from 9.6 billion dollars in 1994 to 41.1 billion dollars in 2016. Within the near future it is expected that over 294 billion dollars are spent on dietary supplements by 2021 [89,108] (Figure 4). The global market value for functional food products was estimated in 168 billion dollars in 2013 and can eventually nearly double in less than a decade, reaching 300 billion dollars by 2020 [109,110] (Figure 5). In japan, the total market for functional foods (FOSHU and New Functional Foods) in 2018 was 8 billion dollars [93].

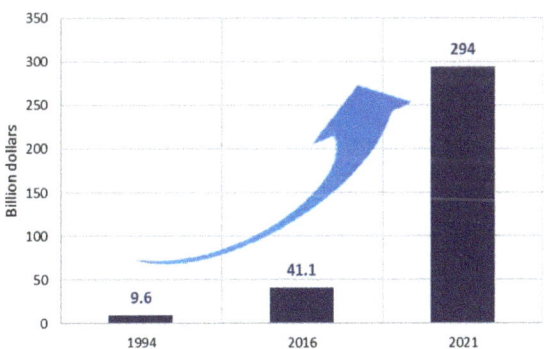

Figure 4. Value of the market of dietary supplements in the US [89,108].

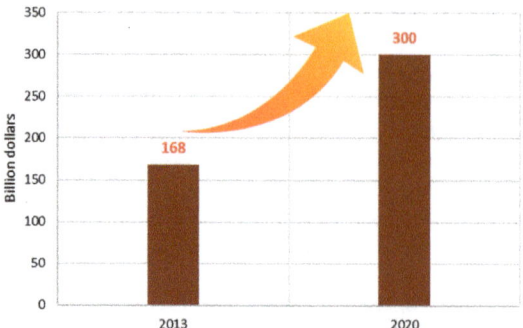

Figure 5. Global market value of functional foods [109,110].

The market share for functional food products is growing due to their benefits for human health and because consumers attribute increasing importance to food as part of a healthy lifestyle. Therefore, functional foods are becoming a part of consumers' regular diets. Notwithstanding the increasing market, the rate of unsuccessful food products is high, and this trend is also observed for the market of functional food products. A high number of the newly introduced products are removed from the market soon after they are launched, and some of the possible reasons that could explain this include an overreliance on technological innovations coupled to an erroneous judgment of consumers' needs and preferences [109–112].

According to different research findings, the willingness to purchase functional foods is influenced by factors of very diverse nature, some associated with the consumer and others with characteristics of the product, such as level of involvement of the consumer with the product, consumer lifestyle, sensory attributes and other characteristics of the product, price, brand, country of origin of the product, possible health claims announced on the packaging, the benefits of the product, among others [109].

In line with Ares et al. [113], consumers perceive functional foods as products belonging to a certain category. Hence, apart from the health benefits and the sensory characteristics, non-sensory factors like package may be determinant to shape consumers' buying decisions. In this context, the authors studied the influence of different package attributes on consumer willingness to purchase chocolate milk desserts in two variations: the regular and an improved functional version. Their results, obtained for consumers in Uruguay, showed that consumers' level of involvement with the product influenced their evaluation of it. Moreover, it was observed that the colour of the package and the presence of a picture on the label were the factors considered most relevant by consumers, regardless of their level of involvement with the product [113].

Romano et al. [114] investigated how Brazilian consumers perceive a non-traditional and innovative pomegranate juice by identifying the role of packaging attributes relevant to the consumer's intention to purchase. In this study, five factors were considered: (1) the technology used in the juice production: HPP (high hydrostatic pressure) is a non-thermal technology that preserves nutritional as well as sensory properties of the products, (2) the antioxidant potential of the juice, (3) price, (4) preservatives, (5) colourings. The obtained results showed that consumers valued information about the technology used and also about the antioxidant properties, as drivers to define purchasing intentions [114].

Szakály et al. [100] evaluated to what extent lifestyle and health behaviour influenced consumption of functional foods in Hungary. The results obtained revealed that consumers make balanced decisions, looking for promotional products and bargains in order to obtain good value for their spent money. Furthermore, the authors were able to identify different segments of consumers: the rational, the uninvolved, the conservative, the careless, and the adventurous. The rational consumers, characterized by health consciousness and moderate price sensitivity, represent the most relevant target group for the functional food market. Moreover, the adventurous food consumers stand out as an equally important target group, because they are eager for novelty. The conservative consumers, characterized by positive health behaviour, also represent an interesting segment. In this way, the authors concluded that lifestyle and health behaviour are importantly linked with the preference for functional food products [100].

In a study with German consumers conducted by Goetzke and Spiller [115], it was observed that consumers who purchase functional foods and those who consume organic foods share some features regarding health and well-being. Nevertheless, they present some differentiating aspects, since the purchase of organic or functional foods is driven by different lifestyles: while purchasing of organic foods is associated to consumers with active lifestyles, the buying of functional foods is linked to consumers with a more passive lifestyle [115].

Cukelj et al. [116] studied the attitudes of Croatian consumers towards innovative flaxseed-enriched cookies, which can act as carriers for functional components like lignans and omega-3 fatty acids. The consumers revealed a high level of interest in the functional cookies, especially the elderly women with higher nutrition knowledge and consciousness [116].

Kraus [117] studied the factors influencing willingness to purchase functional foods in Poland and found that these factors were information on the health benefits and nutritional properties of the product, attributes related to taste, health and safety, practical packaging, freshness, purity and naturalness. In relation to the health benefits, the prevention of health problems and the strengthening of the body and improvement of its functions were identified as valued by consumers. With regards to the functional components, consumers showed more interest in vitamins and minerals, dietary fibre and omega-3 fatty acids. Finally, concerning the carriers, consumers preferred cereal products, dairy products, meat products and mixtures of fruits and vegetables [117].

The market of functional foods also includes products specifically addressed to children. Hence, Annunziata et al. [118] evaluated how the parents' choices for suitable functional foods for their children are shaped, using a sample of Italian participants. The results obtained indicated that parents tend to show a strong interest in functional nutrition when choosing foods for their children, even when they are not very well familiarized with these products. Moreover, the variables that influenced the frequency of purchase were sociodemographic characteristics, parents' nutritional knowledge, trust in those products and familiarity with them [118].

Besides the consumers' willingness to purchase, also the willingness to pay a premium is important in new product development because it helps manufacturers to estimate the amount of profit they can expect from selling their product. This is particularly important having in mind that, nowadays, food manufacturers dedicate important budgets to R&D of new food products, as in the case of functional foods. The willingness to pay has been investigated by applying mathematical/economic models, particularly methods of experimental auction, but also contingent valuation method, choice experiment or others [109,119].

Regarding the functional foods market, it has been reported that willingness to pay can be influenced by variables such as health claims, demographic characteristics, trust in products, trust in the technologies used for their production, previous knowledge about the product or functional ingredient and degree of fitting between the carrier and the functional component [109].

Szakály et al. [120] proposed a new model for the willingness of consumers in Hungary to pay for functional foods, by modifying the Munene model. The results obtained with the modified model suggested that consumers have more positive attitudes towards functional foods and consequently are more willing to pay a premium for those products if they truly believe in their health benefits. The highest influential variables identified were the attitudes towards functional foods, followed by beliefs about the attributes of functional foods, and then by the demographic characteristics of the consumers [120].

Consumers tend to increasingly appreciate novel functional foods because they recognize their role in preventing or reducing the risks of some pathologies and particularly chronic diseases as well as improving other physiological functions, helping to achieve a better global health status. The willingness to pay for two types of functional yogurts, enriched with probiotics and with catechin, was measured by Moro et al. [119] for a sample of Italian consumers using the panel data version of a Random Parameters Logit model. The results obtained indicated that the participants were willing to pay a considerably higher premium for the catechin-enriched yogurt, almost double than that of the probiotic version. Furthermore, the results indicated that the willingness to pay for catechin enrichment was associated with grouping variables such as age, income, health status, lifestyle and education [119]. The work by Vecchio et al. [121] investigated also for Italian consumers the willingness to pay for three types of yogurt (conventional, organic and functional) considering two levels of information provided: basic (participants were presented yogurts labelled conventional, organic or functional) and advanced (participants were given additional information). The experiment was carried out using the Vickrey fifth-price sealed-bid mechanism. The findings indicated that providing additional information by, for example, a specific health claim increased consumer's willingness to pay a premium for the functional yogurt, but a similar relation was nor observed for the organic yogurt, for which additional information on organic regulation did not add much perceived value to the extra expenditure. Moreover, it was observed that specific socio-demographic variables like gender, age, presence of children in the household and the need to follow a specific diet influence the willingness to pay for both functional and organic yogurts [121].

Romano et al. [122] used the contingent valuation method to estimate Brazilian consumer's willingness to pay a premium for an innovative added-value pomegranate juice. The average consumer's willingness to pay more for pomegranate juice was estimated, and the income elasticity coefficient was also calculated, so that a 10% increase in consumer income might be expected to induce a raise of about 2% in the willingness to pay the premium for the innovative pomegranate juice [122].

Roosen et al. [123] analysed how consumers trust in a new food technology, in this specific case nanotechnology. Many different concepts for trust can be found in the scientific literature, but from the economic point of view, trust can cause lower efforts towards self-protecting behaviour. Studies conducted with participants from Canada and Germany confirm that a higher level of trust in novel food products' characteristics (orange juice) increases the willingness to pay for them, and this is also the case when new information about the technology is provided [123].

The effect of information on consumers' preferences and willingness to pay for a functional food product (red ginseng concentrate) in Asia were investigated by Ahn et al. [124]. The results suggested that objective information can lead to discrepant changes in consumers' valuation of different product attributes and increase willingness to pay for the functional product [124].

Pappalardo and Lusk [125] conducted a study that, based on food values and willingness to pay measures, aims to identify consumers' subjective beliefs about functional foods. The study was performed with a sample of participants from Sicily (Italy), and the product evaluated was a new functional snack prepared with white lupine and citrus fibre. The obtained results indicated that there was a willingness to pay a premium for the product at test, and the extra value would depend both on the functional components of the product and also on other characteristics that go beyond intrinsic healthy properties. Moreover, the consumers' willingness to pay for functional foods was clearly influenced by food values related to origin, safety, naturalness and price, among others. This means that consumers present dissimilar subjective beliefs when it comes to functional or non-functional foods [125].

Bruschi et al. [126] evaluated Russian consumers' attitudes towards novel functional bakery products (bread and biscuits) made with purple wheat, naturally rich in anthocyanins. Because anthocyanins are a class of phenolic compounds with high antioxidant activity, they have been reported to exhibit anti-inflammatory, anti-cancer, anti-diabetic and ocular-health-enhancing properties. In this way, bakery products with high amounts of anthocyanins are considered functional foods with benefits for human health. The results obtained indicated that, despite the low level of knowledge about these bioactive compounds, when the participants were provided with information about their health-enhancing properties, most of them actually ended up valuing these products as compared with base products. Finally, the results also allowed verifying that the type of product matters (functional bread was better accepted as compared to biscuits) and the level of information provided also matters (the willingness to pay a premium was higher when information was given about the nature of the purple wheat being an old variety when compared to information about the content in anthocyanins) [126].

The ingestion of functional foods represents a somewhat inexpensive and cost-effective way to access nutritious foods that provide long-term advantages for the wellbeing of individuals and households. However, this has different impacts whether talking about urban or rural areas, in which people rely primarily, if not totally, on purchased food commodities or produced foods, respectively. The use of fortified foods or diversified/modified diets involves consuming a variety of foods that provide the diverse macro-nutrients, micro-nutrients and bioactive compounds beneficial for consumers. Nevertheless, when it comes to low income consumers, it is important to evaluate if they are willing to pay for these improved and nutritious foods, which are recommended as primary intervention to reduce nutritional deficiencies, and especially micro-nutrients, in developing countries. The work by Chege et al. [127] investigated this problematic and also how these consumers value these products, i.e., if they are accepted as the traditional basic foods or if they are regarded as luxurious new food products. For the study, they used as model a porridge flour. Their results indicated that low income consumers in Kenya and Uganda are willing to pay an extra amount for the improved biofortified porridge flour. Besides, it was observed that the willingness to pay was influenced by factors such as providing nutrition information about the product, characteristics of household, economic status of the household and presence of young children (6–59 months old) in the household [127,128].

The perception of TFPs by consumers is related to origin, locality, authenticity and gastronomic heritage of regions or countries that frequently evoke memories of childhood. Furthermore, since the TFPs are primarily appreciated by consumers for their natural nature and distinguishing sensory characteristics, the innovation of these traditional products may be accepted if it preserves the naturalness and the sensory profile of the product [39,129]. Still, other innovations that improve the healthiness and nutritional profile of TFPs are accepted by consumers, as long as they reinforce the traditional and authentic character of the product [130]. However, innovations in traditional foods seem to be more readily accepted by those who frequently consume a particular product [52]. For example, the study of Roselli et al. [55] that evaluated the willingness of consumers to accept an innovative extra virgin olive oil (EVOO) obtained by ultrasound extraction revealed that the consumers who are more keen to accept and purchase the product are those who perceived the product's quality positively after being informed about the pivotal properties of the new product.

Pieniak et al. [131] found that while familiarity and the natural content of food is positively associated with consumption and general attitude toward traditional food, the convenience was negatively related to attitude and consumption of TFPs. However, attitude towards and consumption of TFPs was not correlated with the degree to which consumers valued sensory qualities and price sensitivity.

Molnár et al. [129] conducted a study within the European Union (EU) project TRUEFOOD (Integrated project in 6th Framework Programme; Contract no. FOOD-CT-2006-016264) to examine traditional food chain goals while also exploring the link between those and the generic consumer perceptions and choices in relation to traditional foods. In this study, the aspects identified as more relevant and important to consumers were traditionalism and quality goals.

8. Final Remarks

The food sector is one of the most relevant ones in the present global economy. However, companies related to food production, transformation and services still face many challenges, being one of the most pertinent the high number of unsuccessful new products. Presently, innovation practices in the food industry attribute vital importance to the voice of the consumer, recognized as essential for success. The study of consumer behaviour and attitudes towards food includes measures like preference, choice, purchase or consumption, desire to eat certain foods, buying intentions and frequency of consumption. Moreover, strategies to develop a successful new product include an appropriate sensory evaluation allied to an understanding of the consumers' acceptance criteria. Hence, consumers can be viewed as pivotal agents to develop products with more value and able to fit market needs after launch as well as during the PLC.

Regarding the new foods' acceptance, the incorporation of intrinsic as well as extrinsic factors on novel foods development, such as the sensorial perceptions and cognitive evaluations of consumers, are vital. Moreover, the knowledge of consumer perception helps to develop effective food marketing and communication strategies that influence their choices and behaviours.

Concerning the innovation in traditional foods, the producers still face the challenge to further improve their convenience, safety and healthiness. However, to protect the integrity of traditional products and to include the perceptions and behaviour of consumers, the innovation of TFPs should be considered in terms of specificities and with the involvement of all links in the chain of the traditional food. However, much of the development of new food products is destined to the market of functional foods and nutraceuticals, which has been increasing hugely due to higher consumer demand for these health enhancing products and because consumers are increasingly more informed. The appeal of functional foods and the intention to try and eventually purchase such foods vary according to the type of product and to how the consumer perceives their beneficial effects of their health claim.

Both the consumers' willingness to purchase and the willingness to pay a premium are important in new product development and help food manufacturers to estimate the amount of profit they can expect by selling their products. This is so much more because nowadays food manufacturers spend important budgets on R&D of new food products, as for example in functional foods. It has been reported that the willingness to purchase functional foods is influenced by factors such as level of involvement of the consumer with the product, consumer lifestyle, sensory attributes and other characteristics of the product, price, brand, country of origin, possible health claims announced on the packaging and the benefits of the product, among others. Moreover, the willingness to pay can be influenced by variables such as health claims, demographic characteristics, trust in the products, trust in the technologies used for their production, previous knowledge about the product or functional ingredient and degree of fit between the carrier and the functional component. Concerning traditional foods, the prerequisite for consumers' willingness to purchase and pay a premium for innovation in traditional food products is the preservation and the reinforcement of the traditional and authentic character of the products.

Author Contributions: Conceptualization, R.P.F.G.; methodology, R.P.F.G.; writing—original draft preparation, R.P.F.G., S.G.F., M.J.B., O.A.; writing—review and editing, R.P.F.G., S.G.F., M.J.B., O.A.; visualization, R.P.F.G.; supervision, R.P.F.G.; funding acquisition, R.P.F.G. All authors have read and agreed to the published version of the manuscript.

Funding: FCT-Foundation for Science and Technology, I.P., project Ref^a UIDB/00681/2020.

Acknowledgments: This work is funded by National Funds through the FCT-Foundation for Science and Technology, I.P., within the scope of the project Ref^a UIDB/00681/2020. Furthermore, we would like to thank the CERNAS Research Centre and the Polytechnic Institute of Viseu for their support. Thanks to Project reference POCI-01-0145-FEDER-029305, co-financed by the Foundation for Science and Technology (FCT) and the European Regional Development Fund (ERDF), through Portugal 2020-Competitiveness and Internationalization Operational Program (POCI). Forest Research Centre (CEF) is a research unit funded by Fundação para a Ciência e a Tecnologia I.P. (FCT), Portugal (UIDB/00239/2020).

Conflicts of Interest: The authors declare no conflict of interest.

References

1. Horvat, A.; Behdani, B.; Fogliano, V.; Luning, P.A. A systems approach to dynamic performance assessment in new food product development. *Trends Food Sci. Technol.* **2019**, *91*, 330–338. [CrossRef]
2. Kalluri, V.; Kodali, R. Analysis of new product development research: 1998–2009. *Benchmarking Int. J.* **2014**. [CrossRef]

3. Pinna, C.; Galati, F.; Rossi, M.; Saidy, C.; Harik, R.; Terzi, S. Effect of product lifecycle management on new product development performances: Evidence from the food industry. *Comput. Ind.* **2018**, *100*, 184–195. [CrossRef]
4. Pinna, C.; Plo, L.; Robin, V.; Girard, P.; Terzi, S. An approach to improve implementation of PLM solution in food industry—case study of Poult Group. *Int. J. Prod. Lifecycle Manag.* **2017**, *10*, 151–170. [CrossRef]
5. Ryynänen, T.; Hakatie, A. "We must have the wrong consumers"—A case study on new food product development failure. *Br. Food J.* **2014**. [CrossRef]
6. Bech, S.; Brunoe, T.D.; Nielsen, K.; Andersen, A.-L. Product and process variety management: Case study in the food industry. *Procedia CIRP* **2019**, *81*, 1065–1070. [CrossRef]
7. ElMaraghy, H.; Schuh, G.; ElMaraghy, W.; Piller, F.; Schönsleben, P.; Tseng, M.; Bernard, A. Product variety management. *CIRP Ann.* **2013**, *62*, 629–652. [CrossRef]
8. Huffman, C.; Kahn, B.E. Variety for sale: Mass customization or mass confusion? *J. Retail.* **1998**, *74*, 491–513. [CrossRef]
9. Moskowitz, H.R.; Saguy, I.; Straus, T. *An Integrated Approach to New Food Product Development*; CRC Press, Taylor & Francis Group: Boca Raton, FL, USA, 2009; ISBN 978-1-4200-6553-4.
10. Busse, M.; Siebert, R. The role of consumers in food innovation processes. *Eur. J. Innov. Manag.* **2018**. [CrossRef]
11. Horvat, A.; Granato, G.; Fogliano, V.; Luning, P.A. Understanding consumer data use in new product development and the product life cycle in European food firms—An empirical study. *Food Qual. Prefer.* **2019**, *76*, 20–32. [CrossRef]
12. Janssen, K.L.; Dankbaar, B. Proactive involvement of consumers in innovation: Selecting appropriate techniques. *Int. J. Innov. Manag.* **2008**, *12*, 511–541. [CrossRef]
13. Martinez, M.G. Co-creation of value by open innovation: Unlocking new sources of competitive advantage. *Agribusiness* **2014**, *30*, 132–147. [CrossRef]
14. Zaborek, P.; Mazur, J. Enabling Value Co-Creation with Consumers as a Driver of Business Performance: A Dual Perspective of Polish Manufacturing and Service SMEs. *J. Bus. Res.* **2019**, *104*, 541–551. [CrossRef]
15. Fuller, G.W. *New Food Product Development: From Concept to Marketplace*, 3rd ed.; CRC Press: Boca Raton, FL, USA, 2016; ISBN 978-1-4398-1865-7.
16. Cardello, A.V.; Schutz, H.; Snow, C.; Lesher, L. Predictors of food acceptance, consumption and satisfaction in specific eating situations. *Food Qual. Prefer.* **2000**, *11*, 201–216. [CrossRef]
17. Guiné, R.P.F.; Valente, L.P.; Ramalhosa, E.C.D. New foods, new consumers: Innovation in food product development. *Curr. Nutr. Food Sci.* **2016**, *12*, 175–189. [CrossRef]
18. Cardello, A.V. Consumer concerns and expectations about novel food processing technologies: Effects on product liking. *Appetite* **2003**, *40*, 217–233. [CrossRef]
19. Meiselman, H.L.; Schutz, H.G. History of food acceptance research in the US Army. *Appetite* **2003**, *40*, 199–216. [CrossRef]
20. Guiné, R. Sweet samosas: A new food product in the Portuguese market. *Acad. Res. Int.* **2012**, *2*, 70–81.
21. Cooper, R.G. *Winning at New Products: Accelerating the Process. from Idea to Launch*; Perseus Publishing: Cambridge, MA, USA, 2001; ISBN 978-0-7382-0463-5.
22. Garber, L.L., Jr.; Hyatt, E.M.; Starr, R.G., Jr. Measuring consumer response to food products. *Food Qual. Prefer.* **2003**, *14*, 3–15. [CrossRef]
23. Kotler, P.; Armstrong, G. *Principles of Marketing*, 15th ed.; Prentice Hall: Upper Saddle, NJ, USA, 2013; ISBN 978-0-13-308404-7.
24. Guiné, R.P.F.; Barros, A.; Queirós, A.; Pina, A.; Vale, A.; Ramoa, H.; Folha, J.; Carneiro, R. Development of a solid vinaigrette and product testing. *J. Culin. Sci. Technol.* **2013**, *11*, 259–274. [CrossRef]
25. Henriques, A.S.; King, S.C.; Meiselman, H.L. Consumer segmentation based on food neophobia and its application to product development. *Food Qual. Prefer.* **2009**, *20*, 83–91. [CrossRef]
26. Chen, X.-P.; Li, W.; Xiao, X.-F.; Zhang, L.-L.; Liu, C.-X. Phytochemical and pharmacological studies on Radix Angelica sinensis. *Chin. J. Nat. Med.* **2013**, *11*, 577–587. [CrossRef] [PubMed]
27. Costa-Font, M.; Gil, J.M.; Traill, W.B. Consumer acceptance, valuation of and attitudes towards genetically modified food: Review and implications for food policy. *Food Policy* **2008**, *33*, 99–111. [CrossRef]
28. Koivisto Hursti, U.; Magnusson, M.K.; Algers, A. Swedish consumers' opinions about gene technology. *Br. Food J.* **2002**, *104*, 860–872. [CrossRef]

29. Miles, S.; Ueland, Ø.; Frewer, L.J. Public attitudes towards genetically-modified food. *Br. Food J.* **2005**, *107*, 246–262. [CrossRef]
30. Da Silva, V.M.; Minim, V.P.R.; Ferreira, M.A.M.; de Paula Souza, P.H.; da Silva Moraes, L.E.; Minim, L.A. Study of the perception of consumers in relation to different ice cream concepts. *Food Qual. Prefer.* **2014**, *36*, 161–168. [CrossRef]
31. Verbeke, W.; Liu, R. The impacts of information about the risks and benefits of pork consumption on Chinese consumers' perceptions towards, and intention to eat, pork. *Meat Sci.* **2014**, *98*, 766–772. [CrossRef]
32. Guerrero, L.; Guàrdia, M.D.; Xicola, J.; Verbeke, W.; Vanhonacker, F.; Zakowska-Biemans, S.; Sajdakowska, M.; Sulmont-Rossé, C.; Issanchou, S.; Contel, M.; et al. Consumer-driven definition of traditional food products and innovation in traditional foods. A qualitative cross-cultural study. *Appetite* **2009**, *52*, 345–354. [CrossRef]
33. Anders, S.M.; Caswell, J.A. The benefits and costs of proliferation of geographical labeling for developing countries. *Estey Cent. J. Int. Law Trade Policy* **2009**, *10*, 1–17.
34. Sodano, V. Competitiveness of regional products in the international food market. *Econ. Agro Aliment.* **2002**, *7*, 32–47.
35. Jordana, J. Traditional foods: Challenges facing the European food industry. *Food Res. Int.* **2000**, *33*, 147–152. [CrossRef]
36. Galli, F. Chapter 1—traditional food: Definitions and nuances. In *Case Studies in the Traditional Food Sector*; Cavicchi, A., Santini, C., Eds.; Woodhead Publishing Series in Food Science, Technology and Nutrition; Woodhead Publishing: Chennai, India, 2018; pp. 3–24; ISBN 978-0-08-101007-5.
37. Caputo, V.; Sacchi, G.; Lagoudakis, A. Chapter 3—traditional food products and consumer choices: A review. In *Case Studies in the Traditional Food Sector*; Cavicchi, A., Santini, C., Eds.; Woodhead Publishing Series in Food Science, Technology and Nutrition; Woodhead Publishing: Chennai, India, 2018; pp. 47–87; ISBN 978-0-08-101007-5.
38. Vanhonacker, F.; Lengard, V.; Hersleth, M.; Verbeke, W. Profiling European traditional food consumers. *Br. Food J.* **2010**, *112*, 871–886. [CrossRef]
39. Cerjak, M.; Haas, R.; Brunner, F.; Tomic, M. What motivates consumers to buy traditional food products? Evidence from Croatia and Austria using word association and laddering interviews. *Br. Food J.* **2014**, *116*, 1726–1747. [CrossRef]
40. Grunert, K.G.; Aachmann, K. Consumer reactions to the use of EU quality labels on food products: A review of the literature. *Food Control.* **2016**, *59*, 178–187. [CrossRef]
41. EU. *Council Regulation (EC) No 509/2006 of 20 March 2006 on Agricultural Products and Foodstuffs as Traditional Specialities Guaranteed*; Official Journal of the European Union L 93/1: Brussels, Belgium, 2006.
42. Weichselbaum, E.; Benelam, B.; Costa, H.S. *Synthesis Report No 6—Traditional Foods in Europe*; FOOD-CT-2005-513944, EU6th Framework Food Quality and Safety Programme; EuroFIR: Norwich, UK, 2007.
43. Trichopoulou, A.; Vasilopoulou, E.; Georga, K.; Soukara, S.; Dilis, V. Traditional foods: Why and how to sustain them. *Trends Food Sci. Technol.* **2006**, *17*, 498–504. [CrossRef]
44. Guerrero, L.; Claret, A.; Verbeke, W.; Enderli, G.; Zakowska-Biemans, S.; Vanhonacker, F.; Issanchou, S.; Sajdakowska, M.; Granli, B.S.; Scalvedi, L.; et al. Perception of traditional food products in six European regions using free word association. *Food Qual. Prefer.* **2010**, *21*, 225–233. [CrossRef]
45. European Union. *Regulation (EU) No 1151/2012 of the European Parliament and of the Council of 21 November 2012 on Quality Schemes for Agricultural Products and Foodstuffs*; European Union: Brussels, Belgium, 2012; p. 29.
46. European Union. Quality Schemes Explained. Available online: https://ec.europa.eu/info/food-farming-fisheries/food-safety-and-quality/certification/quality-labels/quality-schemes-explained_en (accessed on 6 September 2020).
47. Kühne, B.; Vanhonacker, F.; Gellynck, X.; Verbeke, W. Innovation in traditional food products in Europe: Do sector innovation activities match consumers' acceptance? *Food Qual. Prefer.* **2010**, *21*, 629–638. [CrossRef]
48. Kizos, T.; Vakoufaris, H. Valorisation of a local asset: The case of olive oil on Lesvos Island, Greece. *Food Policy* **2011**, *36*, 705–714. [CrossRef]
49. Tregear, A.; Arfini, F.; Belletti, G.; Marescotti, A. Regional foods and rural development: The role of product qualification. *J. Rural Stud.* **2007**, *23*, 12–22. [CrossRef]
50. Gellynck, X.; Kühne, B. Innovation and collaboration in traditional food chain networks. *J. Chain Netw. Sci.* **2008**, *8*, 121–129. [CrossRef]

51. Linnemann, A.R.; Benner, M.; Verkerk, R.; van Boekel, M.A.J.S. Consumer-driven food product development. *Trends Food Sci. Technol.* **2006**, *17*, 184–190. [CrossRef]
52. Vanhonacker, F.; Kühne, B.; Gellynck, X.; Guerrero, L.; Hersleth, M.; Verbeke, W. Innovations in traditional foods: Impact on perceived traditional character and consumer acceptance. *Food Res. Int.* **2013**, *54*, 1828–1835. [CrossRef]
53. Kühne, B.; Gellynck, X.; Weaver, R.D. Enhancing innovation capacity through vertical, horizontal, and third-party networks for traditional foods. *Agribusiness* **2015**, *31*, 294–313. [CrossRef]
54. Pittaway, L.; Robertson, M.; Munir, K.; Denyer, D.; Neely, A. Networking and innovation: A systematic review of the evidence. *Int. J. Manag. Rev.* **2004**, *5–6*, 137–168. [CrossRef]
55. Roselli, L.; Cicia, G.; Cavallo, C.; Del Giudice, T.; Carlucci, D.; Clodoveo, M.L.; De Gennaro, B.C. Consumers' willingness to buy innovative traditional food products: The case of extra-virgin olive oil extracted by ultrasound. *Food Res. Int.* **2018**, *108*, 482–490. [CrossRef] [PubMed]
56. Lenssen, K.G.M.; Bast, A.; de Boer, A. Clarifying the health claim assessment procedure of EFSA will benefit functional food innovation. *J. Funct. Foods* **2018**, *47*, 386–396. [CrossRef]
57. Yeung, A.W.K.; Mocan, A.; Atanasov, A.G. Let food be thy medicine and medicine be thy food: A bibliometric analysis of the most cited papers focusing on nutraceuticals and functional foods. *Food Chem.* **2018**, *269*, 455–465. [CrossRef] [PubMed]
58. Bigliardi, B.; Galati, F. Innovation trends in the food industry: The case of functional foods. *Trends Food Sci. Technol.* **2013**, *31*, 118–129. [CrossRef]
59. García-Burgos, M.; Moreno-Fernández, J.; Alférez, M.J.M.; Díaz-Castro, J.; López-Aliaga, I. New perspectives in fermented dairy products and their health relevance. *J. Funct. Foods* **2020**, *72*, 104059. [CrossRef]
60. Guiné, R.P.F.; Rodrigues, A.P.; Ferreira, S.M.; Gonçalves, F.J. Development of yogurts enriched with antioxidants from wine. *J. Culin. Sci. Technol.* **2016**, *14*, 263–275. [CrossRef]
61. Wang, X.; Kristo, E.; LaPointe, G. Adding apple pomace as a functional ingredient in stirred-type yogurt and yogurt drinks. *Food Hydrocoll.* **2020**, *100*, 105453. [CrossRef]
62. Pereira, R.N.; Teixeira, J.A.; Vicente, A.A.; Cappato, L.P.; da Silva Ferreira, M.V.; da Silva Rocha, R.; da Cruz, A.G. Ohmic heating for the dairy industry: A potential technology to develop probiotic dairy foods in association with modifications of whey protein structure. *Curr. Opin. Food Sci.* **2018**, *22*, 95–101. [CrossRef]
63. Verruck, S.; Dantas, A.; Prudencio, E.S. Functionality of the components from goat's milk, recent advances for functional dairy products development and its implications on human health. *J. Funct. Foods* **2019**, *52*, 243–257. [CrossRef]
64. Van Nieuwenhove, C.P.; Moyano, A.; Castro-Gómez, P.; Fontecha, J.; Sáez, G.; Zárate, G.; Pizarro, P.L. Comparative study of pomegranate and jacaranda seeds as functional components for the conjugated linolenic acid enrichment of yogurt. *LWT* **2019**, *111*, 401–407. [CrossRef]
65. Kowaleski, J.; Quast, L.B.; Steffens, J.; Lovato, F.; Rodrigues dos Santos, L.; Zambiazi da Silva, S.; Maschio de Souza, D.; Felicetti, M.A. Functional yogurt with strawberries and chia seeds. *Food Biosci.* **2020**, *37*, 100726. [CrossRef]
66. Novin, D.; van der Wel, J.; Seifan, M.; Ebrahiminezhad, A.; Ghasemi, Y.; Berenjian, A. A functional dairy product rich in Menaquinone-7 and FeOOH nanoparticles. *LWT* **2020**, *129*, 109564. [CrossRef]
67. Di Nunzio, M.; Picone, G.; Pasini, F.; Chiarello, E.; Caboni, M.F.; Capozzi, F.; Gianotti, A.; Bordoni, A. Olive oil by-product as functional ingredient in bakery products. Influence of processing and evaluation of biological effects. *Food Res. Int.* **2020**, *131*, 108940. [CrossRef]
68. Martins, N.; Oliveira, M.B.P.P.; Ferreira, I.C.F.R. Development of functional dairy foods. In *Bioactive Molecules in Food*; Mérillon, J.-M., Ramawat, K.G., Eds.; Reference Series in Phytochemistry; Springer International Publishing: Cham, Switzerland, 2017; pp. 1–19; ISBN 978-3-319-54528-8.
69. Kadam, S.U.; Prabhasankar, P. Marine foods as functional ingredients in bakery and pasta products. *Food Res. Int.* **2010**, *43*, 1975–1980. [CrossRef]
70. Vergara-Valencia, N.; Granados-Pérez, E.; Agama-Acevedo, E.; Tovar, J.; Ruales, J.; Bello-Pérez, L.A. Fibre concentrate from mango fruit: Characterization, associated antioxidant capacity and application as a bakery product ingredient. *LWT Food Sci. Technol.* **2007**, *40*, 722–729. [CrossRef]
71. Agrahar-Murugkar, D. Food to food fortification of breads and biscuits with herbs, spices, millets and oilseeds on bio-accessibility of calcium, iron and zinc and impact of proteins, fat and phenolics. *LWT* **2020**, *130*, 109703. [CrossRef]

72. Alzuwaid, N.T.; Pleming, D.; Fellows, C.M.; Sissons, M. Fortification of durum wheat spaghetti and common wheat bread with wheat bran protein concentrate-impacts on nutrition and technological properties. *Food Chem.* **2020**, *334*, 127497. [CrossRef] [PubMed]
73. Erive, M.O.; Wang, T.; He, F.; Chen, G. Development of high-fiber wheat bread using microfluidized corn bran. *Food Chem.* **2020**, *310*, 125921. [CrossRef] [PubMed]
74. Leialohilani, A.; de Boer, A. EU food legislation impacts innovation in the area of plant-based dairy alternatives. *Trends Food Sci. Technol.* **2020**. [CrossRef]
75. Segura-Badilla, O.; Lazcano-Hernández, M.; Kammar-García, A.; Vera-López, O.; Aguilar-Alonso, P.; Ramírez-Calixto, J.; Navarro-Cruz, A.R. Use of coconut water (*Cocus nucifera* L.) for the development of a symbiotic functional drink. *Heliyon* **2020**, *6*, e03653. [CrossRef] [PubMed]
76. Derkyi, N.S.A.; Acheampong, M.A.; Mwin, E.N.; Tetteh, P.; Aidoo, S.C. Product design for a functional non-alcoholic drink. *S. Afr. J. Chem. Eng.* **2018**, *25*, 85–90. [CrossRef]
77. Hamid; Thakur, N.; Thakur, A. Microencapsulation of wild pomegranate flavedo phenolics by lyophilization: Effect of maltodextrin concentration, structural morphology, functional properties, elemental composition and ingredient for development of functional beverage. *LWT* **2020**, 110077. [CrossRef]
78. Kotilainen, L.; Rajalahti, R.; Ragasa, C.; Pehu, E. *Health Enhancing Foods: Opportunities for Strengthening Developing Countries*; The World Bank: Washington, DC, USA, 2006; p. 1.
79. Spence, J.T. Challenges related to the composition of functional foods. *J. Food Compos. Anal.* **2006**, *19*, S4–S6. [CrossRef]
80. Makinen-Aakula, M. Trends in functional foods dairy market. In Proceedings of the Third Functional Food Net Meeting, Liverpool, UK, 18–19 September 2006.
81. Belwal, T.; Devkota, H.P.; Hassan, H.A.; Ahluwalia, S.; Ramadan, M.F.; Mocan, A.; Atanasov, A.G. Phytopharmacology of Acerola (*Malpighia* spp.) and its potential as functional food. *Trends Food Sci. Technol.* **2018**, *74*, 99–106. [CrossRef]
82. Bolhassani, A. Chapter 10—bioactive components of saffron and their pharmacological properties. In *Studies in Natural Products Chemistry*; Atta-ur-Rahman, Ed.; Elsevier: Amsterdam, The Netherlands, 2018; Volume 58, pp. 289–311.
83. Coman, V.; Teleky, B.-E.; Mitrea, L.; Martău, G.A.; Szabo, K.; Călinoiu, L.-F.; Vodnar, D.C. Bioactive potential of fruit and vegetable wastes. In *Advances in Food and Nutrition Research*; Academic Press: Amsterdam, The Netherlands, 2019; Volume 90, pp. 1–18.
84. Ide, K.; Kawasaki, Y.; Kawakami, K.; Yamada, H. Chapter 5—effects of bioactive components of green tea on alzheimer's disease. In *Studies in Natural Products Chemistry*; Atta-ur-Rahman, Ed.; Elsevier: Amsterdam, The Netherlands, 2018; Volume 56, pp. 151–172.
85. Liu, R.-Z.; Wang, R.; An, H.-M.; Liu, X.-G.; Li, C.-R.; Li, P.; Yang, H. A strategy for screening bioactive components from natural products based on two-dimensional cell membrane chromatography and component-knockout approach. *J. Chromatogr. A* **2019**, *1601*, 171–177. [CrossRef]
86. Nowak, E.; Livney, Y.D.; Niu, Z.; Singh, H. Delivery of bioactives in food for optimal efficacy: What inspirations and insights can be gained from pharmaceutics? *Trends Food Sci. Technol.* **2019**, *91*, 557–573. [CrossRef]
87. European Parliament Regulation (EC) No 1924/2006 of the european parliament and of the council of 20 December 2006 on nutrition and health claims made on foods. *Off. J. Eur. Union* **2006**, *49*, 9–25.
88. NCCIH. *Complementary, Alternative, or Integrative Health: What's In a Name*; National Centre for Complementary and Integrative Health: Bethesda, MD, USA, 2018.
89. Harnett, J.E.; Ung, C.O.L.; Hu, H.; Sultani, M.; Desselle, S.P. Advancing the pharmacist's role in promoting the appropriate and safe use of dietary supplements. *Complement. Ther. Med.* **2019**, *44*, 174–181. [CrossRef] [PubMed]
90. WHO. *WHO Traditional Medicine Strategy: 2014–2023*; World Health Organisation: Geneva, Switzerland, 2014.
91. NIH. *Dietary Supplement Health and Education Act. of 1994 Public Law 103–417 103rd Congress*; National Institutes of Health: Rockville, MD, USA, 1994.
92. Guiné, R.P.F.; Silva, A.C.F. Probiotics, prebiotics and synbiotics. In *Functional Foods: Sources, Health Effects and Future Perspectives*; Nova Publishers: New York, NY, USA, 2017; pp. 143–207.
93. Iwatani, S.; Yamamoto, N. Functional food products in Japan: A review. *Food Sci. Hum. Wellness* **2019**, *8*, 96–101. [CrossRef]

94. Khedkar, S.; Carraresi, L.; Bröring, S. Food or pharmaceuticals? Consumers' perception of health-related borderline products. *PharmaNutrition* **2017**, *5*, 133–140. [CrossRef]
95. Aschemann-Witzel, J.; Grunert, K.G. Influence of 'soft' versus 'scientific' health information framing and contradictory information on consumers' health inferences and attitudes towards a food supplement. *Food Qual. Prefer.* **2015**, *42*, 90–99. [CrossRef]
96. Fenko, A.; Kersten, L.; Bialkova, S. Overcoming consumer scepticism toward food labels: The role of multisensory experience. *Food Qual. Prefer.* **2016**, *48*, 81–92. [CrossRef]
97. Loebnitz, N.; Grunert, K.G. Impact of self-health awareness and perceived product benefits on purchase intentions for hedonic and utilitarian foods with nutrition claims. *Food Qual. Prefer.* **2018**, *64*, 221–231. [CrossRef]
98. Williams, P.; Ridges, L.A.; Batterham, M.; Ripper, B.; Hung, M. Australian consumer attitudes to health claim—food product compatibility for functional foods. *Food Policy* **2008**, *33*, 640–643. [CrossRef]
99. Hunter, D.C.; Jones, V.S.; Hedderley, D.I.; Jaeger, S.R. The influence of claims of appetite control benefits in those trying to lose or maintain weight: The role of claim believability and attitudes to functional foods. *Food Res. Int.* **2019**, *119*, 715–724. [CrossRef]
100. Szakály, Z.; Szente, V.; Kövér, G.; Polereczki, Z.; Szigeti, O. The influence of lifestyle on health behavior and preference for functional foods. *Appetite* **2012**, *58*, 406–413. [CrossRef]
101. Buckland, N.; Dalton, M.; Stubbs, J.; Hetherington, M.; Blundell, J.; Finlayson, G. Associations between nutritional properties of food and consumer perceptions related to weight management. *Food Qual. Prefer.* **2015**, *45*, 18–25. [CrossRef]
102. Lähteenmäki, L. Claiming health in food products. *Food Qual. Prefer.* **2013**, *27*, 196–201. [CrossRef]
103. Song, X.; Pérez-Cueto, F.J.A.; Bølling Laugesen, S.M.; van der Zanden, L.D.T.; Giacalone, D. Older consumers' attitudes towards food carriers for protein-enrichment. *Appetite* **2019**, *135*, 10–19. [CrossRef] [PubMed]
104. van der Zanden, L.D.T.; van Kleef, E.; de Wijk, R.A.; van Trijp, H.C.M. Examining heterogeneity in elderly consumers' acceptance of carriers for protein-enriched food: A segmentation study. *Food Qual. Prefer.* **2015**, *42*, 130–138. [CrossRef]
105. Vella, M.N.; Stratton, L.M.; Sheeshka, J.; Duncan, A.M. Exploration of functional food consumption in older adults in relation to food matrices, bioactive ingredients, and health. *J. Nutr. Gerontol. Geriatr.* **2013**, *32*, 122–144. [CrossRef]
106. Van der Zanden, L.D.T.; van Trijp, H.C.M. Designing New and Functional Foods for the Aging. In *Food for the Aging Population: Second Edition*; Elsevier Inc., Academic Press: Amsterdam, The Netherlands, 2016; pp. 323–347; ISBN 978-0-08-100348-0.
107. De Dienes Alicia, H.; Mónica, M.G.M.; Jorge, J.A.M. Application of Multi-Criteria Decision Methods (MCDM) for the development of functional food products in Venezuela. *Procedia Food Sci.* **2011**, *1*, 1560–1567. [CrossRef]
108. McQuade, J.L.; Meng, Z.; Chen, Z.; Wei, Q.; Zhang, Y.; Bei, W.; Palmer, J.L.; Cohen, L. Utilization of and attitudes towards traditional chinese medicine therapies in a chinese cancer hospital: A survey of patients and physicians. *Evid. Based Complement. Altern. Med.* **2012**, *2012*, 1–12. [CrossRef]
109. Plasek, B.; Temesi, Á. The credibility of the effects of functional food products and consumers' willingness to purchase/willingness to pay–review. *Appetite* **2019**, 104398. [CrossRef]
110. Santeramo, F.G.; Carlucci, D.; De Devitiis, B.; Seccia, A.; Stasi, A.; Viscecchia, R.; Nardone, G. Emerging trends in European food, diets and food industry. *Food Res. Int.* **2018**, *104*, 39–47. [CrossRef]
111. Bleiel, J. Functional foods from the perspective of the consumer: How to make it a success? *Int. Dairy J.* **2010**, *20*, 303–306. [CrossRef]
112. Mellentin, J. *Failures in Functional Foods and Beverages*; New Nutrition Business: London, UK, 2014.
113. Ares, G.; Besio, M.; Giménez, A.; Deliza, R. Relationship between involvement and functional milk desserts intention to purchase. Influence on attitude towards packaging characteristics. *Appetite* **2010**, *55*, 298–304. [CrossRef] [PubMed]
114. Romano, K.R.; Rosenthal, A.; Deliza, R. How do Brazilian consumers perceive a non-traditional and innovative fruit juice? An approach looking at the packaging. *Food Res. Int.* **2015**, *74*, 123–130. [CrossRef] [PubMed]
115. Goetzke, B.I.; Spiller, A. Health-improving lifestyles of organic and functional food consumers. *Br. Food J.* **2014**, *116*, 510–526. [CrossRef]

116. Cukelj, N.; Putnik, P.; Novotni, D.; Ajredini, S.; Voucko, B.; Curic, D. Market potential of lignans and omega-3 functional cookies. *Br. Food J.* **2016**, *118*, 2420–2433. [CrossRef]
117. Kraus, A. Factors influencing the decisions to buy and consume functional food. *Br. Food J.* **2015**. [CrossRef]
118. Azzurra, A.; Massimiliano, A.; Angela, M. Measuring sustainable food consumption: A case study on organic food. *Sustain. Prod. Consum.* **2019**, *17*, 95–107. [CrossRef]
119. Moro, D.; Veneziani, M.; Sckokai, P.; Castellari, E. Consumer willingness to pay for catechin-enriched yogurt: Evidence from a stated choice experiment. *Agribusiness* **2015**, *31*, 243–258. [CrossRef]
120. Szakály, Z.; Kovács, S.; Pető, K.; Huszka, P.; Kiss, M. A modified model of the willingness to pay for functional foods. *Appetite* **2019**, *138*, 94–101. [CrossRef]
121. Vecchio, R.; Loo, E.J.V.; Annunziata, A. Consumers' willingness to pay for conventional, organic and functional yogurt: Evidence from experimental auctions. *Int. J. Consum. Stud.* **2016**, *40*, 368–378. [CrossRef]
122. Romano, K.R.; Dias Bartolomeu Abadio Finco, F.; Rosenthal, A.; Vinicius Alves Finco, M.; Deliza, R. Willingness to pay more for value-added pomegranate juice (*Punica granatum* L.): An open-ended contingent valuation. *Food Res. Int.* **2016**, *89*, 359–364. [CrossRef]
123. Roosen, J.; Bieberstein, A.; Blanchemanche, S.; Goddard, E.; Marette, S.; Vandermoere, F. Trust and willingness to pay for nanotechnology food. *Food Policy* **2015**, *52*, 75–83. [CrossRef]
124. Ahn, B.; Bae, M.-S.; Nayga, R.M. Information effects on consumers' preferences and willingness to pay for a functional food product: The case of red ginseng concentrate. *Asian Econ. J.* **2016**, *30*, 197–219. [CrossRef]
125. Pappalardo, G.; Lusk, J.L. The role of beliefs in purchasing process of functional foods. *Food Qual. Prefer.* **2016**, *53*, 151–158. [CrossRef]
126. Bruschi, V.; Teuber, R.; Dolgopolova, I. Acceptance and willingness to pay for health-enhancing bakery products—Empirical evidence for young urban Russian consumers. *Food Qual. Prefer.* **2015**, *46*, 79–91. [CrossRef]
127. Chege, C.G.K.; Sibiko, K.W.; Wanyama, R.; Jager, M.; Birachi, E. Are consumers at the base of the pyramid willing to pay for nutritious foods? *Food Policy* **2019**, *87*, 101745. [CrossRef]
128. Bouis, H.E.; Hotz, C.; McClafferty, B.; Meenakshi, J.V.; Pfeiffer, W.H. Biofortification: A new tool to reduce micronutrient malnutrition. *Food Nutr. Bull.* **2011**, *32*, S31–S40. [CrossRef]
129. Molnár, A.; Gellynck, X.; Vanhonacker, F.; Gagalyuk, T.; Verbeke, W. Do chain goals match consumer perceptions? The case of the traditional food sector in selected European Union countries. *Agribusiness* **2011**, *27*, 221–243. [CrossRef]
130. Almli, V.L.; Næs, T.; Enderli, G.; Sulmont-Rossé, C.; Issanchou, S.; Hersleth, M. Consumers' acceptance of innovations in traditional cheese. A comparative study in France and Norway. *Appetite* **2011**, *57*, 110–120. [CrossRef]
131. Pieniak, Z.; Verbeke, W.; Vanhonacker, F.; Guerrero, L.; Hersleth, M. Association between traditional food consumption and motives for food choice in six European countries. *Appetite* **2009**, *53*, 101–108. [CrossRef]

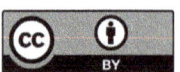

© 2020 by the authors. Licensee MDPI, Basel, Switzerland. This article is an open access article distributed under the terms and conditions of the Creative Commons Attribution (CC BY) license (http://creativecommons.org/licenses/by/4.0/).

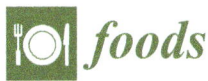

Article

Study about Food Choice Determinants According to Six Types of Conditioning Motivations in a Sample of 11,960 Participants

Raquel P. F. Guiné [1,*], Elena Bartkiene [2], Viktória Szűcs [3], Monica Tarcea [4], Marija Ljubičić [5], Maša Černelič-Bizjak [6], Kathy Isoldi [7], Ayman EL-Kenawy [8], Vanessa Ferreira [9], Evita Straumite [10], Małgorzata Korzeniowska [11], Elena Vittadini [12], Marcela Leal [13], Lucia Frez-Muñoz [14], Maria Papageorgiou [15], Ilija Djekić [16], Manuela Ferreira [17], Paula Correia [1], Ana Paula Cardoso [18] and João Duarte [17]

1. CERNAS Research Centre, Polytechnic Institute of Viseu, 3504-510 Viseu, Portugal; paulacorreia@esav.ipv.pt
2. Department of Food Safety and Quality, Lithuanian University of Health Sciences, 44307 Kaunas, Lithuania; elena.bartkiene@lsmuni.lt
3. Directorate of Food Industry, Hungarian Chamber of Agriculture, H119 Budapest, Hungary; szucs.viktoria@nak.hu
4. Department of Community Nutrition & Food Safety, University of Medicine, Pharmacy, Science and Technology, 540139 Targu-Mures, Romania; monica.tarcea@umfst.ro
5. Department of Pediatrics, General Hospital Zadar, 23000 Zadar, Croatia; marija.ljubicic@zd.t-com.hr
6. Faculty of Health Sciences, University of Primorska, 6310 Izola, Slovenia; Masa.Cernelic@fvz.upr.si
7. Department of Biomedical, Health and Nutrition Sciences, Long Island University, 720 Northern Boulevard, Brookville, New York, NY 11548-1327, USA; kathy.isoldi@liu.edu
8. Department of Molecular Biology, Genetic Engineering and Biotechnology Institute, University of Sadat City, Sadat City 79/22857, Egypt; elkenawyay@yahoo.com
9. Department of Nutrition, School of Nursing, UFMG University, Belo Horizonte 30130-100, Brazil; vanessa.nutr@gmail.com
10. Department of Food Technology, Latvia University of Life Sciences and Technologies, LV 3001 Jelgava, Latvia; evita.straumite@llu.lv
11. Faculty of Food Science, Wrocław University of Environmental and Life Sciences, 51-630 Wrocław, Poland; malgorzata.korzeniowska@upwr.edu.pl
12. School of Biosciences and Veterinary Medicine, University of Camerino, 62032 Camerino, Italy; elena.vittadini@unicam.it
13. School of Nutrition, Faculty of Health Sciences, Maimonides University, Buenos Aires C1405, Argentina; leal.nutricion@gmail.com
14. Food Quality and Design Group, Wageningen University & Research, 6700 HB Wageningen, The Netherlands; lucia.frezmunoz@wur.nl
15. Alexander Technological Educational Institute, Department Food Technology, 57400 Thessaloniki, Thessaloniki, Greece; mariapapage@food.teithe.gr
16. Faculty of Agriculture, University of Belgrade, 11000 Belgrade, Serbia; idjekic@agrif.bg.ac.rs
17. UICISA:E Research Centre, Polytechnic Institute of Viseu, 3504-510 Viseu, Portugal; mmcferreira@gmail.com (M.F.); duarte.johnny@gmail.com (J.D.)
18. CIDEI Research Centre, Polytechnic Institute of Viseu, 3504-510 Viseu, Portugal; a.p.cardoso@esev.ipv.pt
* Correspondence: raquelguine@esav.ipv.pt; Tel.: +351-232-446-641

Received: 8 June 2020; Accepted: 22 June 2020; Published: 7 July 2020

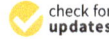

Abstract: Many aspects linked to personal characteristics, society and culture constitute some of the motivators that drive food choice. The aim of this work was to determine in what extent the eating behaviors of individuals are shaped by six different types of determinants, namely: health, emotions, price and availability, society and culture, environment and politics, and marketing and commercials. This is a descriptive cross-sectional study, involving a non-probabilistic sample of 11,960 participants from 16 countries. The objective of this work was to validate the questionnaire, so as to make it suitable for application in different contexts and different countries. For that, six scales were considered for validation by confirmatory factor analysis with structural equation modelling. The obtained results showed that the six individual scales evaluated presented good or very good fitting indices, with saturation in goodness-of-fit index in all cases. The values of chi-square ratio were 6.921 (for health), 0.987 (environment), 0.610 (emotions) and 0.000 in the remaining cases (convenience, society, marketing). Furthermore, the fit was perfect, with saturation for all indices, in three of the six models (convenience, society and marketing). The results of this wok allowed the validation of the six scales, and the assessing of different types of factors that can influence food choices and eating behaviors, namely in the categories: health, emotions, price and availability, society and culture, environment and politics, and marketing and commercials.

Keywords: eating determinants; healthy diet; emotions; feeding behavior; socio-cultural environment; instrument validation

1. Introduction

Dietary patterns depend on everyday food choices, and include aspects like quantity, proportion, variety and combinations or frequencies of consumption. Knowledge about food choices and which factors may determine what people select to consume are important from the social, as well as the health, point of view. The aspects linked to society and culture are some of the motivators that drive food choice [1,2].

The food environment in western societies has been recognized as tending too much and too fast to the unhealthy side of eating, being designated by some as "toxic" [3]. People are constantly exposed to unhealthy food in supermarkets, food shops, restaurants (most especially fast food) or vending machines. This constant appeal of unhealthy food is well known to contribute to unhealthy food choices, which lead to epidemic burdens of obesity, diabetes, heart diseases and other chronic diseases [3–5]. In the opposite trend are the consumers who value their health and food as health-enhancing motors. These individuals tend to make appropriate and careful food choices, opting for a more balanced diet and favoring the consumption of functional foods. It is known that the market of functional foods and nutraceuticals has experienced a very fast growing rate in the past few decades [5]. In this way, health and disease can act as motivators to influence people's food choices [3–8].

Emotions are fundamental in all aspects of life, and eating is not an exception. People tend to be conditioned to some extent in their eating behaviors according to their emotional patterns, or even to make variable food choices according to a momentary mood. Emotional eating corresponds to a tendency to overeat as a response to negative emotions such as anxiety or irritability [9]. On the other hand, sadness, loneliness or depression can impede many people from eating the foods necessary for the correct functioning of their body [10]. Hence the role of emotions in determining food choices is incredibly relevant [9,10].

Furthermore, economic factors have a very marked influence on eating habits, and in countries with a low household income the differences are marked, as compared with the more industrialized, more urbanized and more globalized societies, which undergo a nutritional transition. Besides income, availability issues also contribute to shaping eating behaviors, most especially in today's globalized markets, with goods being traded between many different countries [1,11].

The role of consumption and consumer behavior is increasingly considered in the food supply chain. Sustainable consumption or green consumer behavior corresponds to customers' choices and refusals to buy and consume products harmful to the environment, and as alternatives seek to purchase products that have a minimal impact on the environment, or preferably, that are beneficial for the global sustainability. Because sustainable consumption behaviors can significantly diminish the social and environmental impacts, more and more people are taking these aspects into account when making their food choices [12–14].

The development of a valid and reliable instrument for assessing the factors taken into consideration by consumers when making their food choices is not only a matter of purely academic interest, but it also impacts many different aspects of society, namely health, economy, society, environment, just to name a few. The use of a validated instrument allows for reliability in the data gathered, and guarantees its applicability on a broader scale, particularly when that validation is carried out with data obtained from different sources, like for example different countries [15–18].

Because the factors that may determine the eating behaviors of individuals can be of very differentiated natures, and have variable degrees of influence on people's food choices, this work intended to test six different complementing scales for eating motivations, namely: health, emotions, price and availability, society and culture, environment and politics, and marketing and commercials. As such, the objective was to validate the questionnaire and its six scales, so as to make them suitable for application in different contexts and different countries. The validation process followed was a confirmatory factor analysis with structural equation modelling.

2. Materials and Methods

2.1. Questionnaire

The instrument used for this research was developed by Ferrão et al. [18] with the purpose of addressing different groups of food motivations. The EATMOT project uses a questionnaire that was developed to explore in what way some personal, psychological and social motivations can influence food choices and eating practices. The questionnaire was prepared and previously validated for a study carried out only in Portugal [18], and then it was translated into the native languages of the 15 participating countries, following a back-translation methodology for validation. For the translation process, all the issues related to the possible cultural influences in the interpretation of the questions were verified. The questionnaire structure included different sections, intended to collect information believed relevant for the study, specifically accounting for groups of questions related to six different types of food motivations: Section 1—Health motivations, Section 2—Emotional motivations, Section 3—Economic and Availability motivations, Section 4—Social and Cultural motivations, Section 5—Environmental and Political motivations, Section 6—Marketing and Commercials motivations. All questions in these six sections of the questionnaire are presented in detail in Appendix A.

The participants would express their level of agreement with each statement on the following 5 points hedonic scale: 1—strongly disagree, 2—disagree, 3—neither agree nor disagree, 4—agree and 5—strongly agree. Because some of the questions were in the inverted mode (Q1.5, Q1.9, Q6.1, and Q6.4), the corresponding scores were reversed. In this way, the higher the global scores, the stronger the influence on the food choice and eating processes.

2.2. Data Collection

The questionnaire was applied to adult participants, over 18 years old, who answered it voluntarily, anonymously, and after informed consent. All ethical procedures were strictly followed when designing and applying the questionnaire, and it was ensured that the data provided was kept strictly confidential, i.e., no individual responses could ever be associated with the respondent. The survey was approved by the Ethical Committee of Polytechnic Institute of Viseu, with reference n° 04/2017, and follows national and international protocols for research on humans. The sample was selected by convenience and consisted of 11,960 individuals aged between 18 and 90 years, from which the majority were female (71%). The participants were from 16 countries situated on three continents (Europe, America and Africa), and were distributed as: Argentina (4%), Brazil (6%), Croatia (13%), Egypt (7%), Greece

(4%), Hungary (4%), Italy (5%), Latvia (5%), Lithuania (4%), Netherlands (4%), Poland (5%), Portugal (11%), Serbia (4%), Slovenia (9%), Romania (7%) and United States of America (7%).

2.3. Analysis of the Data

The reliability studies to evaluate the internal consistency were made by means of the Pearson's linear correlation coefficient (r) and the Cronbach's alpha. The values of alpha reported by Marôco [19] were used as references: > 0.9 excellent; 0.8–0.9 very good; 0.7–0.8 good; 0.6–0.7 medium; 0.5–0.6 reasonable; < 0.5 bad. However, the same author admits that in the social sciences the adoption of alpha values above 0.5 is plausible. A good definition of the factor implies that items with correlations to the overall score lower than 0.2 when it contains this particular item should not be considered [20–22].

For each scale, the factorial solution that emerged through confirmatory factorial analysis (CFA) was tested using the AMOS 24 software (Analysis of Moment Structures). The covariance matrix and the maximum likelihood estimation (MLE) algorithm for parameter estimation were considered [23]. The latent variables (exogenous and/or endogenous) are represented by larger circles and the indicators (measures observed) by rectangles, while the errors are represented by small circles. The following parameters were considered for evaluation: (i) factorial weights; (ii) variances and covariates of the individual reliability of the indicators; (iii) variances and covariances of the factors; and (iv) error correlations [24]. Model acceptance was decided according to: (i) the interpretability, (ii) the modification indexes proposed by the AMOS, and (iii) the model adjustment indicators [24].

Regarding the interpretation of the parameters, the reference values considered were: correlation between the factors (Φ)—the higher the coefficients, the better; regression coefficients (λ)—values greater than 0.50; individual reliability of indicators (δ)—coefficients equal to or greater than 0.25; statistical significance—p-value lower than 0.05 [19].

For the indicators of the quality of adjustment of the model, the following reference values were adopted [25,26]:

(a) Values used for absolute fit: Ratio of chi-square and degrees of freedom (χ^2/df)—if (χ^2/df) is equal to 1 the fit is perfect, for values lower than 2 it is good, for values lower than 5 it is acceptable and for values greater than 5 is unacceptable. Root mean square residual (RMR)—the lower the value of RMR the better is the fit, so RMR = 0 indicates a perfect fit. Standardized root mean square residual (SRMR)—a value of zero indicates a perfect fit and values lower than 0.08 are generally considered a good fit. Goodness of fit index (GFI)—values around 0.95 or higher are recommended (with maximum value equal to 1), but values over 0.90 are considered a good fit.

(b) Values for relative fit: Comparative fit index (CFI), which is an additional comparative index of the adjustment to the model—values lower than 0.90 indicate a poor fit, values between 0.90 and 0.95 indicate a good adjustment and above 0.95 a very good adjustment (maximum value of 1 corresponds to perfect fit). This index is independent of the sample size.

(c) Population discrepancy index: Root mean square error of approximation (RMSEA)—reference values for the RMSEA, with a 90% confidence interval, between 0.05 and 0.08 mean the adjustment is good, while it is considered very good when the index is lower than 0.05.

3. Results

3.1. Health Motivations

Structural Equation Modelling has been used by different researchers, such as Guiné et al. [17], for the development of a scale to measure knowledge about dietary fiber, or by Sidali et al. [27], to assess the acceptance of insect-based food coming from the Ecuadorian Amazon rainforest by western students. SEM was also used by Lagerkvist et al. [28] to estimate a construct that could explain consumer confidence in food safety practices along the food supply chain, and Lim et al. [29] used SEM to assess the relationship between food safety knowledge, attitude and behavior among household food preparers. Ting et al. [30] used SEM to model tourists' food consumption intentions at their destination.

Table 1 shows the statistics (mean and standard deviation) and the correlations of each item with the global value. Analyzing the average indices of the items and corresponding standard deviations, it was found that they are well cantered, since all the items have observed average indices higher than the central score.

Table 1. Statistics for the unidimensional model of the scale about health motivations.

Item	Internal Consistency of Items (Original)				
	Mean Score	Standard Deviation	r (Item-Total)	r^2	α Without Item
Q1.1	3.66	1.043	0.407	0.216	0.681
Q1.2	3.21	1.073	0.264	0.127	0.705
Q1.3	3.59	0.930	0.469	0.302	0.672
Q1.4	3.74	0.931	0.489	0.408	0.669
Q1.5	2.89	1.125	0.221	0.280	0.713
Q1.6	3.38	1.017	0.509	0.359	0.663
Q1.7	3.25	1.065	0.338	0.263	0.692
Q1.8	3.95	0.949	0.507	0.412	0.666
Q1.9	2.92	1.154	0.236	0.286	0.712
Q1.10	3.24	1.147	0.329	0.176	0.695
	Global Cronbach's alpha = 0.709				
Fitting Indices of CFA Model [1]		Initial [2]		Final [3]	
χ^2/df		228.0		6.921	
GFI		0.883		1.000	
CFI		0.668		0.999	
RMSEA		0.138		0.022	
RMSR		0.109		0.005	
SRMR		0.090		0.054	

[1] χ^2/df = Ratio of chi-square and degrees of freedom; GFI = Goodness of fit index; CFI = Comparative fit index; RMSEA = Root mean square error of approximation; RMSR = Root mean square residual; SRMR = Standardized root mean square residual. [2] Without modification indices. [3] With modification indices and eliminated items.

Table 1 also shows that the item-total correlation coefficients (r) indicate that item Q1.5 is the most problematic, with r = 0.221s and the maximum correlation is obtained in item Q1.6 (r = 0.509), which accounts for about 36% of its variability. Regarding the values of Cronbach's alpha, these are classified as medium to good since they range from 0.663 in item Q1.6s to 0.713 in item Q1.5, with a global alpha that is also good (α = 0.709). Confirmatory factorial analysis showed that the coefficients of asymmetry and kurtosis presented normal values, oscillating for asymmetry in absolute values between 0.146 and 0.735, and for kurtosis between 0.057 and 0.877, with a Mardia's coefficient of 0.283 for multivariate normality test. The critical ratios are significant, but from Figure 1a it can be observed that items Q1.2, Q1.5 and Q1.9 have saturations lower than 0.40, which was the lower limit considered as recommended by Marôco [26] for the original studies, and therefore they were eliminated from the model. The same type of analysis led successively to the elimination of other items that presented problems of multicollinearity, resulting in the final refined model represented in Figure 1b. Table 1 also presents the global adjustment indices of the one-dimensional model for health motivations. In the first model, all indices revealed poor or inadequate values, but after refinement the indices presented very good values with saturated index for GFI.

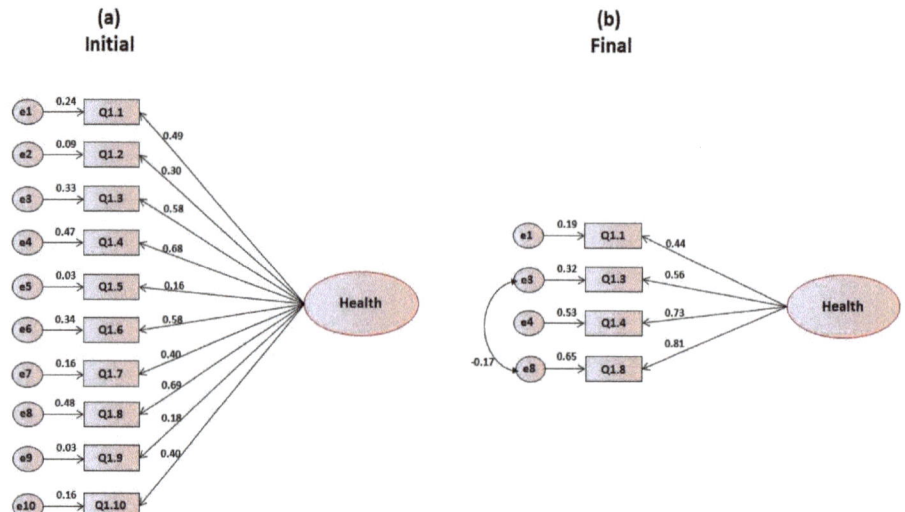

Figure 1. (a) Initial and (b) final models for the health motivations' scale.

3.2. Emotional Motivations

The statistics (mean and standard deviation) and the correlations of each item with the global value are presented in the Table 2. An analysis of the average scores and standard deviations of the items indicates that some items are in the threshold of the central position, which may turn out problematic for the consistency of the scale, since the trend of responses is focused more on the neutral position. The correlation coefficient's (r) item-total shows that item Q2.2 (r = 0.108) should be excluded because it is lower than the reference value (0.20). The maximum correlation is obtained for item Q2.8 (r = 0.669), which explains about 59% of its variability. The values of Cronbach's alpha can be classified as medium to good, as they range from 0.689 in item Q2.8, to 0.774 in item Q2.2, with a value for the overall alpha (α = 0.772) that is considered good. When the unifactorial model was submitted to confirmatory factorial analysis, it was shown that the coefficients of skewness and kurtosis presented absolute values corresponding to normality, ranging from 0.044 to 0.657 for skewness and between 0.241 and 1.158 for kurtosis, with a multivariate Mardia's coefficient of 0.257. The critical ratios are significant, which could lead to the maintenance of all items. However, as indicated in Figure 2a, items Q2.2, Q2.3, Q2.4 and Q2.5 have factorial weights below 0.40, which is the lowest limit recommended by Marôco [26] for original studies, and therefore they have been eliminated, thus giving the final model illustrated in Figure 2b. This final model resulted from the elimination of the aforementioned items plus the refinement through the modification indices proposed by AMOS. It can be observed that in the final model all items have saturations greater than 0.50, and the goodness of fit indices for the overall adjustment can be classified as very good according to Table 2, with GFI and CFI values of 1, which corresponds to perfect fit, and a value of RMSEA of zero, also indicative of a perfect fit.

Table 2. Statistics for the unidimensional model of the scale about emotional motivations.

Item	Internal Consistency of Items (Original)				
	Mean Score	Standard Deviation	r (Item-Total)	r^2	α Without Item
Q2.1	2.98	1.123	0.569	0.359	0.708
Q2.2	3.15	1.075	0.108	0.066	0.774
Q2.3	2.82	1.282	0.290	0.103	0.754
Q2.4	3.14	1.152	0.216	0.085	0.762
Q2.5	3.49	1.100	0.332	0.219	0.744
Q2.6	2.57	1.190	0.663	0.565	0.690
Q2.7	2.98	1.250	0.553	0.415	0.708
Q2.8	2.57	1.182	0.669	0.586	0.689
Q2.9	2.94	1.265	0.507	0.400	0.716
	Global Cronbach's alpha = 0.772				
Fitting Indices of CFA Model [1]		Initial [2]		Final [3]	
χ^2/df		105.0		0.610	
GFI		0.951		1.000	
CFI		0.901		1.000	
RMSEA		0.093		0.000	
RMSR		0.078		0.003	
SRMR		0.058		0.017	

[1] χ^2/df = Ratio of chi-square and degrees of freedom; GFI = Goodness of fit index; CFI = Comparative fit index; RMSEA = Root mean square error of approximation; RMSR = Root mean square residual; SRMR = Standardized root mean square residual. [2] Without modification indices. [3] With modification indices and eliminated items.

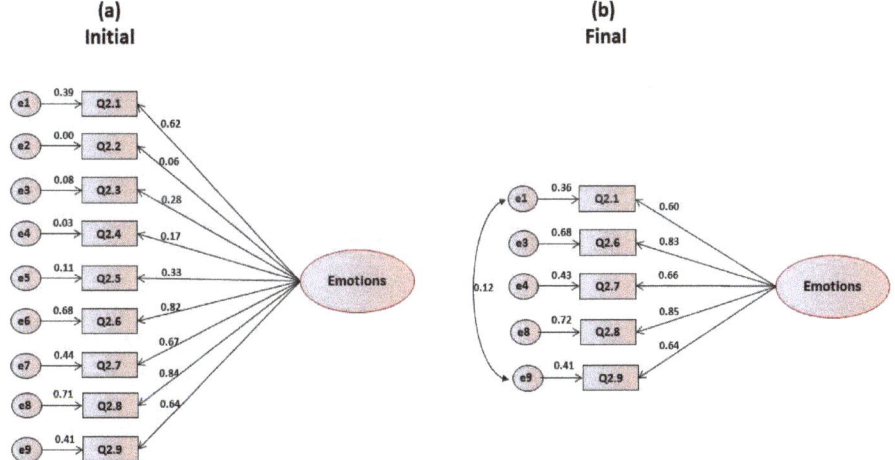

Figure 2. (a) Initial and (b) final models for the emotional motivations' scale.

3.3. Economic and Availability Motivations

By analysis of the mean scores and standard deviations of the items in the scale for economic and availability motivations (Table 3), it is pointed out that only item Q3.7 is below the central threshold, being the most problematic item. Regarding the corrected item-total coefficients, it is observed that items Q3.1, Q3.4 and Q3.7 present correlations lower than 0.20, and therefore, in a more incisive analysis, they should be eliminated. The maximum correlation is obtained for item Q3.6 (r = 0.411), which accounts for 22.6% of its variability. Cronbach's alpha values range from bad to reasonable, varying from 0.383 in item Q3.2 to 0.582 in item Q3.4, also with an acceptable overall alpha of (α = 0.500).

Again, the unifactorial structure was submitted to confirmatory factorial analysis. Analyzing the statistics regarding the normality of the items, it was observed that they all presented absolute values for both asymmetry and kurtosis within the reference values, which were respectively lower than 3.0 and 7.0 for skewness and kurtosis. The multivariate coefficient of Márdia is 0.257, and the critical ratios resulting from the trajectories of the items to the factor are statistically significant. Figure 3a illustrates the initial model, allowing us to verify that items Q3.1, Q3.4, Q3.5 and Q3.6 present saturations lower than 0.40, leading to their elimination. Further, the goodness of fit indices of global adjustment for this model are inadequate (Table 3). By eliminating the items and refining the model, only 3 items remain in the final model because they present saturations higher than the minimum recommended (Figure 3b). For this final model, the goodness of fit indices of global adjustment are all saturated: CFI and GFI are equal to 1, and the remaining values are all equal to zero (Table 3).

Table 3. Statistics for the unidimensional model of the scale about economic and availability motivations.

Item	Internal Consistency of Items (Original)				
	Mean Score	Standard Deviation	r (Item-Total)	r^2	α Without Item
Q3.1	3.62	1.010	0.121	0.246	0.508
Q3.2	2.65	1.134	0.404	0.374	0.383
Q3.3	3.04	1.123	0.372	0.309	0.399
Q3.4	3.87	1.057	−0.072	0.166	0.582
Q3.5	3.17	1.091	0.327	0.155	0.422
Q3.6	2.78	1.079	0.411	0.226	0.384
Q3.7	2.41	1.188	0.164	0.342	0.497
Global Cronbach's alpha = 0.500					
Fitting Indices of CFA Model [1]		Initial [2]		Final [3]	
χ^2/df		404.1		0.000	
GFI		0.867		1.000	
CFI		0.606		1.000	
RMSEA		0.184		0.000	
RMSR		0.141		0.000	
SRMR		0.124		0.000	

[1] χ^2/df = Ratio of chi-square and degrees of freedom; GFI = Goodness of fit index; CFI = Comparative fit index; RMSEA = Root mean square error of approximation; RMSR = Root mean square residual; SRMR = Standardized root mean square residual. [2] Without modification indices. [3] With modification indices and eliminated items.

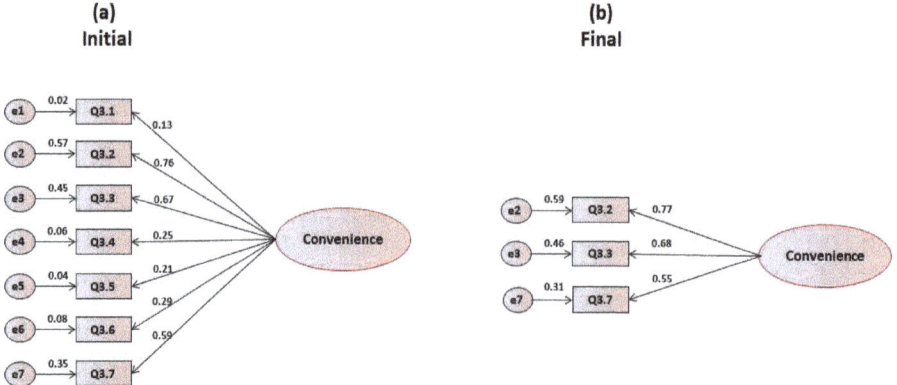

Figure 3. (a) Initial and (b) final models for the economic and availability motivations' scale.

3.4. Social and Cultural Motivations

Regarding items of the social and cultural motivations' scale, as it can be observed in Table 4, the corrected correlation coefficient's item-total shows that items Q4.1, Q4.5 and Q4.8 present correlations lower than 0.20, leading to the recommendation of the elimination of such items. The maximum correlation is obtained for item Q4.4 (r = 0.359), which accounts for 42.6% of its variability. Cronbach's alpha values oscillate between the inadequate and reasonable, ranging from 0.426 in item Q4.4 to 0.548 in item Q4.5, with the global alpha being acceptable (α = 0.504).

Table 4. Statistics for the unidimensional model of the scale about social and cultural motivations.

Item	Internal Consistency of Items (Original)				
	Mean Score	Standard Deviation	r (Item-Total)	r^2	α Without Item
Q4.1	3.74	1.034	0.178	0.219	0.487
Q4.2	3.06	1.107	0.338	0.179	0.433
Q4.3	2.65	1.072	0.273	0.133	0.457
Q4.4	2.44	1.090	0.359	0.194	0.426
Q4.5	2.61	1.131	−0.004	0.164	0.548
Q4.6	3.28	1.108	0.208	0.176	0.478
Q4.7	2.62	1.199	0.260	0.167	0.459
Q4.8	3.47	1.155	0.118	0.170	0.509
Q4.9	2.38	1.080	0.281	0.235	0.454
		Global Cronbach's alpha = 0.504			
Fitting Indices of CFA Model [1]		Initial [2]		Final [3]	
χ^2/df		321.7		0.000	
GFI		0.854		1.000	
CFI		0.348		1.000	
RMSEA		0.164		0.000	
RMSR		0.164		0.000	
SRMR		0.132		0.000	

[1] χ^2/df = Ratio of chi-square and degrees of freedom; GFI = Goodness of fit index; CFI = Comparative fit index; RMSEA = Root mean square error of approximation; RMSR = Root mean square residual; SRMR = Standardized root mean square residual. [2] Without modification indices. [3] With modification indices and eliminated items.

The confirmatory factor analysis of the hypothesized unifactorial structure revealed that all the items present a normal distribution, with asymmetry and kurtosis values within the reference values, respectively, lower than 3.0 and 7.0. The multivariate coefficient of Márdia is 0.231. The critical ratios resulting from the trajectories of the items to the factor are statistically significant, which lead to their maintenance. Figure 4a presents the initial model, which excluded item Q4.6 due to multicollinearity problems, and indicates that items Q4.3, Q4.4, Q4.5, Q4.7 and Q4.9 show saturation below 0.40, leading to their elimination. The goodness of fit indices for the global adjustment are inadequate for this initial model (Table 4). When refining the model and eliminating the unsuitable items, only three items remain in the unifactorial structure (Figure 4b). Although one of the items revealed a saturation of 0.38 (under 0.4 but in the limit of acceptance), it was decided to maintain it due to its importance to the structure of the factor. Table 4 also presents the global adjustment indices for this one-dimensional model, and, while in the initial model all indexes were inadequate, in the final model, after refinement, the indexes are excellent, all being saturated.

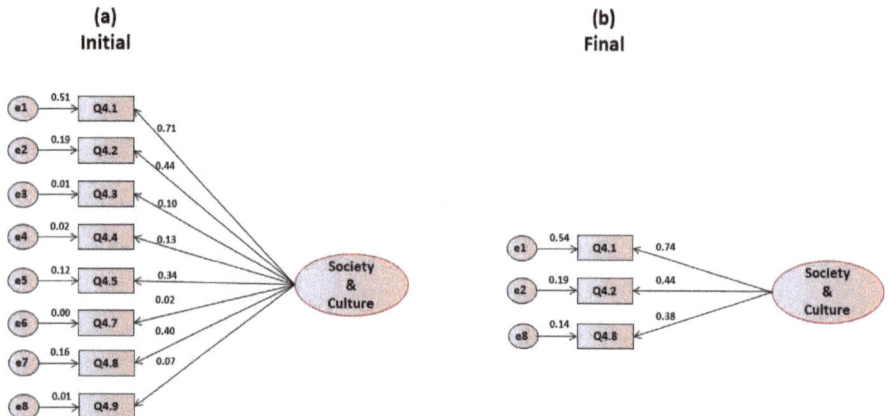

Figure 4. (a) Initial and (b) final models for the social and cultural motivations' scale.

3.5. Environmental and Political Motivations

Regarding the environmental and political motivations, an analysis of the mean scores and standard deviations of the items (Table 5) shows that they are well centered, being above the central score. The correlation coefficient's item-total presents values above 0.20, which leads to the maintenance of all items. Cronbach's alpha values are good for all items, between 0.753 in item Q5.4 and 0.789 in item Q5.2, while the overall alpha is on the threshold of very good ($\alpha = 0.799$). The confirmatory factorial analysis of the proposed unifactorial structure revealed that all items present a normal distribution, with values of asymmetry and kurtosis within the reference values, oscillating in absolute values for skewness between 0.031 and 0.773, and for kurtosis between 0.054 and 0.599. The multivariate coefficient of Márdia is 0.205. The critical ratios are statistically significant, which leads to the maintenance of all items. Figure 5a represents the initial model, from which it can be observed that all items saturate above 0.40, leading to their maintenance. The indices for evaluation of the goodness of global fit in this first model are adequate, with the exception of the χ^2/df, which is too high (Table 5). In Figure 5b, the final model is presented after the refinement of the modification indexes proposed by AMOS. It is important to note that, due to multicollinearity problems, items Q5.6 and Q5.77 have been eliminated when defining the final model. The goodness of fit indices for the global adjustment in the final model are very good. While only the chi-square ratio was inadequate for the initial one-dimensional model, in the final model, after refinement, the indexes are excellent, being saturated for GFI, CFI and RMSEA (Table 5).

3.6. Marketing and Commercials Motivations

The mean scores and corresponding standard deviations of the six items in the marketing and commercials' scale presented in Table 6 show that, in general, they are well cantered, the most problematic item being Q6.2, whose observed value is lower than average. The correlation coefficient's item-total reveals very weak and negative correlations in items Q6.1 and Q6.4, which leads to the rejection of these items in a more refined analysis. Cronbach's alpha values are inadmissible, with an overall alpha value of 0.399. However, it was still decided to perform a confirmatory factor analysis in order to determine the possible performances of the items. The confirmatory factorial analysis carried out on the unifactorial structure revealed that all items present a normal distribution, with values of skewness and kurtosis within the reference values. The multivariate coefficient of Márdia is 0.179. Critical ratios are statistically significant, which leads to the maintenance of all items. Figure 6a corresponds to the initial model, which excluded item Q6.7 due to multicollinearity problems, and shows that items Q6.1, Q6.4 and Q6.6 saturate below 0.40, leading to their elimination.

The goodness of fit indices for the global adjustment in this initial model are only suitable for the GFI and SRMR, being poor for CFI and RMSEA and unsuitable for the chi-square ratio (Table 6). Figure 6b represents the final refined model without the eliminated items. It is observed that all items have saturations greater than 0.60, and individual reliability greater than 0.40. The goodness of fit indices for the overall adjustment are very good. As the results in Table 6 show, for the initial one-dimensional model only the chi-square ratio was inadequate, but in the final model, after refinement, the indices are excellent, saturated for all indices.

Table 5. Statistics for the unidimensional model of the scale about environmental and political motivations.

Item	Internal Consistency of Items (Original)				
	Mean Score	Standard Deviation	r (Item-Total)	r^2	α Without Item
Q5.1	3.48	0.996	0.554	0.326	0.769
Q5.2	3.77	1.013	0.442	0.224	0.789
Q5.3	3.30	1.089	0.459	0.218	0.787
Q5.4	3.43	1.093	0.633	0.429	0.753
Q5.5	3.06	1.045	0.542	0.357	0.771
Q5.6	2.81	0.987	0.519	0.301	0.775
Q5.7	3.20	1.021	0.565	0.338	0.767
	Global Cronbach's alpha = 0.799				
Fitting Indices of CFA Model [1]		Initial [2]		Final [3]	
χ^2/df		93.44		0.987	
GFI		0.969		1.000	
CFI		0.937		1.000	
RMSEA		0.088		0.000	
RMSR		0.042		0.032	
SRMR		0.039		0.026	

[1] χ^2/df = Ratio of chi-square and degrees of freedom; GFI = Goodness of fit index; CFI = Comparative fit index; RMSEA = Root mean square error of approximation; RMSR = Root mean square residual; SRMR = Standardized root mean square residual. [2] Without modification indices. [3] With modification indices and eliminated items.

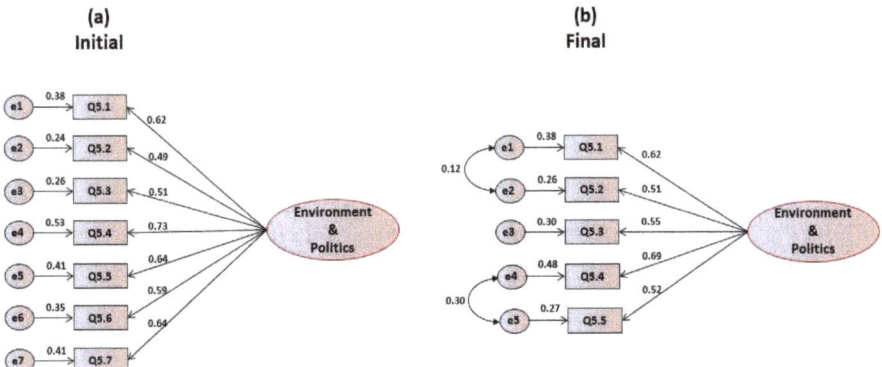

Figure 5. (a) Initial and (b) final models for the environmental and political motivations' scale.

Table 6. Statistics for the unidimensional model of the scale about marketing and commercials motivations.

Item	Internal Consistency of Items (Original)				
	Mean Score	Standard Deviation	r (Item-Total)	r^2	α Without Item
Q6.1	3.18	1.113	−0.049	0.121	0.498
Q6.2	2.30	1.013	0.352	0.301	0.257
Q6.3	2.67	1.130	0.274	0.290	0.299
Q6.4	3.69	1.067	−0.039	0.118	0.487
Q6.5	2.71	1.118	0.329	0.314	0.261
Q6.6	3.04	1.089	0.338	0.117	0.257
Q6.7	3.00	1.071	0.324	0.105	0.310
Global Cronbach's alpha = 0.399					
Fitting Indices of CFA Model [1]		Initial [2]		Final [3]	
χ^2/df		163.8		0.000	
GFI		0.958		1.000	
CFI		0.854		1.000	
RMSEA		0.117		0.000	
RMSR		0.084		0.000	
SRMR		0.071		0.000	

[1] χ^2/df = Ratio of chi-square and degrees of freedom; GFI = Goodness of fit index; CFI = Comparative fit index; RMSEA = Root mean square error of approximation; RMSR = Root mean square residual; SRMR = Standardized root mean square residual. [2] Without modification indices. [3] With modification indices and eliminated items.

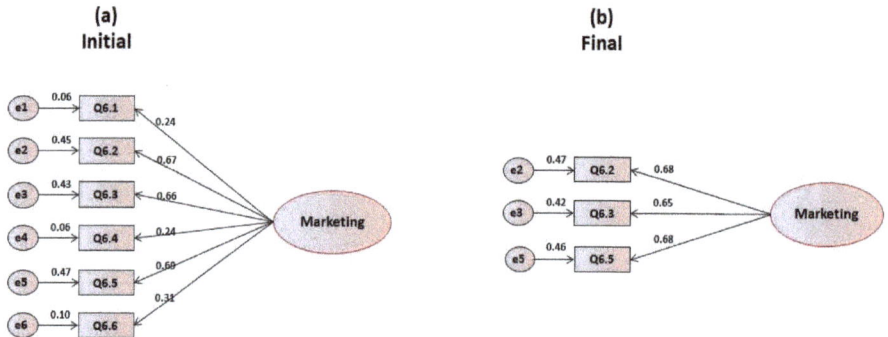

Figure 6. (a) Initial and (b) final models for the marketing and commercials motivations' scale.

4. Discussion

The six dimensions of the EATMOT scale were all validated, thus confirming the adequacy of the selected types of reasons that could influence eating patterns and food choices: health and disease, emotional status, convenience and easiness of access, societal and cultural influences or religious beliefs, environmental concerns or political frameworks, and finally all issues related with marketing, advertising or promotional campaigns.

Regarding the health motivations scale, from the 10 initial questions considered, only 3 were validated, which reflects the fragility of the aspects considered. However, if we look in more detail to the questions validated (Q1.1: "I am very concerned about the hygiene and safety of the food I eat", Q1.4: "It is important for me that my daily diet contains a lot of vitamins and minerals", Q1.8: "It is important for me to eat food that keeps me healthy"), we see that they all focus on health as a general concern, indicating that the participants look upon health more as a general concept than as individual contributions or pathologies. This is expected, since a great deal of scientific evidence has been collected about the close relations between food intake and health status [31–35]. Another factor that may contribute to the importance attributed to some health issues is associated with gender differences. The sample under study was composed of far more women than men, and it has been reported that women tend to be generally more reflective about food and health issues [36,37].

In the original group of nine questions about emotional motivations, there were four items that remained after validation, and they are in fact those questions more directly related with anxiety and negative emotional mood, like stress and depression, which are in fact very strong emotions (Q2.1: "Food helps me cope with stress", Q2.6: "When I feel lonely, I console myself by eating", Q2.8: "For me, food serves as an emotional consolation, Q9.9: "I have more cravings for sweets when I am depressed"). Emotional eating is extremely powerful, and has been associated with the growing epidemic of obesity and related pathologies, owing to the propensity to balance negative emotions through food intake, particularly with unhealthy products such as those rich in sugar or fat [38]. Emotional eating is present among all age groups, although with a higher expression in younger individuals, and could even be considered a pathology that should be handled by mental health practitioners [39].

From the seven questions initially considered concerning convenience aspects that could influence food choices, three were retained, focusing on easiness of access to food, both in terms of facility to acquire and low price, and easiness of preparation (Q3.2: "The main reason for choosing a food is its low price", Q3.3: "I choose the food I consume, because it is convenient to purchase", Q3.7: "I prefer to buy food that is ready to eat or pre-cooked"). In today's society, with "fast" life styles, where people seem to hardly find the time to do everything they wish to, the demand for convenience foods has grown, along with the distance between those who produce food and their consumers [37]. Many factors can justify this growing trend to seek convenience foods, like for example changes in the household structure, intensification of female employment, response of the food industry, marketing campaigns and advertisements, availability of kitchen technology compatible with cooked or pre-cooked meals, individualism, lack of time, or poor cooking skills [40–44].

The social and cultural motivations scale was initially composed of nine items, from which three were validated for the EATMOT scale (Q4.1: "Meals are a time of fellowship and pleasure", Q4.2: "I eat more than usual when I have company", Q4.8: "I like to try new foods to which I am not accustomed"). These focus on eating as a social act and the interaction between people while eating, as well as on the importance given to new foods and gastronomic experiences. According to Nakata [45], food tastes better and people tend to eat higher quantities when they are accompanied than when they are alone. Possible explanations can be assumed to justify this social facilitation of eating, some relying on the positive influence that company has on people by establishing social bounds, and others based on the assumption that people tend to imitate others, and therefore they eat because they see others eating. On the other hand, not only does company influence eating, but the type of social relationships is also considered an important factor for eating facilitation, so that when people are with friends or family they tend to ingest higher quantities of food than when they are in the presence of strangers [46–48].

Regarding environmental concerns and political motivations, from the initial seven items, the majority, four, were retained in the validated scale, which reflects the importance of aspects such as sustainability or human and animals' rights when making food choices (Q5.1: "It is important to me that the food I eat is prepared/packed in an environmental friendly way", Q5.3: "It is important to me that the food I eat comes from my own country", Q5.4: "I prefer to eat food that has been produced in a way that animals' rights have been respected", Q5.5: "I choose foods that have been produced in countries where human rights are not violated"). Food is one of the three consumption domains with greater environmental impact, and therefore food consumption is a central aspect for a sustainable food supply [49,50]. Consumer inclination towards sustainable food purchase can help minimize food waste and residues, as well as packaging materials, and can also minimize the environmental impacts along the production chain, from the farm to the fork. Similarly, informed food choices can have a large impact on the well-being of farm animals [37]. Consumers may also benefit the local economy with their socially responsible choices [51]. However, we must bear in mind that sustainability should not jeopardize food choices in terms of nutritional values. One example is the 'nutritional transition' of dietary patterns, and the consumption of foods with higher content in animal protein, acknowledging that meat is considered as the food product with the greatest environmental impact throughout the food chain [52]. Grunert et al. [53] revealed in their research that sustainability labels still do not play a major role in consumers' food choices. Finally, one of the latest studies on environmental modeling in the food chain revealed the following food related research perspectives: the environmental impacts of novel food processing technologies; innovative food packaging and changes in diets; and food consumption in connection with climate and environmental changes [54].

Finally, the last scale, concerning marketing issues, was initially composed of seven items, from which three were validated to be included in the EATMOT scale (Q6.2: "I eat what I eat, because I recognize it from advertisements or have seen it on TV", Q6.3: "I usually buy food that spontaneously appeals to me", Q6.5: "Food advertising campaigns increase my desire to eat certain foods"), and they confirm the important role of publicity and marketing as influencers on food choice. Food marketing has been identified as such an important determinant for obesity, that in many countries, restrictions have been imposed when advertising foods or beverages for children or adolescents. Further, the role of companies that sponsor many sports is believed to be influential in food consumption [55]. Care must be taken when it comes to advertisements. Although food marketing can be used to incentivize the consumption of healthy foods and beverages, the reality is sometimes different, and marketing is used to promote foods with a high energy density and low nutritional value. This is particularly true when it comes to young people, the demographic for whom food is one the most heavily marketed product categories. On the other hand, promotional campaigns can be an ally in eliciting the purchase of better quality foods at lower prices [56].

5. Conclusions

The results of this work allowed the assessing of six different types of factors that can influence food choices and eating behaviors, in the specific categories: health, emotions, price and availability, society and culture, environment and politics, and marketing and commercials. The results obtained for a wide sample from 16 countries indicated that all the individual scales measured presented good or very good fitting indices, with saturation in GFI in all cases, and values of chi-square ratio of 6.921 (for health), 0.987 (environment), 0.610 (emotions), and 0.000 in the remaining unifactorial models (convenience, society, marketing). Furthermore, the fit was perfect, with saturation for all indices, in three of the six models (convenience, society and marketing).

The scales validated include dimensions that are complementary and help in assessing food choice determinants, which can be very helpful in designing strategies that lead people to adopt better eating habits (those more oriented towards the maintenance of health, rather than having adverse effects). Furthermore, sustainability is a top priority in today's society, and the food supply chain contributes a high impact on the biosystems, increasing water, soil and atmosphere pollution, which will in the end also impact people's health. To understand people's decision processes, and which factors drive them to make some choices instead of others, is pivotal in changing eating behaviors. These results produced six independent scales for assessing eating motivations, which can be applied in future situations with a high degree of confidence, bearing in mind that they were validated for a considerably vast sample, across different countries and with participants from different cultural backgrounds.

Some limitations of this study include the possible biases due to the unequal number of participants, like for example there being more female than male participants, or more participants from countries like Croatia or Portugal, factors that are associated with the use of convenience samples in different countries. These limitations are to some extent counterbalanced by the high number of participants overall.

Author Contributions: Conceptualization, R.P.F.G., J.D.; methodology, R.P.F.G., M.F., J.D., P.C., A.P.C.; software, R.P.F.G., J.D.; validation, R.P.F.G., M.F., J.D., P.C., A.P.C.; formal analysis, R.P.F.G., J.D.; investigation, R.P.F.G., E.B., V.S., M.T., M.L., M.Č.-B., K.I., A.E.-K., V.F., E.S., M.K., E.V., M.L., L.F.-M., M.P., I.D., M.F., P.C., A.P.C., J.D.; resources, R.P.F.G.; data curation, R.P.F.G.; writing—original draft preparation, R.P.F.G., J.D.; writing—review and editing, R.P.F.G., E.B., V.S., M.T., M.L., M.Č.-B., K.I., A.E.-K., V.F., E.S., M.K., E.V., M.L., L.F.-M., M.P., I.D., M.F., P.C., A.P.C., J.D.; visualization, R.P.F.G.; supervision, R.P.F.G.; project administration, R.P.F.G.; funding acquisition, R.P.F.G. All authors have read and agreed to the published version of the manuscript.

Funding: This research was funded by CI&DETS Research Centre (Polytechnic Institute of Viseu, Portugal) grant number PROJ/CI&DETS/CGD/0012. The APC was funded by FCT-Foundation for Science and Technology (Portugal), grant number UIDB/00681/2020.

Acknowledgments: This work supported by National Funds through the FCT-Foundation for Science and Technology, I.P., within the scope of the project Refª UIDB/00681/2020. Furthermore, we would like to thank the CERNAS Research Centre and the Polytechnic Institute of Viseu for their support. This work was prepared in the ambit of the multinational project EATMOT from CI&DETS Research Centre (Polytechnic Institute of Viseu, Portugal) with reference PROJ/CI&DETS/CGD/0012.

Conflicts of Interest: The authors declare no conflict of interest.

Appendix A

The questions included in the questionnaire were distributed across six different sections as follows:

Section 1—Health motivations:
Q1.1. I am very concerned about the hygiene and safety of the food I eat;
Q1.2. It is important for me that my diet is low in fat;
Q1.3. Usually I follow a healthy and balanced diet;
Q1.4. It is important for me that my daily diet contains a lot of vitamins and minerals;
Q1.5. There are some foods that I consume regularly, even if they may raise my cholesterol;
Q1.6. I try to eat foods that do not contain additives;
Q1.7. I avoid eating processed foods, because of their lower nutritional quality;
Q1.8. It is important for me to eat food that keeps me healthy;
Q1.9. There are some foods that I consume regularly, even if they may raise my blood glycaemia;
Q1.10. I avoid foods with genetically modified organisms;

Section 2—Emotional motivations:
Q2.1. Food helps me cope with stress;
Q2.2. I usually eat food that helps me control my weight;
Q2.3. I often consume foods that keep me awake and alert (such as coffee, coke, energy drinks);
Q2.4. I often consume foods that help me relax (such as some teas, red wine);
Q2.5. Food makes me feel good;
Q2.6. When I feel lonely, I console myself by eating;
Q2.7. I eat more when I have nothing to do;
Q2.8. For me, food serves as an emotional consolation;
Q2.9. I have more cravings for sweets when I am depressed;

Section 3—Economic and Availability motivations:
Q3.1. I usually choose food that has a good quality/price ratio;
Q3.2. The main reason for choosing a food is its low price;
Q3.3. I choose the food I consume, because it is convenient to purchase;
Q3.4. I buy fresh vegetables to cook myself more often than frozen;
Q3.5. I usually buy food that is easy to prepare;
Q3.6. I usually buy food that it is on sale;
Q3.7. I prefer to buy food that is ready to eat or pre-cooked;

Section 4—Social and Cultural motivations:
Q4.1. Meals are a time of fellowship and pleasure;
Q4.2. I eat more than usual when I have company;
Q4.3. It is important to me that the food I eat is similar to the food I ate when I was a child;
Q4.4. I eat certain foods because other people (my colleagues, friends, family) also eat it;
Q4.5. I prefer to eat alone;
Q4.6. I choose the foods I eat, because it fits the season;
Q4.7. I eat certain foods because I am expected to eat them;
Q4.8. I like to try new foods to which I am not accustomed;
Q4.9. I usually eat food that is trendy;

Section 5—Environmental & Political motivations:
Q5.1. It is important to me that the food I eat is prepared/packed in an environmentally friendly way;
Q5.2. When I cook I have in mind the quantities to avoid food waste;
Q5.3. It is important to me that the food I eat comes from my own country;
Q5.4. I prefer to eat food that has been produced in a way that animals' rights have been respected;
Q5.5. I choose foods that have been produced in countries where human rights are not violated;
Q5.6. I avoid going to restaurants that do not have a recovery policy of food surplus;
Q5.7. I prefer to buy foods that comply with policies of minimal usage of packaging;

Section 6—Marketing and Commercials motivations:
Q6.1. When I buy food I usually do not care about the marketing campaigns happening in the shop;
Q6.2. I eat what I eat, because I recognize it from advertisements or have seen it on TV;
Q6.3. I usually buy food that spontaneously appeals to me (e.g., situated at eye level, appealing colors, pleasant packaging);
Q6.4. When I go shopping I prefer to read food labels instead of believing in advertising campaigns;
Q6.5. Food advertising campaigns increase my desire to eat certain foods;
Q6.6. Brands are important to me when making food choices;
Q6.7. I try to schedule my shopping for when I know there are promotions or discounts.

References

1. Cabral, D.; Cunha, L.M.; Vaz de Almeida, M.D. Food choice and food consumption frequency of Cape Verde inhabitants. *Appetite* **2019**, *139*, 26–34. [CrossRef] [PubMed]
2. McGuire, S. Scientific Report of the 2015 Dietary Guidelines Advisory Committee. Washington, DC: US Departments of Agriculture and Health and Human Services, 2015. *Adv. Nutr.* **2016**, *7*, 202–204. [CrossRef] [PubMed]
3. Keegan, E.; Kemps, E.; Prichard, I.; Polivy, J.; Herman, C.P.; Tiggemann, M. The effect of the spatial positioning of a healthy food cue on food choice from a pictorial-style menu. *Eat. Behav.* **2019**, *34*, 101313. [CrossRef] [PubMed]
4. Hu, X.F.; Kenny, T.-A.; Chan, H.M. Inuit Country Food Diet Pattern Is Associated with Lower Risk of Coronary Heart Disease. *J. Acad. Nutr. Diet.* **2018**, *118*, 1237.e1–1248.e1. [CrossRef]
5. Iwatani, S.; Yamamoto, N. Functional food products in Japan: A review. *Food Sci. Hum. Wellness* **2019**, *8*, 96–101. [CrossRef]
6. Novak Nicole, L.; Brownell Kelly, D. Role of Policy and Government in the Obesity Epidemic. *Circulation* **2012**, *126*, 2345–2352. [CrossRef]
7. Novak, N.L.; Brownell, K.D. Obesity: A public health approach. *Psychiatr. Clin. N. Am.* **2011**, *34*, 895–909. [CrossRef]
8. Sares-Jäske, L.; Knekt, P.; Lundqvist, A.; Heliövaara, M.; Männistö, S. Dieting attempts modify the association between quality of diet and obesity. *Nutr. Res.* **2017**, *45*, 63–72. [CrossRef]
9. Deroost, N.; Cserjési, R. Attentional avoidance of emotional information in emotional eating. *Psychiatr. Res.* **2018**, *269*, 172–177. [CrossRef]
10. Van den Tol, A.J.M.; Ward, M.R.; Fong, H. The role of coping in emotional eating and the use of music for discharge when feeling stressed. *Arts Psychother.* **2019**, *64*, 95–103. [CrossRef]

11. Bartolini, F. Food Trade and Global Value Chain. In *Encyclopedia of Food Security and Sustainability*; Ferranti, P., Berry, E.M., Anderson, J.R., Eds.; Elsevier: Oxford, UK, 2019; pp. 82–87. ISBN 978-0-12-812688-2.
12. Asian, S.; Hafezalkotob, A.; John, J.J. Sharing economy in organic food supply chains: A pathway to sustainable development. *Int. J. Prod. Econ.* **2019**, *218*, 322–338. [CrossRef]
13. Steg, L.; Vlek, C. Encouraging pro-environmental behaviour: An integrative review and research agenda. *J. Environ. Psychol.* **2009**, *29*, 309–317. [CrossRef]
14. Taghikhah, F.; Voinov, A.; Shukla, N. Extending the supply chain to address sustainability. *J. Clean. Prod.* **2019**, *229*, 652–666. [CrossRef]
15. Wann, D.L. Preliminary Validation of the Sport Fan Motivation Scale. *J. Sport Soc. Issues* **2016**. [CrossRef]
16. Kim, Y.G.; Eves, A. Construction and validation of a scale to measure tourist motivation to consume local food. *Tour. Manag.* **2012**, *33*, 1458–1467. [CrossRef]
17. Guiné, R.; Duarte, J.; Ferreira, M.; Correia, P.; Leal, M.; Rumbak, I.; Baric, I.; Komes, D.; Satalic, Z.; Saric, M.; et al. Knowledge about dietary fibres (KADF): Development and validation of an evaluation instrument through structural equation modelling (SEM). *Public Health* **2016**, *138*, 108–118. [CrossRef]
18. Ferrão, A.C.; Guine, R.P.F.; Correia, P.M.R.; Ferreira, M.; Duarte, J.; Lima, J. Development of A Questionnaire To Assess People's Food Choices Determinants. *Curr. Nutr. Food Sci.* **2019**, *15*, 281–295. [CrossRef]
19. Marôco, J. *Análise Estatística com o SPSS Statistics*, 7th ed.; ReportNumber: Lisbon, Portugal, 2018.
20. Broen, M.P.G.; Moonen, A.J.H.; Kuijf, M.L.; Dujardin, K.; Marsh, L.; Richard, I.H.; Starkstein, S.E.; Martinez–Martin, P.; Leentjens, A.F.G. Factor analysis of the Hamilton Depression Rating Scale in Parkinson's disease. *Parkinsonism Relat. Disord.* **2015**, *21*, 142–146. [CrossRef]
21. Costa, M.G.F.A.; Neves, M.M.J.C.; Duarte, J.C.; Pereira, A.M.S. Conhecimento dos pais sobre alimentação: Construção e validação de um questionário de alimentação infantil. *Rev. Enferm. Ref.* **2012**, *6*, 55–68. [CrossRef]
22. Tanaka, K.; Akechi, T.; Okuyama, T.; Nishiwaki, Y.; Uchitomi, Y. Development and validation of the Cancer Dyspnoea Scale: A multidimensional, brief, self-rating scale. *Br. J. Cancer* **2000**, *82*, 800–805. [CrossRef]
23. Harrington, D. *Confirmatory Factor Analysis*; Oxford University Press: New York, NY, USA, 2009.
24. Brown, T.A. *Confirmatory Factor Analysis for Applied Research*, 2nd ed.; Guilford Press: New York, NY, USA, 2015.
25. Hair, J.F.; Black, W.C.; Babin, B.J.; Anderson, R.E. *Multivariate Data Analysis, 7 ed.*; Prentice Hall: Upper Saddle River, NJ, USA, 2009; ISBN 978-0-13-813263-7.
26. Marôco, J. *Análise de Equações Estruturais. Fundamentos teóricos, Software e Aplicações*; ReportNumber: Lisboa, Portugal, 2014.
27. Sidali, K.L.; Pizzo, S.; Garrido-Pérez, E.I.; Schamel, G. Between food delicacies and food taboos: A structural equation model to assess Western students' acceptance of Amazonian insect food. *Food Res. Int.* **2019**, *115*, 83–89. [CrossRef] [PubMed]
28. Lagerkvist, C.J.; Amuakwa-Mensah, F.; Tei Mensah, J. How consumer confidence in food safety practices along the food supply chain determines food handling practices: Evidence from Ghana. *Food Control* **2018**, *93*, 265–273. [CrossRef]
29. Lim, T.-P.; Chye, F.-Y.; Sulaiman, M.R.; Suki, N.M.; Lee, J.-S. A Structural Modeling on Food Safety Knowledge, Attitude, and Behaviour Among Bum Bum Island community of Semporna, Sabah. *Food Control* **2015**. [CrossRef]
30. Ting, H.; Fam, K.-S.; Jun Hwa, J.C.; Richard, J.E.; Xing, N. Ethnic food consumption intention at the touring destination: The national and regional perspectives using multi-group analysis. *Tourism Manag.* **2019**, *71*, 518–529. [CrossRef]
31. Schäfer, F.; Jeanne, J.-F. Evaluating the effects of food on health in a world of evolving operational challenges. *Contemp. Clin. Trials Commun.* **2018**, *12*, 51–54. [CrossRef] [PubMed]
32. Adewumi, G.A. Health-Promoting Fermented Foods. In *Encyclopedia of Food Chemistry*; Melton, L., Shahidi, F., Varelis, P., Eds.; Academic Press: Oxford, UK, 2019; pp. 399–418. ISBN 978-0-12-814045-1.
33. Shang, N.; Chaplot, S.; Wu, J. 12-Food proteins for health and nutrition. In *Proteins in Food Processing*, 2nd ed.; Yada, R.Y., Ed.; Woodhead Publishing Series in Food Science, Technology and Nutrition; Woodhead Publishing: Cambridge, UK, 2018; pp. 301–336. ISBN 978-0-08-100722-8.

34. Akinmoladun, A.C.; Farombi, T.H.; Farombi, E.O. Food for Brain Health: Flavonoids. In *Encyclopedia of Food Chemistry*; Melton, L., Shahidi, F., Varelis, P., Eds.; Academic Press: Oxford, UK, 2019; pp. 370–386. ISBN 978-0-12-814045-1.
35. Lucan, S.C. When food isn't medicine—A challenge for physicians and health systems. *Prev. Med. Rep.* **2018**, *10*, 62–65. [CrossRef] [PubMed]
36. Behrens, J.; Montes, N.; Silva, M. Effect of nutrition and health claims on the acceptability of soymilk beverages. *Int. J. Food Sci. Technol.* **2007**, *42*, 50–56. [CrossRef]
37. Musto, M.; Cardinale, D.; Lucia, P.; Faraone, D. Creating Public Awareness of How Goats Are Reared and Milk Produced May Affect Consumer Acceptability. *J. Appl. Anim.Welf. Sci.* **2016**, *19*, 217–233. [CrossRef]
38. Mantau, A.; Hattula, S.; Bornemann, T. Individual determinants of emotional eating: A simultaneous investigation. *Appetite* **2018**, *130*, 93–103. [CrossRef]
39. Samuel, L.; Cohen, M. Expressive suppression and emotional eating in older and younger adults: An exploratory study. *Arch. Gerontol. Geriatr.* **2018**, *78*, 127–131. [CrossRef]
40. Scholliers, P. Convenience foods. What, why, and when. *Appetite* **2015**, *94*, 2–6. [CrossRef] [PubMed]
41. Verriet, J. Ready meals and cultural values in the Netherlands, 1950–1970. *Food Hist.* **2013**, *11*, 123–153. [CrossRef]
42. Sheely, M. Global adoption of convenience foods. *Am. J. Agric. Econ.* **2008**, *90*, 1356–1365. [CrossRef]
43. Brunner, T.A.; Horst, K.; Siegrist, M. Convenience food products. Drivers for consumption. *Appetite* **2010**, *55*, 498–506. [CrossRef] [PubMed]
44. Frez-Muñoz, L.; Steenbekkers, B.L.P.A.; Fogliano, V. The Choice of Canned Whole Peeled Tomatoes is Driven by Different Key Quality Attributes Perceived by Consumers Having Different Familiarity with the Product. *J. Food Sci.* **2016**, *81*, S2988–S2996. [CrossRef]
45. Nakata, R.; Kawai, N. The "social" facilitation of eating without the presence of others: Self-reflection on eating makes food taste better and people eat more. *Physiol. Behav.* **2017**, *179*, 23–29. [CrossRef]
46. Baumeister, R.F.; Leary, M.R. The Need to Belong: Desire for Interpersonal Attachments as a Fundamental Human Motivation. *Psychol. Bull.* **1995**, *117*, 497–529. [CrossRef]
47. Sommer, W.; Stürmer, B.; Shmuilovich, O.; Martin-Loeches, M.; Schacht, A. How about Lunch? Consequences of the Meal Context on Cognition and Emotion. *PLoS ONE* **2013**, *8*, e70314. [CrossRef]
48. Salvy, S.J.; Howard, M.; Read, M.; Mele, E. The presence of friends increases food intake in youth. *Am. J. Clin. Nutr.* **2009**, *90*, 282–287. [CrossRef]
49. Azzurra, A.; Massimiliano, A.; Angela, M. Measuring sustainable food consumption: A case study on organic food. *Sustain. Prod. Consum.* **2019**, *17*, 95–107. [CrossRef]
50. Verain, M.C.D.; Sijtsema, S.J.; Antonides, G. Consumer segmentation based on food-category attribute importance: The relation with healthiness and sustainability perceptions. *Food Qual. Prefer.* **2016**, *48*, 99–106. [CrossRef]
51. Colliver, A. Sustainable Food Consumption: A Practice-Based ApproachElizabeth Sargant Wageningen Academic Publishers, Netherlands, 2014, 174 pp., ISBN 9789086862634. *Aust. J. Environ. Educ.* **2015**, *31*, 282–283. [CrossRef]
52. Djekic, I.; Tomasevic, I. Environmental impacts of the meat chain – Current status and future perspectives. *Trends Food Sci. Technol.* **2016**, *54*, 94–102. [CrossRef]
53. Grunert, K.G.; Hieke, S.; Wills, J. Sustainability labels on food products: Consumer motivation, understanding and use. *Food Policy* **2014**, *44*, 177–189. [CrossRef]
54. Djekic, I.; Sanjuán, N.; Clemente, G.; Jambrak, A.R.; Djukić-Vuković, A.; Brodnjak, U.V.; Pop, E.; Thomopoulos, R.; Tonda, A. Review on environmental models in the food chain—Current status and future perspectives. *J. Clean. Prod.* **2018**, *176*, 1012–1025. [CrossRef]
55. Bragg, M.A.; Roberto, C.A.; Harris, J.L.; Brownell, K.D.; Elbel, B. Marketing Food and Beverages to Youth Through Sports. *J. Adolesc. Health* **2018**, *62*, 5–13. [CrossRef]
56. Cairns, G. Evolutions in food marketing, quantifying the impact, and policy implications. *Appetite* **2013**, *62*, 194–197. [CrossRef] [PubMed]

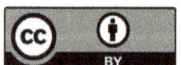

© 2020 by the authors. Licensee MDPI, Basel, Switzerland. This article is an open access article distributed under the terms and conditions of the Creative Commons Attribution (CC BY) license (http://creativecommons.org/licenses/by/4.0/).

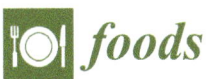

Article

Food Consumption Determinants and Barriers for Healthy Eating at the Workplace—A University Setting [†]

João P. M. Lima [1,2,3,4,*], Sofia A. Costa [5], Teresa R. S. Brandão [6] and Ada Rocha [2,3,7]

[1] Politécnico de Coimbra, ESTeSC, Unidade Científico-Pedagógica de Dietética e Nutrição, Rua 5 de Outubro, S. Martinho do Bispo, 3046-854 Coimbra, Portugal
[2] GreenUPorto—Sustainable Agrifood Production Research Centre, Campus de Vairão Edifício de Ciências Agrárias (FCV2) Rua da Agrária, 747, 4485-646 Vairão, Portugal; adarocha@fcna.up.pt
[3] LAQV-Requimte—R. D. Manuel II, Apartado 55142, 4051-401 Porto, Portugal
[4] ciTechCare—Center for Innovative Care and Health Technology, R. de Santo André 2410, 2410-541 Leiria, Portugal
[5] Instituto de Saúde de Pública da Universidade do Porto, Rua das Taipas 135, 4050-091 Porto, Portugal; sofcosta1@sapo.pt
[6] CBQF—Center for Biotechnology and Fine Chemicals—Associate Laboratory, School of Biotechnology, Catholic University of Portugal, R. de Diogo Botelho 1327, 4169-005 Porto, Portugal; tbrandao@porto.ucp.pt
[7] Faculty of Nutrition and Food Sciences, University of Porto, Rua do Campo Alegre, 823, 4150-180 Porto, Portugal
* Correspondence: joao.lima@estescoimbra.pt
† The work was a part of João Lima's doctoral thesis.

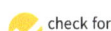

Citation: Lima, J.P.M.; Costa, S.A.; Brandão, T.R.S.; Rocha, A. Food Consumption Determinants and Barriers for Healthy Eating at the Workplace—A University Setting. *Foods* 2021, 10, 695. https://doi.org/10.3390/foods10040695

Academic Editor: Pascal Schlich

Received: 1 March 2021
Accepted: 22 March 2021
Published: 25 March 2021

Publisher's Note: MDPI stays neutral with regard to jurisdictional claims in published maps and institutional affiliations.

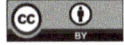

Copyright: © 2021 by the authors. Licensee MDPI, Basel, Switzerland. This article is an open access article distributed under the terms and conditions of the Creative Commons Attribution (CC BY) license (https://creativecommons.org/licenses/by/4.0/).

Abstract: Background: A wide variety of social, cultural and economic factors may influence dietary patterns. This work aims to identify the main determinants of food consumption and barriers for healthy eating at the workplace, in a university setting. Methods: A cross-sectional observational study was conducted with 533 participants. Data were obtained through the application of a self-administered questionnaire that included socio-demographic information, food consumption determinants and the main perceived barriers for healthy eating at the workplace. Results: The respondents identified "price" (22.5%), "meal quality" (20.7%), and "location/distance" (16.5%). For women, the determinant "availability of healthy food options" was more important than for men ($p < 0.001$). The food consumption determinants at the workplace most referred to by respondents were related to the nutritional value. Smell, taste, appearance and texture, and good value for money, were also considered important for choosing food at the workplace. Respondents referred to work commitments and lack of time as the main barriers for healthy eating at the workplace. Conclusions: Identification of determinants involved in food consumption, and the barriers for healthy eating, may contribute to a better definition of health promotion initiatives at the workplace aiming to improve nutritional intake.

Keywords: food choice; food consumption; university; workplace; determinants; barriers

1. Introduction

Globalization has caused drastic changes in food patterns within the last decade. These changes resulted in a reduction in the prevalence of malnutrition along with a widespread increase in prevalence of overweight and obesity [1]. An unhealthy lifestyle is one of the major risk factors for chronic diseases in developed countries [2]. Consumer behaviors play a prominent role in the etiology of several chronic non-communicable diseases, including obesity, diabetes mellitus, and cardiovascular diseases, among others, whose prevalence tends to stand still, or even increase [1,3,4].

Sedentary habits and unhealthy eating behaviors are responsible for a significant economic burden through absenteeism and presenteeism [5–8]. Additionally, for employees, unhealthy lifestyle behaviors and obesity might lead to negative effects related to work [9].

Research has shown that unhealthy employees and those with an unhealthy lifestyle are less productive at work and have decreased work ability [10–14].

The workplace is recognized as an opportune and fruitful setting for health promotion because of the presence of natural social networks, the possibility of reaching a large number of people, and the amount of time people spend at work [15,16]. Promotion of healthy lifestyles, namely healthy nutritional behavior at the workplace, improves workers' health and productivity [17].

The workplace also offers an interesting context for studying eating behaviors. There is often a high level of consistency in people's working lives, with many workers (particularly those who are office-based, as in this sample) spending most of their time in the same location surrounded by the same group of colleagues [18]. Partly for this reason, a number of eating-related research studies have been conducted at the workplace [19–21].

A wide variety of social, cultural, and economic factors may influence dietary patterns. Intra-individual determinants, such as physiological and psychological factors, acquired food preferences, and knowledge about nutrition can be distinguished from interpersonal or social factors, such as family and partners influence [21].

Food choice determinants are frequently presented in four groups:

(a) Biologically determined behavioral predispositions, related to an individual's innate abilities related to food, namely the preference for sweet and salty foods; the mechanisms that control hunger and satiety; and the sensory experience provided by food. These are the most basic determinants of food choice, meaning when choosing food or drinks, people firstly follow their preferences [21];

(b) Sensory-affective factors—those related to feelings and emotions in relation to food—acquired familiarity and ability to learn how to like something are at the second level [21];

(c) Intrapersonal factors, defined by an individual's beliefs, attitudes, knowledge, skills and social norms, follow the previous factors in determining the choice of food, just like the interpersonal ones, which involve family, friends and other social networks [21]. The culture in which each individual was born and raised influences general behavior and food habits [21]. Interpersonal factors theoretical framework was also described by Rothschild, 1999 [22], and applied, for example, in Bos, 2016 [23]. Several authors have ascertained that choices depend on the surrounding environment, and are based on one's knowledge and experience [21];

(d) Environmental factors are the last level determining food consumption. Even though they are the most distant from the individual, environmental factors are the easiest to influence. They include availability and accessibility to food; social, environmental and cultural practices; resources; economic environment; and food marketing practices [21]. For example, resources and economic environment determine food consumption through food cost or individual income [21]. According to the literature, low-income population groups are more likely to adopt unbalanced diets [21].

In addition to the determinants described above, the individual's psychological state is also assumed as one of the major determinants of the act of eating. Situations of emotional difficulty, states of anxiety and stress, situations of rejection, or loneliness, in more vulnerable individuals, can lead to changes in eating behavior [21].

Several studies concluded that individuals who identified a higher number of barriers for healthier eating habits correspond to those with worse habits [23,24]. The main factors identified by consumers as barriers for healthy eating were lack of time, poor cooking skills, food price, or the lack of healthy choices at food service units [23–26].

Meals eaten at the workplace represent a large contribution to the daily energy intake and influence the balance of the diet [27]. The study "Food and Portuguese Population Lifestyle" [28], identified the factors that influence the food choices of Portuguese adults, and their relationship with socio-demographic and health features [29]. The attribute of "Taste" was the most important factor determining food choice, followed by the "Price" and the "Intention of healthy eating", according to Poínhos et al. [29].

Previous research conducted at different workplaces related to food consumption determinants and perceived barriers, identified that structures and systems within the workplace have a significant role in dietary behaviors. These include the facilities available [30–32], training of staff [33], long hours worked as a result of high workloads and work pressures, and a culture that encourages working through breaks [34,35]. Lack of time for lunch can affect both health and productivity [36,37]. The conflict between promoting a greater range of healthier foods and business constraints has also been previously identified [38].

In order to develop effective workplace interventions for healthy eating, researchers must first consider all the known determinants of eating behavior as potential targets for intervention, such as distinct features of working conditions. In a recent systematic review of factors affecting healthy eating among nurses, the majority of studies found that workplaces often create barriers for healthy eating [20]. Therefore, to define appropriate health promotion initiatives, it is necessary to characterize the determinants involved in food choice, in order to influence food consumption at the workplace. Additionally, to identify perceived barriers for healthier eating habits it is also important for the implementation and assessment of interventions in different scenarios [39,40].

To the best of our knowledge, there are no studies that identify and characterize the determinants involved in food choice in Portugal, especially at the workplace, and it becomes relevant to develop research to better understand this subject. Therefore, this study intends to identify the perceived barriers for healthy eating, and the main determinants of food consumption at the workplace, among university employees.

2. Materials and Methods

2.1. Study Design and Sample

A cross-sectional observational study was conducted at a Portuguese university through face-to-face interviews by a trained researcher at the participants' workplace. This university had 3307 employees: 1750 teachers and researchers (academic), 1551 non-teaching staff (non-academic) [41]. A convenience sample was used, stratified by organic units, aiming to represent the study population, allowing researchers to infer conclusions for the study population. Given that the sample corresponds to approximately 15% of the population, it was stratified into teaching and researcher staff, and non-teaching and non-researcher staff; 533 employees were selected. Data collection was performed during labor hours.

2.2. Ethical Issues

The project was approved by Ethical Commission of the University of Porto, with the number CEFADE 25.2014. The principles of the Helsinki Declaration were respected and the workers under analysis accepted participation in the study through informed consent, after having the purpose and methods involved in the study explained to them individually.

2.3. Questionnaires for Data Collection

Data were obtained through the application of a self-administered questionnaire. It included socio-demographic information and food consumption determinants at the workplace, and a list of barriers for healthy eating at the workplace. The questionnaire included questions such as the employee's age, gender and marital status. Academic qualifications were also questioned, through a closed answer format composed of nine levels of response (between primary school and PhD or Post-Doc). Employees with academic qualifications higher than bachelor's degree were asked about the training area. Concerning work practices, respondents were asked about the amount of time they spend working at this institution, and the work regime (full-time or part-time). They were asked about the professional category, function performed, with discrimination between teaching and non-teaching activity, and the establishment where they work.

To assess food consumption determinants, a section of the questionnaire was developed through the adaptation of the Food Choice Questionnaire, developed by Steptoe et al. [42] after translation and validation for the Portuguese population by Cardoso and Vale [43]. Steptoe et al. also contributed to the questions of the Food Choice Questionnaire. A Likert Scale of 5 points, from strongly disagree (1) to strongly agree (5) was used in the questions related to determinants. Questions used in the studies "Food and Portuguese Population Lifestyle" and "Food and Portuguese Population Lifestyle" [28,29] were included in the questionnaire. The determinants of the choice of location for lunch in the workplace were also evaluated. Respondents were invited to select the three main factors affecting their choice from a predefined list presented in our results [29,44–47].

The barriers presented to respondents were selected from the literature, and others were added considering individual perceptions of the researchers. Respondents could select as many options from the list as they wanted.

Food offer, quality of meals, prices and food and nutritional intake of employees were analyzed and published in previous research papers [48,49].

2.4. Statistical Analysis

Data were analyzed using the Statistical Package for Social Sciences version 21.0 ® for Windows. Descriptive analysis was performed, and normality of cardinal variables was tested with Shapiro-Wilk Test. Association between nominal variables was analyzed by chi-square test. Association between ordinals and nominal variables was performed with Kruskal-Wallis tests. Between ordinal variables, or between ordinal and cardinal non-normal, Spearman correlation was performed. Taking into consideration the differentiation of the sample in terms of age, results were analyzed by age groups, through splitting the sample by the median age (43 years old) to identify younger and older respondents. Cut-off of 0.05 was used as the level of statistical significance. Data were also analyzed according to Multiple Correspondence Analysis (MCA) procedures, which allows for exploring the pattern of relationships of several categorical variables and representing them in few dimensions of homogeneous variables. For this model, sociodemographic variables were included, namely gender, educational level, and professional occupation; lunch setting (lunch brought from home, university food services, restaurants and go home), determinants for the lunch place choice and determinants of food consumption identified from Food Choice Questionnaire [42,43].

3. Results

3.1. Sample Characterization

From 533 assessed individuals, 513 were considered valid answers. Participants were aged between 21 and 80 years old (mean 43.3 ± 10.6), mostly females (65.5%) and married (63.4%). About 94% of respondents were full-time workers. Most workers (80.3%) had a university degree and about 35% had a PhD or a Post-Doc diploma. Only 3.3% of respondents did not complete high school education. Of respondents, 34.2% were Teachers, 63.0% were Non-Academic Staff/Researchers and 2.8% had both activities.

The majority of workers had a sedentary activity since 81.5% of them reported spending most of their time seated, and 74.5% characterized their work as not being "very physically demanding".

Only 23.1% of respondents reported following an unhealthy diet at the workplace. Hence, only these workers were asked to point out the barriers for adopting a healthier diet.

3.2. Determinants of Choosing the Place for Having Lunch

The majority (96.7%) of respondents had lunch every day, however, only 36.1% of them attended the university food service. Of the respondents, 28% had lunch in local restaurants. About 52% of workers brought lunch from home and only 16.2% had lunch at home.

The respondents identified "price" (22.5%), "meal quality" (20.7), "location/distance" (16.5%), "healthy food options" (13.1%) and "lead time" (10.6%) as the most important determinants used to choose the place for having lunch. For women, the option of having "healthy food options" ($p < 0.001$) was more important than for men. Additionally, "location" ($p < 0.001$) and "noise" ($p = 0.016$) were more important for women than for men (Figure 1).

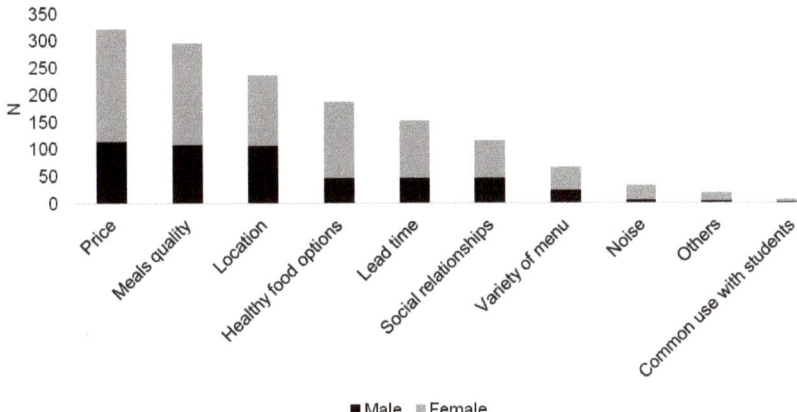

Figure 1. Food consumption determinants to choose the place for having lunch per gender. N: Number of individuals

"Price" as a determinant for choosing the place for having lunch was more important in younger respondents (Table 1). This determinant was also more important for those with a lower academic degree ($p < 0.001$) than for those with a higher level of education. Respondents with a higher academic degree referred more frequently to "Location/Distance" of places for having lunch as a determinant of choice. "Meal quality" ($p = 0.002$) and "healthy food options" ($p = 0.049$) were considered determinants for choosing the lunch setting more frequently by teaching staff.

Table 1. Food consumption determinants to choose the place for having lunch per age group.

Determinants for Place Choosing	Youngers (%)	Olders (%)	p-Value
Price	24.1	20.4	0.006 [1]
Meal quality	21.0	20.4	0.457
Location	15.2	18.3	0.104
Healthy food options	13.1	13.2	0.859
Lead time	11.0	9.7	0.298
Social relationships	7.4	8.9	0.354
Variety of menu	4.8	4.3	0.561
Noise	1.9	2.8	0.282
Others	1.1	1.6	0.439
Common use with students	0.4	0.5	0.765

[1] Differences with statistical significance.

Based on results of MCA three main dimensions were identified that explained 33.4% of data variability. The following homogeneous groups of variables were obtained (Figure 2).

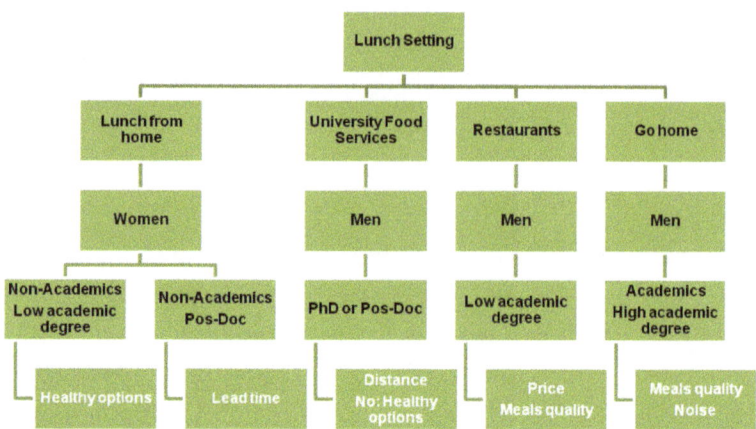

Figure 2. Food consumption determinants to choose the setting for having lunch (Multiple Correspondence Analysis (MCA) analysis).

3.3. Determinants of Food Consumption at the Workplace

Determinants of food consumption at the workplace most referred to by respondents (more than 70%) were related to foods rich in vitamins, minerals and fiber, nutritionally balanced, with natural ingredients and no additives, and that contribute to health and weight control. Smell, taste, appearance, texture, and a good value for money were also considered important for choosing food at the workplace.

Based on the results of MCA, two main dimensions were identified that explained 59.9% of data variability, and the following homogeneous groups of variables were obtained (Figure 3).

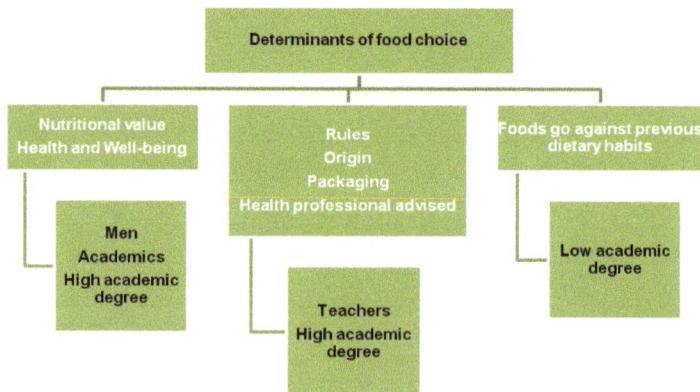

Figure 3. Food consumption determinants at the workplace (MCA analysis).

3.4. Barriers for Healthy Eating at the Workplace

The participants referred mostly to work commitments and lack of time as barriers for healthy eating at the workplace (Figure 4). From the barriers under analysis, differences between genders were only observed related to knowledge about nutrition. Males identified "Lack of knowledge about nutrition/healthy eating" as a barrier for healthy eating more frequently than women (Table 2). No differences were observed between age groups related to perceived barriers for healthy eating (Table 3).

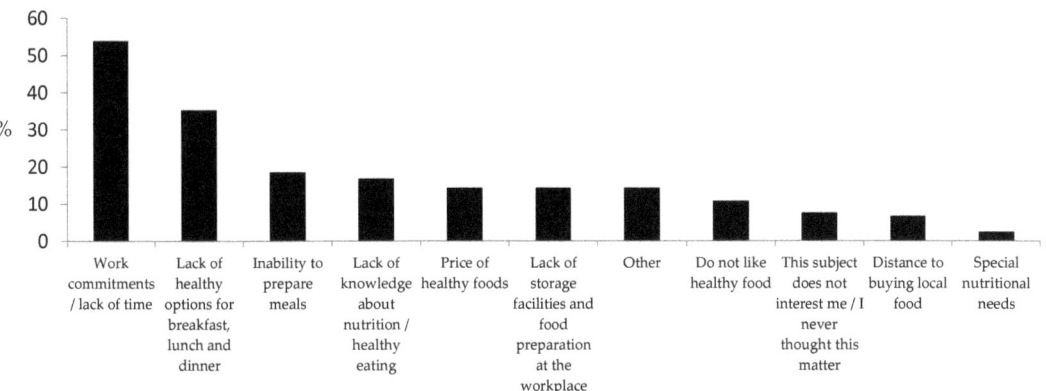

Figure 4. Frequency of perceived barriers for healthy eating at the workplace.

Table 2. Perceived barriers for healthy eating at the workplace by gender.

Barriers for Healthier Eating	Male (%)	Female (%)	p-Value
Do not like healthy food	3.7	6.7	0.449
Price of healthy foods	8.3	6.7	0.420
Inability to prepare meals	10.2	9.2	0.526
Lack of knowledge about nutrition/healthy eating	12.0	5.0	0.019 [1]
Distance to food stores	5.6	1.7	0.067
Work commitments/lack of time	22.2	31.9	0.222
Lack of storage facilities and food preparation at the workplace	5.6	9.2	0.436
Lack of healthy options for breakfast, lunch and dinner	19.4	16.8	0.244
Special nutritional needs	0.9	1.7	0.707
This subject does not interest me/I never though this matter	4.6	3.4	0.466
Others	7.4	7.6	0.781

[1] Differences with statistical significance.

Table 3. Perceived barriers for healthy eating at the workplace by age group.

Barriers for Healthier Eating	Youngers (%)	Olders (%)	p-Value
Do not like healthy food	6.1	4.2	0.288
Price of healthy foods	5.3	10.5	0.308
Inability to prepare meals	11.4	7.4	0.104
Lack of knowledge about nutrition/healthy eating	9.8	6.3	0.131
Distance to food stores	3.8	3.2	0.561
Work commitments/lack of time	28.0	26.3	0.101
Lack of storage facilities and food preparation at the workplace	7.6	7.4	0.577
Lack of healthy options for breakfast, lunch and dinner	17.4	18.9	0.575
Special nutritional needs	0.8	2.1	0.499
This subject does not interest me/I never though this matter	1.5	7.4	0.058
Others	8.3	6.3	0.279

In comparing academic with non-academic respondents, significant differences for two distinct barriers were found. It seems that food price is a prohibitive factor for having a healthy diet, essentially for non-academic staff in relation to other individuals ($p = 0.004$). Lack of healthy options for breakfast, lunch and dinner were identified by academic staff more frequently than by non-academics ($p = 0.012$) (Table 4). Concerning other parameters assessed, ranges of age and marital status did not seem to influence the barriers for healthier eating at the workplace.

Table 4. Perceived barriers for healthy eating at the workplace by professional occupation.

Barriers for Healthier Eating	Academics (%)	Non-Academics (%)	p-Value
Do not like healthy food	3.5	6.6	0.406
Price of healthy foods	1.2	10.9	0.004 [1]
Inability to prepare meals	7.1	10.9	0.307
Lack of knowledge about nutrition/healthy eating	5.9	10.2	0.314
Distance to food stores	5.9	2.2	0.147
Work commitments/lack of time	32.9	24.8	0.054
Lack of storage facilities and food preparation at the workplace	5.9	6.6	0.826
Lack of healthy options for breakfast, lunch and dinner	25.9	14.6	0.012 [1]
Special nutritional needs	1.2	1.5	0.856
This subject does not interest me/I never though this matter	5.9	2.9	0.272
Others	4.7	8.8	0.236

[1] Differences with statistical significance.

4. Discussion

Major determinants for choosing a place to have lunch were related to "meal quality", "price", and "location". Working at higher education institutes determines an increased burden of work and responsibilities, most of them extra classes [50], which contributes to work commitments and lack of time to take breaks, prepare, and have healthy meals. Additionally, sensory aspects of food consumption can influence the choice of lunch place. Sensory aspects are usually observed as determinant of food consumption. The cost of meals is more relevant for younger respondents as observed in a previous study [51].

Younger, non-teaching female employees with lower academic qualifications are the group who most frequently bring lunch from home. Bringing food from home is likely associated with higher level cooking skills—more common in the female gender [25]. Additionally, this group also has lower disposable income and hence, bringing food from home allows for more savings.

Lunch location is also determined by other factors. According to other authors, meals outside the home often have a higher energy value and a poorer nutritional profile [27]. Indeed, of the women who bring lunch from home, some do so to ensure a healthier lunch.

On the other hand, teachers with PhD or Post-Doc Diplomas mentioned waiting time as a key decision driver. This is likely associated with a higher level of responsibility, strong focus on work, and consequently, shorter lunch breaks.

In this study, food availability was identified more frequently by academic staff than other respondents. On the other hand, non-academics reported a higher concern, and identified the lack of storage facilities and food preparation areas at the workplace as a barrier. This parallelism on identified barriers could indicate that academics more frequently use university cafeterias, and non-academics bring food from home and use storage and preparation facilities, when available at the workplace, more frequently. These results are in line with the identification of a third barrier, significantly the difference between individuals with different professional occupations. Effectively, non-academics identified the price of healthy food options as a barrier for healthy eating more frequently than academics. Differences in salary between them could explain this result. The perception of these factors could influence the choice of place for having meals—cafeterias, or storage and preparation facilities.

Attending to the wide availability of information about healthy eating, the number of respondents that identify the lack of knowledge about nutrition or healthy eating as a barrier is unexpected. Men identified this barrier more frequently than women. In addition, Yahia observed that men identified the barrier, lack of knowledge about nutrition or healthy eating, more frequently than women, among university students [52].

Universities are a captive environment where staff is restricted to a campus where offices, classes and study facilities are located, and where there is limited choice for food provision [53,54]. The workplace can be a strong determinant of food consumption behavior as it provides convenient access to healthy and/or unhealthy food choices. In a population experiencing time constraints having good food choices at the workplace provides an easy option for refueling [37,48]. Food available at, or near workplaces, is more convenient, low in cost, and sells well [21]. Similar findings were reported by Pinhão et al. in a representative sample of the Portuguese population, where "taste" was the most selected factor, followed by "price" and "trying to eat healthy" [29] as determinants of food choice.

Our results are in accordance with those found by Kjøllesdal in Norwegian adults, showing that people with higher educational levels and in higher income groups ate in staff canteens more frequently than others [55].

According to previous literature, access to healthy foods in the workplace is often limited, compared with an abundance of unhealthy foods present in workplace canteens, onsite shops, and vending machines [46,48,56,57]. According to literature, workers desire a greater variety of healthy and fresh foods compared with the current offerings [46,57–59], which is identified in this research as a barrier for healthy eating. Healthy options also determined workers food choice. Interestingly, some employees felt that food served in the canteen is not balanced with their nutritional needs. The factors that influence food consumption of employees related to healthy options, nutritional value of foods, meal quality, and health and well-being, may be associated with employees' perception of canteen' meals being too high in calories and tailored for physically demanding roles [46].

However, employees also reported that the lunch provided by the work canteen is the only opportunity to have a "proper meal" each day [58]. In the same way, the workplace could be a provider of healthy foods (such as vegetables and fruit) and increase intake of those foods [59,60]. Availability at the workplace is a determinant for food choice and a barrier for healthy eating, the reasons why the availability of facilities where food can be prepared was considered to be an important facilitator of healthy eating [46,59]. On the other hand, the higher cost of healthy options compared with unhealthy options was identified as one of the most significant barriers to healthy eating [46].

The determinants that most influence food choice at the workplace in this study are related to the individual. The identification of knowledge about the health benefits of food is commonly observed, followed by biological determinants such as taste, smell, or the texture of the food, and finally, of an environmental nature related to the quality-price ratio of the food.

Food choices of men, with higher academic qualifications and belonging to the teaching staff, are determined by food taste and texture, and by availability and price-quality relationship. Additionally, they value the potential benefits of food, and their food choice is determined by them. The influence that foods can have on well-being is also important, such as choosing foods that help maintain alertness and support emotional health.

Regardless of gender, among professors with higher academic qualifications, food choice is determined by cultural, religious or ethnic beliefs, political ideologies, the clarity and environmental responsibility of packaging products, and medical advice regarding the intake of certain foods. On the other hand, among individuals with lower academic qualifications, these determinants have a reduced importance.

In fact, food choice is a complex result of preferences for sensory characteristics, combined with the influence of non-sensory factors, including food-related expectations and attitudes, health claims, price, ethical concerns and mood, as already reported by other authors [47,61]. Regarding these concerns, the availability of healthy food options at the workplace, namely in cafeterias, is very important. On the other hand, the inability to prepare meals was also identified as a barrier for healthy eating, pointing to a need to improve cooking skills, for example, by the inclusion of this topic in the school curriculum.

Only a small proportion of respondents perceived barriers for adoption of a healthy diet. Other authors observed similar results [25,26,62]. Healthier environments should be promoted to facilitate healthy eating and fighting chronic diseases such as obesity [63]. However, of all variables tested, only the price and lack of knowledge about nutrition/healthy eating showed significant differences between respondents. Some studies have shown that people that identify a higher number of barriers are those that follow unhealthy eating habits more frequently [24,63].

The barriers identified in this research are related only to individuals that are considered as having unhealthy eating at the workplace. Future works should also include those who are considered as having healthy habits.

Strategies to promote healthier food habits aim at reducing barriers to access healthy options and increasing opportunities for employees to make healthier food choices. Implementation includes provision of healthier options, improved accessibility, and establishment of mandatory policies to provide healthy options or restrict less healthy offerings at the workplace [16].

Some limitations were identified in this study. Lack of information concerning income that impair conclusions potentially explained by this. Another limitation was related to the usage of different tools to access food determinants for choosing the place to have lunch, and the determinants of food consumption in general. However, the fact that the tool used to access the determinants for choosing the place to have lunch was used in another Portuguese study with a national representative sample, motivates the researchers to that procedure. The use of a convenience sample determined a higher proportion of non-academic staff as they were more available for data collection.

5. Conclusions

The most important determinants identified by respondents choosing the place for having meals were "meal quality", "price", and "location/distance". For women, the availability of "healthy food options" was more important than for men.

Our results seem to demonstrate that gender, marital status, academic degree and main professional occupation, are related to the choice of the place for having lunch. Differences were found between gender, marital status and age ranges, in terms of factors-affecting food choice at the workplace. A higher concern with nutritional value of food was observed for younger respondents, individuals living alone, and women.

Gender and academic degree are relevant in food choice. Factors influencing individuals with a low academic degree were previous food habits, price, and quality of meals, in determining the choice of place for having lunch at restaurants or at home. On the other hand, women with a high academic degree prefer to bring meals from home as they find them healthier.

Related to determinants of food choice in general, MCA analysis reported the major differences related to academic degree and main occupation, with lower academic degree individuals being not influenced by external determinants, since their food choice was mainly influenced by previous food habits. Higher academic degree employees in general are influenced by nutritional value of food and its relationship to health and well-being, packaging, and health professional advice, the reason why strategies to promote healthy eating in these scenarios are necessarily different. If we could design a healthy eating program based on information about the nutrition value of food and health, namely through packaging, our results would show clearly that this option could be adequate for teachers and other employees with high academic degrees, but not for others that probably need personal counseling to change previous food habits.

This work also identified lack of time, work commitments, and lack of healthy options for having meals at the workplace as barriers for healthy eating. Educational level, professional occupation, and gender were the socio-economic characteristics evaluated that influenced the perception of barriers for healthy eating.

These results may contribute to a better definition of strategies to promote healthy eating in these scenarios and show that different strategies are needed for different target groups to reduce barriers once they are perceived differently by individuals.

Author Contributions: Conceptualization, J.P.M.L. and A.R.; formal analysis, S.A.C. and T.R.S.B.; investigation, J.P.M.L. and A.R.; writing—original draft preparation, J.P.M.L.; writing—review and editing, A.R. All authors have read and agreed to the published version of the manuscript.

Funding: This research was supported by national funds through FCT—Foundation for Science and Technology within the scope of UIDB/05748/2020 and UIDP/05748/2020.

Institutional Review Board Statement: The study was conducted according to the guidelines of the Declaration of Helsinki, and approved by the Ethical Commission of the University of Porto (protocol code CEFADE 25.2014 at 22/10/2014).

Informed Consent Statement: Informed consent was obtained from all subjects involved in the study.

Data Availability Statement: The work was a part of João Lima's doctoral thesis.

Acknowledgments: Authors thank Graça Neto, English Professional, for English grammar and structure revision of the manuscript.

Conflicts of Interest: The authors declare no conflict of interest.

References

1. Popkin, B.; Adair, L.S.; Ng, S.W. Now and then: The global nutrition transition: The pandemic of obesity in developing countries. *Nutr. Rev.* **2012**, *70*, 3–21. [CrossRef]
2. WHO. *Diet, Nutrition and the Prevention of Chronic Diseases: Report of a Joint WHO/FAO Expert Consultation*; WHO: Geneva, Switzerland, 2003.
3. Loureiro, I. A importância da educação alimentar na escola. In *Promoção da Saúde: Modelos e Práticas de Intervenção nos Âmbitos da Actividade Física, Nutrição e Tabagismo*; Edições FMH: Lisboa, Portugal, 2000; pp. 57–84.
4. WHO. *Obesity: Preventing and Managing the Global Epidemic*; World Health Organization: Geneva, Switzerland, 2004.
5. Ding, D.; Lawson, K.D.; Kolbe-Alexander, T.L.; Finkelstein, E.A.; Katzmarzyk, P.T.; Van Mechelen, W.; Pratt, M. The economic burden of physical inactivity: A global analysis of major non-communicable diseases. *Lancet* **2016**, *388*, 1311–1324. [CrossRef]
6. Dohrn, M.; Kwak, L.; Oja, P.; Sjöström, M.; Hagströmer, M. Replacing sedentary time with physical activity: A 15-year follow-up of mortality in a national cohort. *Clin. Epidemiol.* **2018**, *10*, 179. [CrossRef] [PubMed]
7. Burton, W.N.; Conti, D.J.; Chen, C.Y.; Schultz, A.B.; Edington, D.W. The role of health risk factors and disease on worker productivity. *J. Occup. Environ. Med.* **1999**, *41*, 863–877. [CrossRef]
8. Schultz, A.B.; Chen, C.Y.; Edington, D.W. The cost and impact of health conditions on presenteeism to employers: A review of the literature. *Pharmacoeconomics* **2009**, *27*, 365–378. [CrossRef]
9. Schmier, J.K.; Jones, M.L.; Halpern, M.T. Cost of obesity in the workplace. *Scand. J. Work Environ. Health* **2006**, *32*, 5–11. [CrossRef]
10. Robroek, S.J.; van den Berg, T.I.; Plat, J.F.; Burdorf, A. The role of obesity and lifestyle behaviours in a productive workforce. *Occup. Environ. Med.* **2011**, *68*, 134–139. [CrossRef]
11. Proper, K.I.; van den Heuvel, S.G.; De Vroome, E.M.; Hildebrandt, V.H.; Vander Beek, A.J. Dose-response relation between physical activity and sick leave. *Br. J. Sports Med.* **2006**, *40*, 173–178. [CrossRef]
12. van Duijvenbode, D.C.; Hoozemans, M.J.; van Poppel, M.N.; Proper, K.I. The relationship between overweight and obesity, and sick leave: A system-atic review. *Int. J. Obes.* **2009**, *33*, 807–816. [CrossRef]
13. Alavinia, S.M.; Molenaar, D.; Burdorf, A. Productivity loss in the work-force: Associations with health, work demands, and individual characteristics. *Am. J. Ind. Med.* **2009**, *52*, 49–56. [CrossRef] [PubMed]
14. Williden, M.; Schofield, G.; Duncan, S. Establishing links between health and productivity in the New Zealand workforce. *J. Occup. Environ. Med.* **2012**, *54*, 545–550. [CrossRef]
15. Dishman, R.K.; Oldenburg, B.; O'Neal, H.; Shephard, R.J. Worksite physical activity interventions. *Am. J. Prev. Med.* **1998**, *15*, 344–361. [CrossRef]
16. Hutchinson, A.D.; Wilson, C. Improving nutrition and physical activity in the workplace: A meta-analysis of intervention studies. *Health Promot. Int.* **2012**, *27*, 238–249. [CrossRef]
17. Grimani, A.; Aboagye, E.; Kwak, L. The effectiveness of workplace nutrition and physical activity interventions in improving productivity, work performance and workability: A systematic review. *BMC Public Health* **2019**, *19*, 1676. [CrossRef]
18. Smedslund, G.; Fisher, K.; Boles, S.; Lichtenstein, E. The effectiveness of workplace smoking cessation programmes: A meta-analysis of recent studies. *Tob Control.* **2004**, *13*, 197–204. [CrossRef]
19. Allan, J.; Querstret, D.; Banas, K.; de Bruin, M. Environmental interventions for altering eating behaviours of employees in the workplace: A systematic review. *Obes. Rev.* **2017**, *18*, 214–226. [CrossRef]
20. Nicholls, R.; Perry, L.; Duffield, C.; Gallagher, R.; Pierce, H. Barriers and facilitators to healthy eating for nurses in the workplace: An integrative review. *J. Adv. Nurs.* **2017**, *73*, 1051–1065. [CrossRef] [PubMed]
21. Contento, I.R. *Overview of Determinants of Food Choice and Dietary Change: Implications for Nutrition Education*; Jones & Bartlett Learning, LLC: Burlington, MA, USA, 2011.
22. Rothschild, M.L. Carrots, sticks, and promises: A conceptual framework for the management of public health and social issue behaviors. *J. Mark.* **1999**, *63*, 24–37. [CrossRef]

23. Bos, C.; van der Lans, I.A.; van Rijnsoever, F.J.; van Trijp, H.C. Heterogeneity in barriers regarding the motivation, the opportunity and the ability to choose low-calorie snack foods and beverages: Associations with real-life choices. *Public Health Nutr.* **2016**, *19*, 1584–1597. [CrossRef]
24. Lara, J.; McCrum, L.-A.; Mathers, J.C. Association of Mediterranean diet and other health behaviours with barriers to healthy eating and perceived health among British adults of retirement age. *Maturitas* **2014**, *79*, 292–298. [CrossRef]
25. Kearney, J.M.; McElhone, S. Perceived barriers in trying to eat healthier—Results of a pan-EU consumer attitudinal survey. *Br. J. Nutr.* **2007**, *81*, S133–S137. [CrossRef]
26. de Mestral, C.; Stringhini, S.; Marques-Vidal, P. Barriers to healthy eating in Switzerland: A nationwide study. *Clin. Nutr.* **2016**, *35*, 1490–1498. [CrossRef] [PubMed]
27. Orfanos, P.; Naska, A.; Rodrigues, S.; Lopes, C.; Freisling, H.; Rohrmann, S.; Sieri, S.; Elmadfa, I.; Lachat, C.; Gedrich, K.; et al. Eating at restaurants, at work or at home. Is there a difference? A study among adults of 11 European countries in the context of the HECTOR project. *Eur. J. Clin. Nutr.* **2017**, *71*, 407–419. [CrossRef]
28. Poínhos, R.; Franchini, B.; Afonso, C.; Correia, F.; Teixeira, V.H.; Moreira, P.; Durão, C.; Pinho, O.; Silva, D.; Lima Reis, J.P.; et al. Alimentação e estilos de vida da população portuguesa: Metodologia e resultados preliminares. *Alim. Hum.* **2009**, *15*, 43–60.
29. Poínhos, R.; Franchini, B.; Afonso, C.; Correia, F.; de Almeida, M.D.V. The SPCNA Directorate. Factors perceived by Portuguese adults as influent in food consumption (abstract). *Public Health Nutr.* **2010**, *13*, 270.
30. Faugier, J.; Lancaster, J.; Pickles, D.; Dobson, K. Barriers to healthy eating in the nursing profession: Part 1. *Nurs. Stand.* **2001**, *15*, 33–36. [PubMed]
31. Faugier, J.; Lancaster, J.; Pickles, D.; Dobson, K. Barriers to healthy eating in the nursing profession: Part 2. *Nurs. Stand.* **2001**, *15*, 33–35.
32. Sorensen, G.; Linnan, L.; Hunt, M. Worksite-based research and initiatives to increase fruit and vegetable consumption. *Prev. Med.* **2004**, *39*, S94–S100. [CrossRef]
33. Holdsworth, M.; Haslam, C. A review of point of choice nutrition labelling schemes in the workplace, public eating places and universities. *J. Hum. Nutr. Diet.* **1998**, *11*, 423–445. [CrossRef]
34. Devine, C.; Connors, M.; Sobal, J.; Bisogni, C. Sandwiching it in: Spillover of work onto food choices and family roles in low and moderate income urban households. *Soc. Sci. Med.* **2003**, *56*, 617–630. [CrossRef]
35. Devine, C.; Nelson, J.; Chin, N.; Dozier, A.; Fernandez, I. "Pizza is cheaper than salad": Assessing workers' views for an environmental food intervention. *Obesity* **2007**, *15*, 57S–68S. [CrossRef] [PubMed]
36. Wanjek, C. *Food at Work. Workplace Solutions for Malnutrition and Chronic Disease*; International Labour Office: Geneva, Switzerland, 2005.
37. Jabs, J.; Devine, C.M. Time scarcity and food choices: An overview. *Appetite* **2006**, *47*, 196–204. [CrossRef] [PubMed]
38. Steenhuis, I.; van Assema, P.; Reubsaet, A.; Kok, G. Process evaluation of two environmental nutrition programmes and an educational nutrition programme conducted at supermarkets and worksite cafeterias in the Netherlands. *J. Hum. Nutr. Diet.* **2004**, *17*, 107–115. [CrossRef]
39. Hilger, J.; Loerbroks, A.; Diehl, K. Eating behaviour of university students in Germany: Dietary intake, barriers to healthy eating and changes in eating behaviour since the time of matriculation. *Appetite* **2017**, *109*, 100–107. [CrossRef]
40. Munt, A.E.; Partridge, S.R.; Allman-Farinelli, M. The barriers and enablers of healthy eating among young adults: A missing piece of the obesity puzzle: A scoping review. *Obes Rev.* **2017**, *18*, 1–17. [CrossRef]
41. Universidade do Porto. *Recursos Humanos da U. Porto*; Reitoria da Universidade do Porto: Porto, Portugal, 2013.
42. Steptoe, A.; Pollard, T.M.; Wardle, J. Development of a Measure of the Motives Underlying the Selection of Food: The Food Choice Questionnaire. *Appetite* **1995**, *25*, 267–284. [CrossRef]
43. Cardoso, P.; Vale, S.P. Avaliação de critérios de escolha alimentar—Uma aplicação do Food Choice Questionnaire. *Rev. Fac. Ciênc. Saúde* **2010**, *7*, 62–72.
44. Pridgeon, A.; Whitehead, K. A qualitative study to investigate the drivers and barriers to healthy eating in two public sector workplaces. *J. Hum. Nutr. Diet.* **2013**, *26*, 85–95. [CrossRef]
45. Larson, N.; Story, M. A Review of Environmental Influences on Food Choices. *Ann. Behav. Med.* **2009**, *38*, S56–S73. [CrossRef]
46. Blanck, H.M.; Yaroch, A.L.; Atienza, A.A.; Yi, S.L.; Zhang, J.; Masse, L.C. Factors Influencing Lunchtime Food Choices among Working Americans. *Health Educ. Behav.* **2009**, *36*, 289–301. [CrossRef]
47. Prescott, J.; Young, O.; O'Neil, L.; Yau, N.J.N.; Stevens, R. Motives for food choice: A comparison of consumers from Japan, Taiwan, Malaysia and New Zealand. *Food Qual. Prefer.* **2002**, *13*, 489–495. [CrossRef]
48. Lima, J.P.M.; Costa, S.; Rocha, A. How do workers eat at the workplace? *Nutr. Food Sci.* **2018**, *48*, 194–205. [CrossRef]
49. Lima, J.P.M.; Costa, S.A.; Rocha, A. Nutritional intake of university employees'. *Br. Food J.* **2018**, *120*, 483–489. [CrossRef]
50. Navarro, M.; Más, M. Job stress and burnout syndrome at university: A descriptive analysis of the current situation and review of the principal lines of research. *Annu. Clin. Health Psychol.* **2010**, *6*, 67–72.
51. Blanck, H.; Yaroch, A.; Atienza, A.; Yi, S.; Zhang, J.; Masse, L. Factors influencing lunchtime food choices among working Americans. *Soc. Pub. Health Educ.* **2007**, *36*, 289–301. [CrossRef] [PubMed]
52. Yahia, N.; Wang, D.; Rapley, M.; Dey, R. Assessment of weight status, dietary habits and beliefs, physical activity, and nutritional knowledge among university students. *Perspect. Public Health* **2015**, *136*, 231–244. [CrossRef] [PubMed]

53. Bevan, A.; Hartwell, H.; Hemingway, A.; Proença, R. An exploration of the fruit and vegetable "foodscape" in a university setting for staff A preliminary study. *Br. Food J.* **2015**, *117*, 37–49. [CrossRef]
54. Mikkelsen, B. Images of foodscapes: Introduction to foodscapes studies and their application in the study of healthy eating out-of-home environments. *R. Soc. Public Health* **2011**, *131*, 209–216. [CrossRef]
55. Kjøllesdal, M.R.; Holmboe-Ottesen, G.; Wandel, M. Frequent use of staff canteens is associated with unhealthy dietary habits and obesity in a Norwegian adult population. *Public Health Nutr.* **2011**, *14*, 133–141. [CrossRef] [PubMed]
56. Baskin, E.; Gorlin, M.; Chance, Z.; Novemsky, N.; Dhar, R.; Huskey, K.; Hatzis, M. Proximity of snacks to beverages increases food consumption in the workplace: A field study. *Appetite* **2016**, *103*, 244–248. [CrossRef]
57. Freedman, M.R.; Rubinstein, R.J. Obesity and food choices among faculty and staff at a large urban university. *J. Am. Coll. Health* **2010**, *59*, 205–210. [CrossRef] [PubMed]
58. Payne, N.; Jones, F.; Harris, P.R. Employees' perceptions of the impact of work on health behaviours. *J. Health Psychol.* **2013**, *18*, 887–899. [CrossRef]
59. Lake, A.A.; Smith, S.A.; Bryant, C.E.; Alinia, S.; Brandt, K.; Seal, C.J.; Tetens, I. Exploring the dynamics of a free fruit at work intervention. *BMC Public Health* **2016**, *16*, 839. [CrossRef] [PubMed]
60. Thorsen, A.V.; Lassen, A.D.; Tetens, I.; Hels, O.; Mikkelsen, B.E. Long-term sustainability of a worksite canteen intervention of serving more fruit and vegetables. *Public Health Nutr.* **2010**, *13*, 1647–1652. [CrossRef] [PubMed]
61. The Determinants of Food Choice. European Food Information Council. 2005. Available online: https://www.eufic.org/en/healthy-living/article/the-determinants-of-food-choice (accessed on 6 June 2006).
62. Stankevitz, K.; Dement, J.; Schoenfisch, A.; Joyner, J.; Clancy, S.M.; Stroo, M.; Østbye, T. Perceived Barriers to Healthy Eating and Physical Activity among Participants in a Workplace Obesity Intervention. *J. Occup. Environ. Med.* **2017**, *59*, 746–751. [CrossRef] [PubMed]
63. Mackenbach, J.D.; Lakerveld, J.; Van Lenthe, F.J.; Teixeira, P.J.; Compernolle, S.; De Bourdeaudhuij, I.; Charreire, H.; Oppert, J.-M.; Bárdos, H.; Glonti, K.; et al. Interactions of individual perceived barriers and neighbourhood destinations with obesity-related behaviours in Europe. *Obes. Rev.* **2016**, *17*, 68–80. [CrossRef] [PubMed]

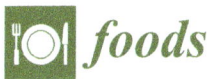

Article

Demographic, Anthropometric and Food Behavior Data towards Healthy Eating in Romania

Anca Bacârea [1], Vladimir Constantin Bacârea [2,*], Cristina Cînpeanu [3], Claudiu Teodorescu [3], Ana Gabriela Seni [3], Raquel P. F. Guiné [4] and Monica Tarcea [3]

1. Department of Pathophysiology, University of Medicine, Pharmacy, Science and Technology "George Emil Palade", 540139 Targu Mures, Romania; anca.bacarea@umfst.ro
2. Department of Scientific Research Methodology, University of Medicine, Pharmacy, Science and Technology "George Emil Palade", 540139 Targu Mures, Romania
3. Department of Community Nutrition and Food Safety, University of Medicine, Pharmacy, Science and Technology "George Emil Palade", 540139 Targu Mures, Romania; cristina.cinpeanu@outlook.com (C.C.); claudiu.teodorescu4@gmail.com (C.T.); gabrielaseni@gmail.com (A.G.S.); monica.tarcea@umfst.ro (M.T.)
4. CI&DETS/CERNAS Research Centres, Campus Politécnico, Polytechnic Institute of Viseu, 3500-606 Viseu, Portugal; raquelguine@esav.ipv.pt
* Correspondence: vladimir.bacarea@umfst.ro

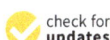

Citation: Bacârea, A.; Bacârea, V.C.; Cînpeanu, C.; Teodorescu, C.; Seni, A.G.; Guiné, R.P.F.; Tarcea, M. Demographic, Anthropometric and Food Behavior Data towards Healthy Eating in Romania. *Foods* **2021**, *10*, 487. https://doi.org/10.3390/foods10030487

Academic Editor: Mari Sandell

Received: 14 January 2021
Accepted: 19 February 2021
Published: 24 February 2021

Publisher's Note: MDPI stays neutral with regard to jurisdictional claims in published maps and institutional affiliations.

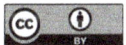

Copyright: © 2021 by the authors. Licensee MDPI, Basel, Switzerland. This article is an open access article distributed under the terms and conditions of the Creative Commons Attribution (CC BY) license (https://creativecommons.org/licenses/by/4.0/).

Abstract: Background: Each country has specific social, cultural, and economic characteristics regarding the motivations for improving health. The aim of this study was to evaluate demographic characteristics, anthropometric data, and elements related to food behavior and health, as well as Romanians' motivations towards healthy eating. Methods: This is a descriptive cross-sectional questionnaire based study enrolling 751 Romanian participants, which was carried out in in 2017–2018. Results: We obtained a positive correlation between age and Body Mass Index, and this was maintained also when we analyzed the two genders separately, being, however, even stronger for women. The number of hours/day spent watching TV or in front of the computer was positively correlated with both age and BMI. In general, with aging, there is an increasing concern regarding the practice of a healthy diet. The higher education level was significantly associated with healthier choices. Conclusions: The study of the three dietary dimensions, food properties, health attitudes, and dietary behavior, vis-à-vis various disorders revealed that the group most concerned of their diet was those who suffered from cardiovascular disorders.

Keywords: health; motivation; BMI; food behavior; education

1. Introduction

There have been various studies regarding the impact of social and cultural factors upon different communities' food behavior [1]. There is substantial evidence that social norms regarding food consumption strongly effect food choice, quality, and quantity consumed [2].

The globalization of agrifood systems has increased the availability and variety of foods through in food production and distribution changes. On one side, agricultural priorities rely on production and processing systems, markets, and livelihoods, with more concern for food safety and less care about general public health issues. Conversely, traditional public health focuses on agricultural issues that affect food security and the potential role of agriculture in preventing food-related diseases. We need to consider multidisciplinary aspects and the complex relationship between agribusiness, food consumption patterns, and health [3].

Adopting healthy diets can improve the nutritional behaviors and the status of population health. The guidelines released by the World Health Organization (WHO) establish a substantial reduction in the consumption of dairy products (by 28%), animal fats (by 30%), meat (13%), and sugar (by 24%) and a substantial increase in the consumption of cereals

Software, La Jolla, CA, the USA) and Epi Info version 7 (Centers for Disease Control and Prevention, Atlanta, GA, USA) and SPSS Statistics v.25 for statistical analyses. We used statistical methods to provide mean and SD for continuous variables or median and range for discrete variables, and absolute and relative frequency counts for categorical variables. The Student T-test and Mann–Whitney U test were used as appropriate statistical tests to compare continuous variables between the groups (normal or non-Gaussian distribution); for correlations, we used the Pearson or the Spearman test according to variables distribution. To establish a mean difference between several continuous variables, we used the ANOVA test for Gaussian distributions and the Kruskal–Wallis test for non-Gaussian distributions [29]. A p-value under 0.05 was considered statistically significant. The item analysis was performed using the Pearson correlation coefficients, and the associations were interpreted as not existing (r = 0), very weak (0.00 < r < 0.10), weak (0.10 $\leq$ r < 0.30), moderate (0.30 $\leq$ r < 0.50), strong (0.50 $\leq$ r < 0.70), very strong (0.70 $\leq$ r < 1), or perfect (r = 1), according to the value of r [6]. The internal consistency of the scales was evaluated by using Cronbach's alpha, according to Marôco [30], as follows: over 0.9: excellent, 0.8–0.9: very good, 0.7–0.8: good, 0.6–0.7: medium, 0.5–0.6: reasonable, below 0.5: bad.

3. Results

The characteristics of the studied population: socio-demographic data, environment, professional areas, physical activity, and medical history can be found in Table 1.

Table 1. Demographic, anthropometric data, and elements related to food behavior and health status of the studied population.

Parameter		N [1]	(%)
Age (years)		751	100%
	18–29	260	34.62%
	30–39	128	17.04%
	40–49	187	24.90%
	50–59	132	17.58%
	$\geq$60	44	5.86%
Gender			
	Female	511	68.04%
	Male	240	31.96%
Education			
	General school	3	0.40%
	High school	167	22.24%
	College	581	77.36%
Environment			
	Urban	623	82.96%
	Suburban	26	3.46%
	Rural	102	13.52%
Marital status			
	Single	211	28.10%
	Married/living together	480	63.91%
	Divorced/separated	50	6.66%
	Widow	10	1.33%
Employee status			
	Employed	542	72.17%
	Unemployed	31	4.13%
	Retired	29	3.86%
	Working student	149	19.84%

Table 1. Cont.

Parameter	N [1]	(%)
Professional area		
Nutrition	97	12.92%
Food	48	6.39%
Agriculture	13	1.73%
Sports	33	4.39%
Psychology	35	4.66%
Health-related activities	332	44.21%
Professional activity is not related to any of the above areas	269	35.82%
You are responsible for what you eat		
Yes	699	93.08%
No	52	6.92%
Physical activity		
Never	52	6.92%
Sporadic (<1 time/week)	253	33.69%
Occasionally (1 time/week)	229	30.49%
Moderate (2–3 times/week)	170	22.64
Intense (>3 times/week)	47	6.29%
How often do you think you are on a healthy/balanced diet?		
Never	55	7.32%
Rarely	118	15.71%
Sometimes	203	27.03%
Frequently	343	45.67%
Always	32	4.26%
Chronic diseases		
Cardiovascular disease	27	3.60%
Diabetes mellitus	25	3.33%
High cholesterol	47	6.26%
High blood pressure	47	6.26%
Gastric disorders	41	5.46%
Intestinal disorders	21	2.80%
Obesity	50	6.66%
Other chronic diseases	32	4.26%

[1] N = number of participants.

The BMI values were calculated for the whole sample and varied between 15.05 and 43.57 kg/m^2, being on average 24.59 ± 4.34 kg/m^2. In Table 2, we evaluated our subjects' BMI and age in relation to the studied parameters.

We obtained a positive correlation between age and BMI, and this was also maintained when we analyzed the two genders separately, this correlation being stronger in women. When analyzing the marital status, we obtained statistically significant differences between single vs. married ($p < 0.0001$) and between single vs. divorced ($p = 0.0382$), but not between single vs. widow ($p = 0.2386$). A continuation of this study to include a higher number of subjects in the widowed category is needed to confirm this result. This was also the case of agricultural worker as a subcategory of professional activity, for which we obtained significantly higher BMI, but the number of cases for this category was lower.

Regarding the number of hours/day spent r in front of the TV or computer, we obtained positive correlations for both age and BMI.

Table 2. The relationship among BMI, age, and studied parameters.

Parameter (N [1] = 751)	Age (years) Mean ± SD Min, Max	BMI [2] (kg/m²) Mean ± SD Min, Max	P Value [3]
Age (years)	38.02 ± 13.42 18, 80	24.60 ± 4.34 15.05, 43.57	
18–29	23.18 ± 3.27	22.58 ± 3.67 16.13, 34.47	$p < 0.0001$ [4] r [5] $= 0.3948$
30–39	34.38 ± 2.79	24.15 ± 3.93 15.05, 40.81	
40–49	44.28 ± 2.86	25.85 ± 4.38 17.82, 43.57	
50–59	52.78 ± 2.71	26.75 ± 4.38 19.19, 40.40	
≥ 60	65.38 ± 4.75	25.88 ± 3.60 18.36, 38.6	
Gender			
Female	36.60 ± 12.80 18, 80	23.97 ± 4.43 15.05, 43.57	$p < 0.0001$ [6] r [7] $= 0.4223$
Male	41.04 ± 14.21 18, 80	25.91 ± 3.85 16.48, 40.81	$p = 0.0061$ [6] r [7] $= 0.1765$
General school	22 ± 3.46 18, 24	19.24 ± 0.89 18.28, 20.07	NA [8]
High school	29.83 ± 12.71 18, 69	23.80 ± 3.90 17.14, 39.06	$t(746) = 2.792$ $p = 0.0054$ [9]
College	40.46 ± 12.65 21, 80	24.85 ± 4.44 15.05, 43.57	
Environment			
Urban	38.49 ± 12.94 18, 80	24.65 ± 4.34 15.05, 43.57	$H(3) = 3.503$ $p = 0.1735$ [10]
Suburban	38.61 ± 16.31 18, 77	25.36 ± 4.35 18.42, 35.15	
Rural	35.00 ± 15.16 18, 69	24.00 ± 4.34 17.00, 40.40	
Marital status			
Single	26.72 ± 9.79 18, 65	23.18 ± 4.05 15.05, 37.20	$H(4) = 39.360$ $p < 0.0001$ [10]
Married/living together	41.44 ± 12.01 18, 80	25.21 ± 4.39 16.13, 43.57	
Divorced/separated	48.86 ± 7.81 27, 69	24.57 ± 4.06 18.06, 39.97	
Widow	58.20 ± 6.76 42, 64	24.93 ± 2.31 22.32, 30.29	
Employee status			$F(2, 599) = 0.026$ $p = 0.9734$ [11]
Employed	41.39 ± 10.66 19, 77	25.19 ± 4.38 15.05, 43.57	
Unemployed	33.41 ± 10.11 21, 55	25.07 ± 4.62 16.40, 35.23	
Retired	64.20 ± 7.46 50, 80	25.28 ± 3.37 18.36, 35, 41	
Working student	21.61 ± 3.84 18, 47	22.19 ± 3.44 17.10, 33.56	

Table 2. *Cont.*

Parameter (N [1] = 751)	Age (years) Mean ± SD Min, Max	BMI [2] (kg/m²) Mean ± SD Min, Max	P Value [3]
Professional area			H(7) = 25.67 p = 0.0003 [10]
Nutrition	30.14 ± 11.36 19, 55	23.23 ± 3.72 17.09, 37.20	
Food	34.16 ± 13.44 19, 77	24.23 ± 5.15 17.04, 35.23	
Agriculture	37.77 ± 17.81 20, 77	28.62 ± 6.13 18.36, 39.06	
Sports	30.18 ± 9.93 18, 52	23.74 ± 2.67 18.33, 29.45	
Psychology	35.80 ± 14.27 19, 69	23.22 ± 3.91 17.10, 37.63	
Health-related activities	40.58 ± 12.68 18, 80	24.97 ± 4.14 17.00, 43.57	
Professional activity is not related to any of the above areas	38.23 ± 13.66 18, 74	24.61 ± 4.54 15.05, 40.81	
You are responsible for what you eat			U = 16,780 p = 0.3430 [12]
Yes	37.97 ± 13.36 18, 80	24.56 ± 4.36 15.05, 43.57	
No	38.63 ± 14.34 18, 66	25.01 ± 4.07 17.10, 35.23	
Physical activity			H(4) = 6.0958 p = 0.1921 [10]
Never	39.00 ± 11.33 21, 63	23.90 ± 4.69 16.40, 40.81	
Sporadic (<1 time/week)	40.57 ± 12.89 18, 69	25.10 ± 4.65 16.13, 43.57	
Occasionally (1 time/week)	36.35 ± 13.92 18, 80	24.57 ± 4.42 15.05, 39.06	
Moderate (2–3 times/week)	36.75 ± 13.50 18, 74	24.11 ± 3.79 17.00, 37.24	
Intense (>3 times/week)	35.93 ± 13.92 19, 80	24.39 ± 3.51 18.33, 32.43	
Hours/day spent watching TV or in front of the computer	4.81 ± 3.17 2, 20		p < 0.0001 [4] r^x [5] = 0.1540 p = 0.001 [4] r^y [5] = 0.1202
How often do you think you are on a healthy/balanced diet?			H(4) = 19.166 p = 0.0007 [10]
Never	37.47 ± 12.14 18, 58	25.03 ± 4.34 16.90, 40.40	
Rarely	37.91 ± 13.18 18, 77	25.77 ± 5.48 16.40, 43.57	
Sometimes	35.20 ± 12.18 18, 65	25.04 ± 4.36 17.04, 39.06	
Frequently	39.81 ± 13.85 18, 74	24.07 ± 3.79 16.13, 37.20	
Always	38.03 ± 16.58 19, 80	22.26 ± 3.46 15.05, 29.21	

Table 2. Cont.

Parameter (N [1] = 751)	Age (years) Mean ± SD Min, Max	BMI [2] (kg/m^2) Mean ± SD Min, Max	P Value [3]
Chronic disease			N.P. [12]
Cardiovascular disease	57.25 ± 12.15 32, 80	26.12 ± 4.53 18.36, 37.24	
Diabetes mellitus	45.40 ± 13.51 20, 64	28.54 ± 5.46 20.76, 40.40	
High cholesterol	51.72 ± 12.26 24, 77	27.17 ± 4.57 20.06, 37.63	
High blood pressure	48.82 ± 15.29 19, 80	28.52 ± 5.43 19.19, 43.57	
Gastric disorders	38.00 ± 13.68 19, 64	24.97 ± 5.02 15.05, 35.05	
Intestinal disorders	39.71 ± 13.65 19, 61	23.90 ± 3.97 16.48, 31.23	
Obesity	43.60 ± 12.91 19, 77	32.30 ± 4.17 29.74, 43.57	
Other chronic diseases	41.43 ± 11.31 19, 65	24.87 ± 4.24 15.05, 35.23	

[1] N = number of participants; [2] BMI = body mass index; [3] $p < 0.05$ is considered significant; [4] Spearman test; [5] Spearman correlation; [6] Pearson test; [7] r = Pearson correlation; [8] NA = not applicable; this group was excluded from the analysis due to low number of cases; [9] T-test; [10] Kruskal–Wallis test; [11] ANOVA test; [12] Mann–Whitney test; r^x = correlation between hours/day spent watching TV or in front of the computer and age; r^y = correlation between hours/day spent watching TV or in front of the computer and BMI; [12] N.P. = not performed, because it is not relevant for the current research to compare BMI according to different pathologies (obesity is included, and there are subjects with more than one of the conditions asked).

We obtained no significant associations among BMI, environment, current professional activity, responsibility for eating, and physical activity.

We displayed in Table 3 the results of participants' answers to questions regarding motivations towards healthy eating.

Table 3. Results of options regarding the motivations for health.

Question	1 n (%)	2 n (%)	3 n (%)	4 n (%)	5 n (%)
Q1	6 (0.80%)	20 (2.66%)	123 (16.38%)	300 (39.95%)	302 (40.21%)
Q2	28 (3.73%)	125 (16.64%)	274 (36.48%)	188 (25.03%)	136 (18.11%)
Q3	9 (1.20%)	49 (6.52%)	174 (23.17%)	333 (44.34%)	186 (24.77%)
Q4	8 (1.07%)	22 (2.93%)	160 (21.30%)	290 (38.62%)	271 (36.09%)
Q5	53 (7.06%)	125 (16.64%)	186 (24.77%)	257 (34.22%)	130 (17.31%)
Q6	16 (2.13%)	46 (6.13%)	181 (24.10%)	361 (48.07%)	147 (19.57%)
Q7	22 (2.93%)	147 (19.57%)	212 (28.23%)	251 (33.42%)	119 (15.85%)
Q8	6 (0.80%)	19 (2.53%)	100 (13.32%)	286 (38.08%)	340 (45.27%)
Q9	54 (7.19%)	188 (25.03%)	197 (26.23%)	259 (34.49%)	53 (7.06%)
Q10	45 (5.99%)	65 (8.66%)	188 (25.03%)	189 (25.17%)	264 (35.15%)

1—totally disagree, 2—disagree, 3—neither agree nor disagree, 4—agree, 5—totally agree.

Except for Q2, where the highest percentage was obtained for the item "neither agree nor disagree", for the other questions, the highest percentage was registered for items "agree" and "totally agree".

Table 4 shows item–item correlations for the group of questions investigating participants' attitudes toward food properties. The results indicate moderate correlations. The value of Cronbach alpha was 0.689, which is a medium value, based on which we accepted all three questions in composite scale for food properties.

Table 4. Item–item correlations for the composite scale investigating food properties [1].

Item	Q1	Q6	Q10
Q1	1.000		
Q6	0.434 **	1.000	
Q10	0.410 **	0.430 **	1.000

[1] Cronbach alpha = 0.689, ** Correlation is significant at the 0.01 level (2-tailed).

Table 5 shows item-item correlations for the group of questions investigating health attitudes and motivations. Because of the negative, very weak, and weak associations between the reversed Q5 and Q2, Q4, and Q7, between Q7 and Q4 and Q5R, and between the reversed Q9 and Q2, Q4, Q5R, Q7, and Q8, we considered eliminating Q5, Q7, and Q9. Q5 and Q9 are negative questions, and the answers were probably inconsistent due to the participants' lack of attention.

Table 5. Item–item correlations for the composite scale investigating health status and motivations [1].

Item	Q2	Q4	Q5R [2]	Q7	Q8	Q9R [3]
Q2	1.000					
Q4	0.357 **	1.000				
Q5R [2]	−0.251 **	−0.182 **	1.000			
Q7	−0.021	0.230 **	0.255 **	1.000		
Q8	0.341 **	0.656 **	−0.133 **	0.320 **	1.000	
Q9R [3]	0.150 **	0.108 **	0.259 **	0.040	0.144 **	1.000

[1] Cronbach alpha = 0.517; [2] Q5R = reversed Q5; [3] Q9R = reversed Q9, ** Correlation is significant at the 0.01 level (2-tailed).

When eliminating these three questions, the Cronbach alpha increased to 0.712, which was interpreted as a good value.

The associations between composite scale for food properties, refined scale for health attitudes, reported dietary behavior (Q3), and investigated variables (p values) are shown in Table 6.

With aging, there was an increasing concern for a healthy and balanced diet, but this was not reflected when analyzing food properties in relation to age, perhaps because of lack of knowledge, especially for Q10. However, there was a positive correlation between aging and the three studied dimensions (for food properties and aging $r = 0.1408$, $p = 0.0001$; for health attitudes and aging $r = 0.1643$, $p = 0.0001$; for dietary behavior and aging $r = 0.1490$, $p = 0.0001$). The age category of 18–29 was the most interested in food properties, although this was statistically not significant. The age category ≥ 60 was the most concerned age group about their health and a healthy and balanced diet compared to the other four age groups. The low number of subjects included in the age category ≥ 60 (N = 44) was a limitation of our study, and our results should be confirmed by including a larger population in the study. Women answered more with "agree" and "totally agree" to health attitudes and dietary behavior (Q3) questions than men. Regarding food properties, there was no difference between men and women.

We obtained significantly more "agree" and "totally agree" answers for item Q3 in the case of participants who came from urban environments. For composite scale investigating food properties and health attitudes, respondents from urban environments answered more with "agree" and "totally agree", even if this was statistically not significant.

College education level was significantly associated with health motivations for items investigating health attitudes (college education 52.84% vs. high school 39.52%) and dietary behavior (college education 48.02% vs. high school 31.14%). Even if this was statistically not significant, persons with a college education were more preoccupied with food properties than the persons belonging to the other educational groups.

There were no correlations between BMI, food properties, and attitudes toward health. For Q3, there was a weak negative correlation with BMI.

Table 6. Associations between food properties, health attitudes, and reported dietary behavior related to the investigated variables (p-value [1]).

Parameter	Food Properties	Health Attitudes	Dietary Behavior
Age [2]	$X^2(16, N = 751) = 26.03$ $p = 0.0535$	$X^2(16, N = 751) = 26.60$ $p = 0.0353$	$X^2(16, N = 751) = 28.57$ $p = 0.0270$
Gender [2]	$X^2(4, N = 751) = 2.8726$ $p = 0.5794$	$X^2(4, N = 751) = 11.07$ $p = 0.0258$	$X^2(4, N = 751) = 13.47$ $p = 0.0092$
Environment [2]	$X^2(8, N = 751) = 13.05$ $p = 0.1099$	$X^2(8, N = 751) = 13.08$ $p = 0.109$	$X^2(8, N = 751) = 15.53$ $p = 0.0496$
Education level [2]	$X^2(8, N = 751) = 4.42$ $p = 0.8174$	$X^2(8, N = 751) = 16.18$ $p = 0.0399$	$X^2(8, N = 751) = 33.89$ $p = 0.0000$
BMI [3]	$r = 0.0261$ $p = 0.4738$	$r = 0.0683$ $p = 0.0612$	$r = -0.0038$ $p = 0.292$
Physical activity [2]	$X^2(16, N = 751) = 43.27$ $p = 0.0003$	$X^2(16, N = 751) = 33.13$ $p = 0.0071$	$X^2(16, N = 751) = 52.06$ $p = 0.0000$
Hours/day watching TV/PC [3]	$r = -0.0337$ $p = 0.3551$	$r = 0.0901$ $p = 0.0134$	$r = 0.0230$ $p = 0.5291$
Cardiovascular disease [2]	$X^2(4, N = 751) = 4.14$ $p = 0.3869$	$X^2(4, N = 751) = 15.01$ $p = 0.0047$	$X2(4, N = 751) = 6.84$ $p = 0.1445$
Diabetes mellitus [2]	$X^2(4, N = 751) = 2.40$ $p = 0.6618$	$X^2(4, N = 751) = 2.55$ $p = 0.6345$	$X^2(4, N = 751) = 0.86$ $p = 0.9300$
High cholesterol [2]	$X^2(4, N = 751) = 0.67$ $p = 0.9546$	$X^2(4, N = 751) = 4.59$ $p = 0.3315$	$X^2(4, N = 751) = 1.37$ $p = 0.8488$
High blood pressure [2]	$X^2(4, N = 751) = 5.56$ $p = 0.2340$	$X^2(4, N = 751) = 3.86$ $p = 0.4240$	$X^2(4, N = 751) = 2.96$ $p = 0.5632$
Gastric disorders [2]	$X^2(4, N = 751) = 13.85$ $p = 0.0078$	$X^2(4, N = 751) = 11.85$ $p = 0.0185$	$X^2(4, N = 751) = 16.15$ $p = 0.0028$
Intestinal disorders [2]	$X^2(4, N = 751) = 9.95$ $p = 0.0411$	$X^2(4, N = 751) = 6.98$ $p = 0.1366$	$X^2(4, N = 751) = 8.01$ $p = 0.0911$
Obesity [2]	$X^2(4, N = 751) = 3.09$ $p = 0.5416$	$X^2(4, N = 751) = 4.45$ $p = 0.3485$	$X^2(4, N = 751) = 26.47$ $p = 0.0000$
Other [2]	$X^2(4, N = 751) = 3.86$ $p = 0.4240$	$X^2(4, N = 751) = 6.90$ $p = 0.4100$	$X^2(4, N = 751) = 10.85$ $p = 0.8863$

[1] $p < 0.05$ was considered significant; [2] Chi square test for n x m table; [3] Spearman test.

Most of the respondents practicing occasional and moderate physical activity answered agree or totally agree for all three investigated dimensions.

TV/computer hours were not correlated with food properties, healthy attitudes (very weak correlation $r = 0.0901$), or dietary behavior.

People with cardiovascular disorders were more often preoccupied with a healthy diet (92.59% of those who reported cardiovascular disorders answered "agree" and "totally agree" to the questions investigating health attitude). Although statistically not significant, people with cardiovascular disorders answered more often "agree" and "totally agree" for both composite scales: food properties and dietary behavior (Q3). Of those who reported cardiovascular diseases, 7.41% also reported hypercholesterolemia.

People reporting gastric disorders were preoccupied with all three studied dimensions, and those having intestinal disorders were especially concerned about food properties. This finding is not maintained for composite scales investigating health attitudes and dietary behavior, where the individuals without intestinal disorders are more concerned about healthier choices, although statistically not significant.

Persons who reported obesity show a lack of interest regarding all three investigated dimensions, which was significant for reported dietary behavior and not significant for food properties or heath attitudes. We did not interpret the category including other disorders because of the low number of subjects in this group.

We found a significant relationship ($p = 0.0000$) between reported dietary behavior and health attitudes: 224 subjects answered "agree" and 116 subjects answered "totally agree" for both composite scale investigating health attitudes and for Q3, investigating dietary behavior. Analyzing the different age groups, we obtained the following percentages, showing the concordance in responses "agree" and "totally agree" for these two dimensions: 36.53% for the age category 18–29 years old, 46.87% for the age category 30–39 years old, 50.80% for the age category 40–49 years old, 48.48% for the age category 50–59 years old, and 59.09% for the age category $\geq$60 years old. In other words, with aging, participants' answers are consistent with healthier choices.

4. Discussion

Modern lifestyle induces harmful behavior regarding eating and physical activity [31]. Altered behaviors are a growing problem in Romania, such as in other countries. Obesity is one important disease associated with unhealthy eating behaviors, and the fact that Romania is a middle-income country can contribute to the obesity epidemic spreading [32]. As our results indicated, obesity was the most frequent health problem reported by the participants in this study (6.66%). Since we have already shown a significant positive association between BMI and glycaemia in the age category older than 22 [33], we consider it appropriate to evaluate the BMI in relation to demographic, anthropometric data, and elements related to behavior and health. Similar to the results of Abdella et al. [34], age positively correlated to BMI. We also demonstrated a positive correlation among BMI, age and the number of hours spent in front of the TV or computer. In their study, Martínez-Moyá et al. [35] proved that the number of hours spent watching television and lower physical activity were significantly associated with a higher BMI in young adults [35]. Other studies showed that an increased screen time spent was significantly associated with the risk of obesity, but not the physical activity level [36], and watching television is the leading sedentary activity in association with obesity [37]. This relation was also found in children; according to Golshevsky et al. [38], higher BMI was associated with more hours spent watching television, and less time spent in organized sports activities. The increased number of hours spent in front of the TV with aging can be related to life cycle changes. When we separately analyzed the relationships between the two genders, the correlation was stronger for women, possibly because of the hormonal changes related to aging. When comparing the BMI between the two genders, women had lower mean BMI values than men (23.97 vs. 25.91), possibly because women's mean age was lower than men's (36.6 vs. 41.04).

Many studies emphasized the role of education in BMI control [39,40]. However, we obtained higher BMI values for the group with college education compared to the group with high school. Some explanations for this finding could be easy access to college education and the lack of physical activity. On the other hand, the group with a college education has the highest mean age, so the BMI can be attributed to aging. Strategies to improve knowledge about healthy eating must be developed to have a better weight control and focus on different age categories.

There was no correlation between the environment and BMI, and this is quite normal considering the people's migration and easy access to information regardless of the native environment.

The marital status also influenced the BMI, married persons having higher BMI values compared to single persons. This is in concordance with the results of other studies [41,42]. It is unclear how marital status affects BMI, probably by changing the body weight-related perceptions and eating behaviors [42]. Some studies indicated that increased BMI affects the status of the employee because of health problems or because it decreases the chances to be employed [43,44]. We did not find BMI differences between employed and unemployed participants, probably because in Romania many young adults prefer not to work because of low income, and they benefit from social assistance (33.41 vs. 41.39 years).

Normally, professional activity is associated with different knowledge regarding health and with different physical activity level. The highest mean BMI value was obtained for those working in agriculture, but the result is debatable due to the small number of subjects in this group.

Even if we did not find a statistical difference for BMI between the different categories of physical activity, we must notice that the mean age of subjects performing intense and moderate physical activity is lower than in those with no or sporadic physical activity. This is a good aspect, showing the concern of younger adults for their health. Many studies showed the benefits of physical activity upon health, associated with a decreased risk of cardiovascular events [45] and better control of blood glucose level [46]. Carraça et al. [47], in their recent study, identified a behavioral pattern showing that adults who are not interested in physical activity are women, have a higher BMI, have been less educated, and are unemployed. Their eating habits are more likely to be less healthy, and they perceive more barriers when it comes to physical activity [47]. Another study shows that barriers to healthy eating and/or physical activity significantly influenced BMI, the level of physical activity, stress, and fruit and vegetable intake [48].

Consumers' beliefs and knowledge about healthy foods are variable. A food is considered healthy in general if it is low in total fats and saturated fats, and meets certain requirements regarding cholesterol and certain vitamins or minerals content [2,49,50]. In his study, Lusk identifies four categories on how healthy food should be defined: based on food nutrients, the entire composition of the food, nutrients from the whole diet, and based on holistic consumption patterns, and the respondents were almost equally distributed among these categories [28].

The fact that a person has adequate knowledge and answers the questions accordingly, does not always mean that this knowledge is applied in everyday life. In a study, the participants showed adequate nutrition knowledge, but eating behavior was strongly influenced by social and physical environmental factors [51]. Mete et al. [52] underline the role of social media in improving healthy food choices by promoting healthy eating information.

This is the motivation for our analysis of the questions in three dimensions—food properties, health attitudes, and separately the general question for dietary behavior (Q3). Looking at food properties (hygiene, additives, and genetically modified organisms) in relationship with the studied parameters, we can see that more physically active people and those having gastric and intestinal disorders were more preoccupied with these parameters. The associations were also statistically significant between physical activity, health attitudes, and dietary behavior (Q3), indicating that these people were concerned and motivated to maintain their health. Genetically modified food is a controversial subject and involves important knowledge [53]. People with gastric and intestinal disorders relate food properties to their disease. We assume that this is why they were more preoccupied with healthy diets compared with other people suffering from other pathologies.

With aging, people were more preoccupied with making healthier choices (significant associations between age and refined composite scales regarding health attitudes and Q3), probably because of changes related to aging and occurring pathologies. This is similar to the results of Whitelock et al. [54], where the participants described efforts focusing on avoiding foods high in fats and sugar content. More women than men had perceptions compliant with a healthy diet, possibly because they have better nutritional knowledge and interest for it [27,55,56].

We obtained significantly more answers compliant with a healthy and balanced diet in general for urban areas. However, this difference was not maintained concerning food properties and health attitudes. This can be due to an increased general interest in a healthy diet that is not translated into specific choices. Education level is essential in connection with BMI and various metabolic diseases [40,57]. As expected, we obtained more correct answers in the college group regarding healthy diet and fat, vitamins, and minerals content, but these answers were not reflected in the case of a lower BMI.

In one study about the perception of healthy eating in Romania, it was shown that tradition is very much related to eating behavior, and was correlated with BMI [31]. Lotrean et al. [58] performed a study among Romanian students and revealed three main dietary structures: two of them protective against becoming overweight, but different regarding physical activity, and the third one (fast food diet) associated with higher BMI and lack of daily physical activity [58]. We believe that people have somewhat imbalanced attitudes about food and healthy eating, which could significantly affect the transposition of beliefs, knowledge about healthy eating, and attitudes into behavior. The study subjects having different disorders showed lack of interest regarding healthy eating choices, which can be a contributing key factor to the evolution of their diseases.

According to Nagata et al., after a seven-year follow-up of young adults with overweight/obesity and unhealthy weight control behaviors at baseline, they still had higher BMI than those without unhealthy weight control behaviors [59].

We found a significant association between health attitudes and cardiovascular disorders, which is logical. People with cardiovascular diseases are more preoccupied to have a particularly low-fat diet.

Traditionally, recommendations were made for individual nutrients consumption such as saturated fats, sugar, sodium, and cholesterol in the diet, because they are usually over-consumed by many people and are linked to the development of chronic diseases. These can also lead to erroneous effects [60–62]. One controversial topic was the association between saturated fats and cardiovascular diseases without considering substitute nutrients and cholesterol, and another one is the association between cholesterol and cardiovascular diseases, which is confused with the intake of saturated fats [63]. The contemporary dietary guide recommends healthy dietary models, with an emphasis on food-based recommendations. The diet as a whole, meaning the combinations and the amounts of food (nutrients) we eat daily, is an essential determinant of health [63].

Our study has some limitations because of gender differences (more women than men) and low number of participants in some categories (e.g., agriculture as a field of activity, age group ≥ 60 years old). Additionally, the participants were not from all counties of the country, so the study is not 100% country representative. We calculated the BMI based on the self-reported values for weight and height, so some bias occurred.

We showed that with aging, people were more preoccupied with making healthier choices. However, it is not only the occurrence of various diseases that should make people aware of healthier choices. Hence, there is a need for an intensive national strategy for health motivations. According to age groups, this strategy should be addressed differently, knowing that radical changes in lifestyle are difficult to accept with age. Another important aspect is the translation of information about healthy choices into real choices. According to our findings, obesity was the most frequent health problem reported by the participants in this study, and despite our expectations, we obtained higher BMI values for the college education group, although they chose the correct answers for their health when asked. This indicates the need for a long-term strategy to motivate people to make healthy eating choices, starting with children and involving also their families [58].

5. Conclusions

We obtained a positive correlation between demographic parameters and the BMI in the Romanian population; also their healthy food behaviors were stronger for women. The number of hours/day spent watching TV or in front of the computer was positively correlated with age and BMI. The higher education level was significantly associated with healthier choices regarding nutrition practices and motivations. Regarding the associations between the sociodemographic characteristics and different disorders, we observed that the subjects with cardiovascular disorders were more preoccupied with healthier diets in most cases.

Nutritionists, specialists in medicine, and food stakeholders should promote healthy diets through adequate sources of information aimed at target groups. They should develop a more efficient strategy to motivate people to make healthy eating choices and improve Romanian food behavior.

Author Contributions: Conceptualization: A.B. and R.P.F.G.; methodology: A.B. and V.C.B.; software: V.C.B.; validation: A.B., V.C.B., and R.P.F.G.; formal analysis: A.B. and V.C.B.; investigation: A.B., V.C.B., M.T., C.C., C.T., A.G.S., and R.P.F.G.; resources: R.P.F.G.; data curation: A.B. and V.C.B.; writing—original draft preparation: A.B.; writing—review and editing: A.B., V.C.B., M.T., and R.P.F.G.; visualization: A.B. supervision: A.B. and R.P.F.G.; project administration: R.P.F.G.; funding acquisition: R.P.F.G. All authors have read and agreed to the published version of the manuscript.

Funding: This research was funded by the Research Center CI&DETS (Polytechnic Institute of Viseu, Portugal) with grant n.º PROJ/CI&DETS/CGD/0012. The APC was funded by FCT-Foundation for Science and Technology (Portugal), scholarship number UIDB/00681/2020.

Institutional Review Board Statement: Not applicable.

Informed Consent Statement: Informed consent was obtained from all subjects involved in the study.

Data Availability Statement: Data are available from the corresponding author upon reasonable request.

Acknowledgments: This work was prepared in the ambit of the multinational project EATMOT from CI&DETS Research Centre (IPV—Viseu, Portugal) with reference PROJ/CI&DETS/CGD/0012. This work is supported by Portuguese National Funds through the FCT—Foundation for Science and Technology, I.P., within the scope of the project Refª UIDB/00681/2020. Furthermore, we would like to thank the CERNAS Research Centre and the Polytechnic Institute of Viseu for their support.

Conflicts of Interest: The authors declare no conflict of interest.

References

1. Pelletier, J.E.; Graham, D.J.; Laska, M.N. Social Norms and Dietary Behaviors among Young Adults. *Am. J. Heal. Behav.* **2014**, *38*, 144–152. [CrossRef] [PubMed]
2. Higgs, S. Social norms and their influence on eating behaviors. *Appetite* **2015**, *86*, 38–44. [CrossRef]
3. Lock, K.; Smith, R.D.; Dangour, A.D.; Keogh-Brown, M.; Pigatto, G.; Hawkes, C.; Fisberg, R.M.; Chalabi, Z. Health, agricultural, and economic effects of adoption of healthy diet recommendations. *Lancet* **2010**, *376*, 1699–1709. [CrossRef]
4. Conklin, A.I.; Forouhi, N.G.; Surtees, P.; Khaw, K.-T.; Wareham, N.J.; Monsivais, P. Social relationships and healthful dietary behavior: Evidence from over-50s in the EPIC cohort, UK. *Soc. Sci. Med.* **2014**, *100*, 167–175. [CrossRef]
5. Cornelsen, L.; Green, R.; Turner, R.; Dangour, A.D.; Shankar, B.; Mazzocchi, M.; Smith, R.D. What Happens to Patterns of Food Consumption when Food Prices Change? Evidence from A Systematic Review and Meta-Analysis of Food Price Elasticities Globally. *Heal. Econ.* **2014**, *24*, 1548–1559. [CrossRef] [PubMed]
6. Ferrão, A.C.; Guiné, R.P.; Correia, P.; Ferreira, M.; Duarte, J.; Lima, J. Development of a Questionnaire to Assess People's Food Choices Determinants. *Curr. Nutr. Food Sci.* **2019**, *15*, 281–295. [CrossRef]
7. Guiné, R.P.F.; Ferrão, A.C.; Correia, P.; Cardoso, A.P.; Ferreira, M.; Duarte, J. Influence of emotional determinants on the food choices of the portuguese. *EUREKA Soc. Humanit.* **2019**, *5*, 31–44. [CrossRef]
8. Liang, A.R.-D.; Lim, W.M. Exploring the online buying behavior of specialty food shoppers. *Int. J. Hosp. Manag.* **2011**, *30*, 855–865. [CrossRef]
9. Mayén, A.-L.; De Mestral, C.; Zamora, G.; Paccaud, F.; Marques-Vidal, P.; Bovet, P.; Stringhini, S. Interventions promoting healthy eating as a tool for reducing social inequalities in diet in low- and middle-income countries: A systematic review. *Int. J. Equity Heal.* **2016**, *15*, 205. [CrossRef] [PubMed]
10. Simmons, A.L.; Schlezinger, J.J.; Corkey, B.E. What Are We Putting in Our Food That Is Making Us Fat? Food Additives, Contaminants, and Other Putative Contributors to Obesity. *Curr. Obes. Rep.* **2014**, *3*, 273–285. [CrossRef] [PubMed]
11. Montagnese, C.; Santarpia, L.; Buonifacio, M.; Nardelli, A.; Caldara, A.R.; Silvestri, E.; Contaldo, F.; Pasanisi, F. European food-based dietary guidelines: A comparison and update. *Nutrition* **2015**, *31*, 908–915. [CrossRef] [PubMed]
12. Vandevijvere, S.; MacKenzie, T.; Ni Mhurchu, C. Indicators of the relative availability of healthy versus unhealthy foods in supermarkets: A validation study. *Int. J. Behav. Nutr. Phys. Act.* **2017**, *14*, 53. [CrossRef]
13. Temple, N.J. Front-of-package food labels: A narrative review. *Appetite* **2020**, *144*, 104485. [CrossRef] [PubMed]
14. Bialkova, S.; Sasse, L.; Fenko, A. The role of nutrition labels and advertising claims in altering consumers' evaluation and choice. *Appetite* **2016**, *96*, 38–46. [CrossRef]
15. Steinhauser, J.; Janssen, M.; Hamm, U. Who Buys Products with Nutrition and Health Claims? A Purchase Simulation with Eye Tracking on the Influence of Consumers' Nutrition Knowledge and Health Motivation. *Nutrients* **2019**, *11*, 2199. [CrossRef]
16. Waterlander, W.E.; Steenhuis, I.H.; de Boer, M.R.; Schuit, A.J.; Seidell, J.C. Effects of different discount levels on healthy products coupled with a healthy choice label, special offer label or both: Results from a web-based supermarket experiment. *Int. J. Behav. Nutr. Phys. Act.* **2013**, *10*, 59. [CrossRef] [PubMed]

17. Cecchini, M.; Warin, L. Impact of food labelling systems on food choices and eating behaviors: A systematic review and meta-analysis of randomized studies. *Obes. Rev.* **2016**, *17*, 201–210. [CrossRef] [PubMed]
18. Hammer, B.A.; Vallianatos, H.; Nykiforuk, C.I.J.; Nieuwendyk, L.M. Perceptions of healthy eating in four Alberta communities: A photovoice project. *Agric. Hum. Values* **2015**, *32*, 649–662. [CrossRef]
19. Harris, J.L.; Bargh, J.A. The relationship between television viewing and unhealthy eating: Implications for children and media interventions. *Health Commun.* **2009**, *24*, 660–673. [CrossRef] [PubMed]
20. Elliston, K.G.; Ferguson, S.G.; Schüz, N.; Schüz, B. Situational cues and momentary food environment predict everyday eating behavior in adults with overweight and obesity. *Heal. Psychol.* **2017**, *36*, 337–345. [CrossRef]
21. Alesin, K.C.; Franklin, B.A.; Miller, W.M.; Peterson, E.D.; McCullough, P.A. Impact of obesity on cardiovascular disease. *Endocrinol. Metab. Clin. N. Am.* **2008**, *37*, 663–684. [CrossRef]
22. American Diabetes Association Addendum. 8. Obesity Management for the Treatment of Type 2 Diabetes: Standards of Medical Care in Diabetes-2020. *Diabetes Care* **2020**, *42* (Suppl. 1), 81–89. [CrossRef]
23. Meurling, I.J.; Shea, D.O.; Garvey, J.F. Obesity and sleep: A growing concern. *Curr. Opin. Pulm. Med.* **2019**, *25*, 602–608. [CrossRef] [PubMed]
24. Lopresti, A.L.; Drummond, P.D. Obesity and psychiatric disorders: Commonalities in dysregulated biological pathways and their implications for treatment. *Prog. Neuro-Psychopharmacol. Biol. Psychiatry* **2013**, *45*, 92–99. [CrossRef] [PubMed]
25. Avgerinos, K.I.; Spyrou, N.; Mantzoros, C.S.; Dalamaga, M. Obesity and cancer risk: Emerging biological mechanisms and perspectives. *Metabolism* **2019**, *92*, 121–135. [CrossRef] [PubMed]
26. Bacârea, A.; Bacârea, V.C.; Tarcea, M. The relation between prepregnancy maternal body mass index and total gestational weight gain with the characteristics of the newborns. *J. Matern. Neonatal Med.* **2020**, 1–6. [CrossRef]
27. Ferrão, A.C.; Correia, P.; Ferreira, M.; Guiné, R.P.F. Perceptions towards healthy diet of the Portuguese according to area of work or studies. *Slov. J. Public Heal.* **2019**, *58*, 40–46. [CrossRef] [PubMed]
28. Lusk, J.L. Consumer beliefs about healthy foods and diets. *PLoS ONE* **2019**, *14*, e0223098. [CrossRef]
29. Marusteri, M.; Bacârea, V. Comparing groups for statistical differences: How to choose the right statistical test? *Biochem. Medica* **2010**, *20*, 15–32. [CrossRef]
30. Marôco, J. *Análise Estatística com o SPSS Statistics*, 7th ed.; Report Number: Lisbon, Portugal, 2018.
31. Cînpeanu, O.-C.; Tarcea, M.; Cojan, P.; Iorga, D.; Olah, P.; Guiné, R.P. Perception of Healthy Eating among Romanian Adults. *J. Interdiscip. Med.* **2019**, *4*, 77–86. [CrossRef]
32. Cecchini, M.; Sassi, F.; Lauer, J.A.; Lee, Y.Y.; Guajardo-Barron, V.; Chisholm, D. Tackling of unhealthy diets, physical inactivity, and obesity: Health effects and cost-effectiveness. *Lancet* **2010**, *376*, 1775–1784. [CrossRef]
33. Bacârea, A.; Tarcea, M.; Boțianu, P.V.H.; Ruță, F.; Bacârea, V. Age cut-off for type 2 diabetes mellitus screening amongst young adults from Mures District, Romania—A pilot study. *Obes. Res. Clin. Pr.* **2015**, *9*, 527–530. [CrossRef] [PubMed]
34. Abdella, H.M.; El Farssi, H.O.; Broom, D.R.; Hadden, D.A.; Dalton, C.F. Eating Behaviors and Food Cravings; Influence of Age, Sex, BMI and FTO Genotype. *Nutrition* **2019**, *11*, 377. [CrossRef]
35. Martínez-Moyá, M.; Navarrete-Muñoz, E.M.; García de la Hera, M.; Giménez-Monzo, D.; González-Palacios, S.; Valera-Gran, D.; Sempere-Orts, M.; Vioque, J. Asociación entre horas de televisión, actividad física, horas de sueño y exceso de peso en población adulta joven [Association between hours of television watched, physical activity, sleep and excess weight among young adults]. *Gac Sanit.* **2014**, *28*, 203–208. [CrossRef] [PubMed]
36. Shin, J. Joint Association of Screen Time and Physical Activity with Obesity: Findings from the Korea Media Panel Study. *Osong Public Heal. Res. Perspect.* **2018**, *9*, 207–212. [CrossRef]
37. Patel, V.C.; Spaeth, A.M.; Basner, M. Relationships between time use and obesity in a representative sample of Americans. *Obesity* **2016**, *24*, 2164–2175. [CrossRef]
38. Golshevsky, D.M.; Magnussen, C.; Juonala, M.; Kao, K.-T.; Harcourt, B.E.; Sabin, M.A. Time spent watching television impacts on body mass index in youth with obesity, but only in those with shortest sleep duration. *J. Paediatr. Child. Heal.* **2019**, *56*, 721–726. [CrossRef]
39. Sánchez, C.N.; Maddalena, N.; Penalba, M.; Quarleri, M.; Torres, V.; Wachs, A. Relación entre nivel de instrucción y exceso de peso en pacientes de consulta externa. Estudio transversal [Relationship between level of education and overweight in outpatients. A transversal study]. *Medicina [B Aires]* **2017**, *77*, 291–296. [PubMed]
40. Boing, A.F.; Subramanian, S.V. The influence of area-level education on body mass index, waist circumference and obesity according to gender. *Int. J. Public Heal.* **2015**, *60*, 727–736. [CrossRef] [PubMed]
41. Liao, C.; Gao, W.; Cao, W.; Lv, J.; Yu, C.; Wang, S.; Li, C.; Pang, Z.; Cong, L.; Dong, Z.; et al. Association of Educational Level and Marital Status With Obesity: A Study of Chinese Twins. *Twin Res. Hum. Genet.* **2018**, *21*, 126–135. [CrossRef]
42. Klos, L.A.; Sobal, J. Marital status and body weight, weight perception, and weight management among U.S. adults. *Eat. Behav.* **2013**, *14*, 500–507. [CrossRef]
43. Kinge, J.M. Body mass index and employment status: A new look. *Econ. Hum. Biol.* **2016**, *22*, 117–125. [CrossRef]
44. Feigl, A.B.; Goryakin, Y.; Devaux, M.; Lerouge, A.; Vuik, S.; Cecchini, M. The short-term effect of BMI, alcohol use, and related chronic conditions on labour market outcomes: A time-lag panel analysis utilizing European SHARE dataset. *PLoS ONE* **2019**, *14*, e0211940. [CrossRef] [PubMed]

45. Chughtai, M.; Gwam, C.U.; Mohamed, N.; Khlopas, A.; Sodhi, N.; Sultan, A.A.; Bhave, A.; Mont, M.A. Impact of Physical Activity and Body Mass Index in Cardiovascular and Musculoskeletal Health: A Review. *Surg. Technol. Int.* **2017**, *31*, 213–220. [PubMed]
46. Mainous, A.G., 3rd; Tanner, R.J.; Anton, S.D.; Jo, A.; Luetke, M.C. Physical Activity and Abnormal Blood Glucose Among Healthy Weight Adults. *Am. J. Prev. Med.* **2017**, *53*, 42–47. [CrossRef] [PubMed]
47. Carraça, E.V.; MacKenbach, J.D.; Lakerveld, J.; Rutter, H.; Oppert, J.-M.; De Bourdeaudhuij, I.; Compernolle, S.; Roda, C.; Bárdos, H.; Teixeira, P.J. Lack of interest in physical activity—Individual and environmental attributes in adults across Europe: The SPOTLIGHT project. *Prev. Med.* **2018**, *111*, 41–48. [CrossRef] [PubMed]
48. Ashton, L.M.; Hutchesson, M.J.; Rollo, M.E.; Morgan, P.J.; Collins, C.E. Motivators and Barriers to Engaging in Healthy Eating and Physical Activity. *Am. J. Mens. Health* **2017**, *11*, 330–343. [CrossRef] [PubMed]
49. Food and Drug Administration. "Part 101 –Food Labeling, Subpart D—Specific Requirements for Nutrient Content Claims." Code of Federal Regulation. Title 21, Volume 2, Chapter 1, Subchapter B, Part 101, Subpart, D. 21CFR101.65. 1 April 2018. Available online: https://www.accessdata.fda.gov/scripts/cdrh/cfdocs/cfcfr/cfrsearch.cfm?fr=101.65 (accessed on 5 February 2021).
50. Shepherd, R. Resistance to Changes in Diet. In *Proceedings of the Nutrition Society*; CABI Publishing: Wallingford, UK, 2002; Volume 61, pp. 267–272.
51. van der Velde, L.A.; Schuilenburg, L.A.; Thrivikraman, J.K.; Numans, M.E.; Kiefte-de Jong, J.C. Needs and perceptions regarding healthy eating among people at risk of food insecurity: A qualitative analysis. *Int. J. Equity Health* **2019**, *18*, 184. [CrossRef] [PubMed]
52. Mete, R.; Shield, A.; Murray, K.; Bacon, R.; Kellett, J. What is healthy eating? A qualitative exploration. *Public Heal. Nutr.* **2019**, *22*, 2408–2418. [CrossRef]
53. Wunderlich, S.M.; Gatto, K.A. Consumer Perception of Genetically Modified Organisms and Sources of Information. *Adv. Nutr.* **2015**, *6*, 842–851. [CrossRef] [PubMed]
54. Whitelock, E.; Ensaff, H. On Your Own: Older Adults' Food Choice and Dietary Habits. *Nutrition* **2018**, *10*, 413. [CrossRef]
55. Ahmadi, A.; Torkamani, P.; Sohrabi, Z.; Ghahremani, F. Nutrition knowledge: Application and perception of food labels among women. *Pak. J. Biol. Sci.* **2013**, *16*, 2026–2030. [CrossRef] [PubMed]
56. Putnoky, S.; Banu, A.M.; Moleriu, L.C.; Putnoky, S.; Șerban, D.M.; Niculescu, M.D.; Șerban, C.L. Reliability and validity of a General Nutrition Knowledge Questionnaire for adults in a Romanian population. *Eur. J. Clin. Nutr.* **2020**, *74*, 1576–1584. [CrossRef] [PubMed]
57. Blomster, J.; Zoungas, S.; Woodward, M.; Neal, B.; Harrap, S.; Poulter, N.; Marre, M.; Williams, B.; Chalmers, J.; Hillis, G. The impact of level of education on vascular events and mortality in patients with type 2 diabetes mellitus: Results from the ADVANCE study. *Diabetes Res. Clin. Pr.* **2017**, *127*, 212–217. [CrossRef] [PubMed]
58. Lotrean, L.M.; Stan, O.; Codruta, L.; Laza, V. Dietary patterns, physical activity, body mass index, weight-related behaviors and their interrelationship among Romanian university students-trends from 2003 to 2016. *Nutr. Hosp.* **2018**, *35*, 375–383.
59. Nagata, J.M.; Garber, A.K.; Tabler, J.; Murray, S.B.; Vittinghoff, E.; Bibbins-Domingo, K. Disordered eating behaviors and cardiometabolic risk among young adults with overweight or obesity. *Int. J. Eat. Disord.* **2018**, *51*, 931–941. [CrossRef]
60. Liu, A.G.; Ford, N.A.; Hu, F.B.; Zelman, K.M.; Mozaffarian, D.; Kris-Etherton, P.M. A healthy approach to dietary fats: Understanding the science and taking action to reduce consumer confusion. *Nutr. J.* **2017**, *16*, 1–15. [CrossRef]
61. Azairs-Braesco, V.; Sluik, D.; Maillot, M.; Kok, F.; Moreno, L.A. A review of total & added sugar intakes and dietary sources in Europe. *Nutr. J.* **2017**, *16*, 6.
62. Ha, S.K. Dietary Salt Intake and Hypertension. *Electrolytes Blood Press.* **2014**, *12*, 7–18. [CrossRef]
63. Bowen, K.J.; Sullivan, V.K.; Kris-Etherton, P.M.; Petersen, K.S. Nutrition and Cardiovascular Disease—an Update. *Curr. Atheroscler. Rep.* **2018**, *20*, 8. [CrossRef]

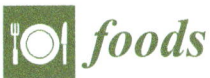

Article

Food Choice Determinants and Perceptions of a Healthy Diet among Italian Consumers

Rungsaran Wongprawmas [1], Cristina Mora [1,*], Nicoletta Pellegrini [2], Raquel P. F. Guiné [3], Eleonora Carini [1], Giovanni Sogari [1] and Elena Vittadini [4]

1. Department of Food and Drug, University of Parma, Parco Area delle Scienze 47/A, 43124 Parma, Italy; rungsaran.wongprawmas@unipr.it (R.W.); eleonora.carini@unipr.it (E.C.); giovanni.sogari@unipr.it (G.S.)
2. Department of Agricultural, Food, Environmental and Animal Sciences, University of Udine, via Sondrio 2/A, 33100 Udine, Italy; Nicoletta.pellegrini@uniud.it
3. CERNAS Research Centre, Polytechnic Institute of Viseu, 3504-510 Viseu, Portugal; raquelguine@esav.ipv.pt
4. School of Biosciences and Veterinary Medicine, University of Camerino, Via Gentile III da Varano, 62032 Camerino, Italy; elenagiovanna.vittadini@unicam.it
* Correspondence: cristina.mora@unipr.it

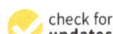

Citation: Wongprawmas, R.; Mora, C.; Pellegrini, N.; Guiné, R.P.F.; Carini, E.; Sogari, G.; Vittadini, E. Food Choice Determinants and Perceptions of a Healthy Diet among Italian Consumers. *Foods* **2021**, *10*, 318. https://doi.org/10.3390/foods10020318

Academic Editor: Koushik Adhikari
Received: 30 December 2020
Accepted: 30 January 2021
Published: 3 February 2021

Publisher's Note: MDPI stays neutral with regard to jurisdictional claims in published maps and institutional affiliations.

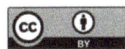

Copyright: © 2021 by the authors. Licensee MDPI, Basel, Switzerland. This article is an open access article distributed under the terms and conditions of the Creative Commons Attribution (CC BY) license (https://creativecommons.org/licenses/by/4.0/).

Abstract: Healthy food choices are crucial for a healthy lifestyle. However, food choices are complex and affected by various factors. Understanding the determinant factors affecting food choices could aid policy-makers in designing better strategies to promote healthy food choices in the general public. This study aims to evaluate the food choice motivations and to segment consumer groups, according to their food choice motivations, in a sample of 531 Italian consumers (collected by convenience sampling), through offline and online survey platforms. K-means cluster analysis was applied to identify consumer groups using six food choice motivation categories (health, emotional, economic and availability, social and cultural, environmental and political, and marketing and commercial). The results suggest that the strongest determinants for the food choices of Italian consumers are Environmental factors and Health. Two consumer profiles were identified through the segmentation analysis: Emotional eating and Health-driven consumers. The respondents were found to have a good awareness of what comprises a healthy diet. There is a potential market for healthy and sustainable food products, especially products with minimal or environmentally friendly packages. Food labels and information strategies could be promoted as tools to assist consumers to make healthy food choices.

Keywords: food choices; eating determinants; healthy diet; emotions

1. Introduction

The food that we consume affects our future health. Diet-related non-communicable diseases (NCDs), such as obesity, type 2 diabetes, cardiovascular disease, hypertension, stroke, and some types of cancer, have been increasingly causing health problems in both developing and developed countries [1,2]. Policy-makers have been trying to introduce several different tools to encourage populations to consume healthier foods and reduce their intake of unhealthy foods, through initiatives such as nutritional education programs and fiscal programs (i.e., sugar drink taxes), among others. Despite these attempts, obesity has greatly risen in the past two decades, even in countries where the rates have been historically low, such as Italy [3].

In Italy, obesity among adults increased from 9% in 2003 to 11% in 2017. Although obesity in adult remained below than the EU average (15%), nearly one in five 15-year-olds in Italy (18%) were overweight or obese in 2013–2014, a share close to the EU average [4]. This raised public policy concern, as excess weight among children and adolescents could affect the population's health in the long run. In order to design appropriate policy tools to increase healthy eating, the motivation behind food choices should be understood and defined.

Food choices are complex and are affected by a combination of various factors, including biological determinants (e.g., hunger, appetite, and taste), psychological social determinants (e.g., mood, stress, and guilt), physiological determinants (e.g., access, education, and time), social determinants (e.g., culture, family, and peers), and economic determinants (e.g., cost, income, and availability). Attitudes, beliefs, and knowledge about food also have an influence on food choices [5]. However, these factors could affect people differently, depending upon their context, personality, social groups, and socio-cultural position.

In the literature it has been discussed that health, mood, convenience, price, familiarity, social norms, natural and ethical concerns, and taste are prime issues considered by consumers when making food choices [6–10]. Eertmans et al. (2006) conducted a survey using the food choice questionnaire (FCQ) in different countries and found that in Italy, health and nature content, convenience and mood were the most important issues Italian consumer concerned in making their food choices [11]. Guiné et al. (2019) studied food choice determinants in Mediterranean countries and found that, in Italy, the food choices were influenced by environmental and political motivation, following by health and emotional reasons [12].

In order to determine the eating patterns of individuals in relation to their choices, particularly in the Mediterranean region, a large project entitled "Psycho-social motivations associated with food choices and eating practices" (EATMOT) was carried out. In this framework, a questionnaire was developed to define food choices, according to six types of conditioning motivations (health, emotional, economic and availability, social and culture, environment and politics, and marketing and commercial) [12]. This study was part of the project and its purpose was twofold: (1) To evaluate the food choice motivations in a sample in Italy; and (2) to segment consumer groups and provide consumer profiling, according to their food choice motivations.

2. Materials and Methods

2.1. Questionnaire

A questionnaire was developed specifically for the EATMOT project by the Center for Education, Technology and Health Studies (CI & DETS Research Center) in Portugal [13]. The questionnaire was prepared in English, then translated into Portuguese for the pre-test and validation of the questionnaire before the actual survey was carried out in 16 countries. The initial scale validity and internal reliability of the questionnaire were assessed only in Portugal (i.e., for the Portuguese version; see details in [13]). After validation, the questionnaire was modified and subsequently translated into English. The final version of the questionnaire was translated into Italian, following a back-translation methodology for validation [14]. During the translation process, the questions were slightly adjusted, in order to be more coherent with Italian culture, while the original meanings were retained. The questionnaire structure included five sections: Part 1—Socio-demographic data; Part 2—Anthropometric data and behavioral- and health-related elements; Part 3—Attitudes relating to healthy food; Part 4—Sources of information about a healthy diet; and Part 5—Food choice motivations (M1: Healthy motivations, M2: Emotional motivations, M3: Economic and availability motivations, M4: Social and cultural motivations, M5: Environmental and political motivations, and M6: Marketing and commercial motivations). The individual items and type of scale for all measures are provided in Appendix A (Table A1).

The questionnaire comprised both closed- and open-ended questions. In the perception of healthy eating and the food choice motivation sections, respondents were asked to give their opinion toward statements according to a 5-point Likert-like scale, ranging from 1 (Strongly disagree) to 5 (Strongly agree); while in the sources of information section, participants were asked to indicate the frequency at which they found information about healthy diets from different sources, on a scale from 1 (Never) to 5 (Always).

2.2. Data Collection

The questionnaire was administered both offline and online (Google forms) using a convenience sample of the Italian population through the personal connections of the authors. The online survey link was distributed through personal emails. Offline data collection was conducted in the North and Central parts of Italy. The interviews were carried out face-to-face with randomly selected consumers in different parts of the town (e.g., grocery stores and supermarkets) by experienced researchers/graduate students under the supervision of the authors of this paper. Data was collected between January and September 2017. The target respondents were adults aged over 18 years old, who voluntarily provided their consent to participate in the study.

All ethical procedures were strictly followed when designing and applying the questionnaire, and it was ensured that the data provided were kept strictly confidential (i.e., such that no individual response could ever be associated with the respondent). The study was conducted in accordance with the Declaration of Helsinki and the protocol was approved by the Ethics Committee of Polytechnic Institute of Viseu (reference n° 04/2017); furthermore, national and international protocols for research on humans were followed.

In total, 585 individuals participated in the survey. Through the validation process (i.e., elimination of incomplete questionnaires, leaving out outliers, and replacing invalid values with the mean), 531 questionnaires were considered valid and used in data analysis phase.

2.3. Data Analysis

Data were analyzed through both univariate and multivariate techniques using the IBM SPSS 26.0 software. A basic descriptive approach was used to describe Italian consumer characteristics, in terms of socio-demographics, anthropometrics, health-related behaviors, and information sources about healthy diets, including perceptions about healthy eating. Body mass index (BMI) was calculated using self-reported height (m) and weight (kg) data. The BMI results were classified according to International Classification Standards [15], as follows: underweight (BMI < 18.50 kg/m^2), normal weight ($18.50 \leq$ BMI ≤ 24.99 kg/m^2), overweight ($25.00 \leq$ BMI ≤ 29.99 kg/m^2), and obese (BMI ≥ 30.00 kg/m^2).

In the food choice motivations section, the median, mean, and standard deviation (SD) values of each item were calculated. Note that, to calculate the global scores, the inverted scores of M1.5 ("There are some foods that I consume regularly even if they may raise my cholesterol"), M1.9 ("There are some foods that I consume regularly even if they may raise my blood glycaemia"), M4.5 ("I prefer to eat alone"), M6.1 ("When I buy food I usually do not care about the marketing campaigns happening in the shop"), and M6.4 ("When I go shopping I prefer to read food labels instead of believing in advertising campaigns") were used, as they were negative questions (according to the motivations). Hence, the higher the global score, the stronger the influence of the motivations on food choices.

Consumer groups were identified using data of the food choice motivations section. Cronbach's alpha was used to test the internal validity of the 49 food motivation items (Cronbach's $\alpha = 0.755$). Then, all 49 items from the six food choice motivations were used for consumer segmentation (10 healthy items, 9 emotional items, 7 economic and availability items, 9 social and cultural items, 7 environmental and political items, and 7 marketing and commercial items). First, Hierarchical cluster analysis (HCA) with Squared Euclidean distances and Ward's method was applied to the items, in order to define the optimum number of clusters. The agglomeration schedule suggested that 2 clusters were suitable for the collected data. Then, K-mean cluster analysis was applied to identify the final clusters. Finally, the resulting clusters were evaluated, according to socio-demographics, anthropometrics, health-related behaviors, information sources, and perception about healthy eating, using the Pearson Chi-square, Student t-tests, and Mann–Whitney U test for independent samples.

3. Results

3.1. Sample Characteristics

3.1.1. Socio-Demographic and Anthropometric Data and Behavioral and Health Aspects

The sample included 531 Italian participants, of whom 65% were female. Their age ranged from 18 to 75 years, with a large group of respondents aged between 35 and 44 years old (27.7%), followed by respondents aged between 25 and 34 (23.9%). The average age was 42 years (SD = 13.47). The majority of respondents were higher educated and held a university degree (50%), while 45% possessed a secondary school diploma and around 5% of respondents had completed primary school. In terms of residences, 61% of the respondents lived in urban areas, 29% lived in suburban areas, and 10% lived in rural areas. Considering their civil status, 66% of respondents were married/living together, while 26% were single, 6% were divorced or separated, and 2% were widowed. The majority of respondents were employed (56%), while 19% were housewives, 9% were retired, 6% were unemployed, 6% were students, and 4% were working students. Most respondents were responsible for buying food for their household (85%).

Based on the self-reported weight and height, the majority of respondents were of normal weight (63.8%), whereas overweight and obese individuals comprised 24.5% and 5.8% of the study sample, respectively. Two hundred responders (37.7%) described themselves as being physically active, 54.8% of the sample declared having a healthy diet, and 76% of responders were not dieting or following a particular dietary regimen. A total of 72.3% of participants declared not having chronic diseases, while only a few suffered from allergies and/or intolerances (16.6%) or experienced eating disorders (9.2%).

3.1.2. Information Sources

Respondents were asked to indicate the frequency at which they found information about eating a healthy diet from different sources of information. They frequently used the internet and magazines, books and newspapers, and sometimes family or friends, television, and doctors. They found information at school or on the radio sporadically (Table 1).

Table 1. Sources of information for the total sample (n = 531).

Source of Information	Median	Mean	SD
Internet	4	3.43	1.07
Magazines, books, newspapers	4	3.41	0.93
Family, friends	3	3.13	0.87
Television	3	2.84	1.03
Health center, hospitals, family doctor (General Practitioner, GP)	3	2.67	1.11
School	2	2.45	1.15
Radio	2	2.33	1.01

Note: Respondents were asked to indicate the frequency at which they found information about eating a healthy diet, on the following scale: 1 = never, 2 = sporadically, 3 = sometimes, 4 = frequently, 5 = always.

3.2. Perceptions about Healthy Eating

The median and average scores of the respondent's perceptions about healthy eating are displayed in Table 2 and Figure 1. Almost all respondents strongly agreed that a healthy diet should be balanced, varied, complete, and should include fruit and vegetables. They also agreed that it is important to eat everything, although in small quantities. Disagreement was observed for inverted questions related to totally avoiding sugary and fatty products and having cravings for sweets, for some people. For questions related to the price of a healthy diet, the value of tradition for healthy patterns, a healthy diet being based on calorie count, or organically produced foods being healthier than their conventional counterparts, the responders neither agreed nor disagreed; in fact, their scores were quite variable.

Table 2. Perceptions about healthy eating (n = 531).

	Statement	Median	Mean	SD
P.4	A healthy diet should be balanced, varied and complete	5	4.66	0.73
P.3	Fruit and vegetables are very important to healthy eating	5	4.65	0.70
P.5	We can eat everything, as long as it is in small quantities	4	3.44	1.03
P.9	I believe that organically produced food is healthier	3	3.20	1.11
P.1	A healthy diet is based on calorie count	3	2.95	1.02
P.8	I believe that tradition is very important to a healthy diet	3	2.82	0.95
P.6	I believe that a healthy diet is not cheap	3	2.70	1.13
P.2	We should never consume sugary products	2	2.55	1.11
P.10	We should never consume fat products	2	2.38	0.97
P.7	In my opinion, it is strange that some people have cravings for sweets	2	2.25	0.92

Note: Respondents were asked to indicate their opinion on the statements, based on a 5-point semantic scale: 1 = strongly disagree, 2 = disagree, 3 = neither agree nor disagree, 4 = agree, 5 = strongly agree.

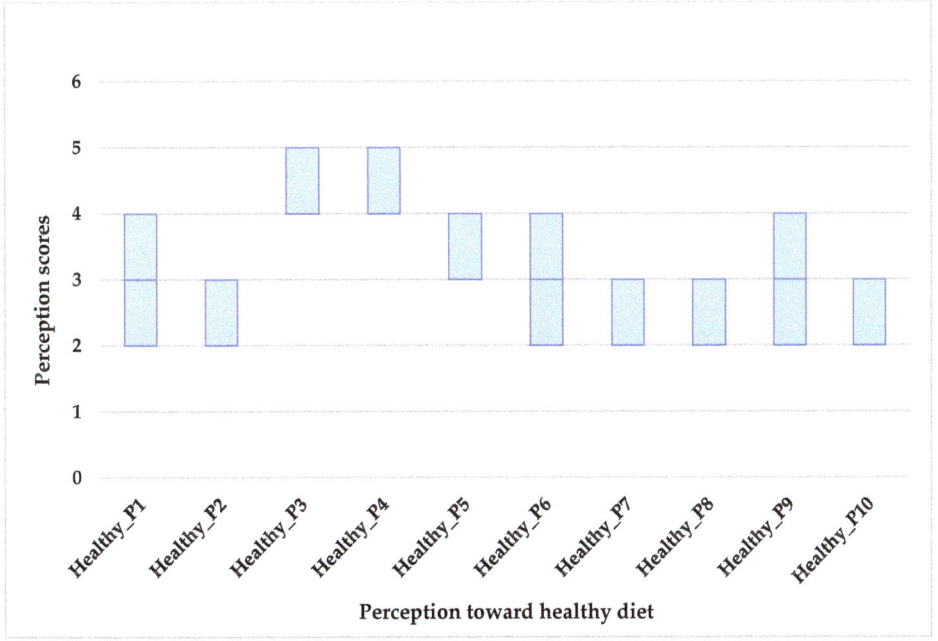

Figure 1. Box plot showing perception scores toward healthy diet (1 = strongly disagree, 2 = disagree, 3 = neither agree nor disagree, 4 = agree, 5 = strongly agree).

We tested the correlations between the different variables recorded in Part 2 of the questionnaire and perceptions toward healthy eating. The following results are those that were correlated and differed among groups at a significance level of 95%. A Kruskal–Wallis test provided strong evidence of a difference (H = 9.866, p = 0.02, df = 3) among the BMI classes toward the statement "A healthy diet should be balanced, varied and complete". The Dunn–Bonferroni post-hoc method was carried out. Normal weight respondents rated the highest score for this statement, and there was evidence that it was significantly higher than those of obese (p = 0.05) and underweight (p = 0.015) respondents, which indicates that this statement could be key to staying healthy and maintaining a normal weight.

Underweight respondents rated the statement "We can eat everything, as long as it is in small quantities" significantly lower than normal weight ($p = 0.013$), overweight ($p = 0.007$), and obese ($p = 0.002$) respondents. Underweight respondents also rated the statement "We should never consume fat products" significantly lower than overweight ($p = 0.028$) and obese ($p = 0.008$) respondents. These results meant that underweight respondents were very concerned about the types of food they consumed, but they disagreed that fatty products should be avoided, while overweight and obese respondents were very concerned about consuming fatty products.

The Mann–Whitney U-test was used to assess the following relations. Respondents who stated that they frequently/always followed a healthy diet scored the statements "Fruit and vegetables are very important to healthy eating" ($z = -2.998, p = 0.003$) and "A healthy diet should be balanced, varied and complete" ($z = -3.193, p = 0.001$) significantly higher than those who reported that they did not follow a healthy diet. Respondents who stated that they moderately/intensively did physical activities scored the statement "A healthy diet should be balanced, varied and complete" significantly higher than those who did not ($z = -2.597, p = 0.009$). Respondents who had chronic diseases scored significantly higher than those who had not on the statements "We should never consume sugary products" ($z = -2.225, p = 0.026$) and "We should never consume fat products" ($z = -2.956, p = 0.003$), indicating that chronic disease affects the perception of a healthy diet. Respondents who had experienced an eating disorder scored the statement "In my opinion, it is strange that some people have cravings for sweets" significantly lower than those who had never experienced one ($z = -2.088, p = 0.037$), showing that, for those who had ever experienced an eating disorder, cravings for sweets were normal. Respondents who followed a voluntary food regimen rated the following statements lower than those who did not follow any food regimen: "We should never consume sugary products" ($z = -4.931, p < 0.001$), "We should never consume fat products" ($z = -3.143, p = 0.002$), and "I believe that organically produced food is healthier" ($z = -2.741, p = 0.006$); while they rated the statement "I believe that tradition is very important to a healthy diet" significantly higher than those who did not follow any food regimen ($z = -3.432, p = 0.001$).

In summary, the statistical analysis demonstrated that BMI class and being active significantly affect the perception of a healthy diet as balanced, varied, and complete. Having a chronic disease significantly affects perceptions related to avoiding fatty and sweet products. Respondents who followed a voluntary food regimen had significantly different perceptions about a healthy diet than those who did not follow any regimen, regarding fat and sugar consumption, the role of tradition, and the healthiness of organically produced foods.

3.3. Food Motivations

The items associated with food choice motivations are shown in Figure 2 and Table 3. Environmental and political motivations (mean = 3.64, SD = 0.57), as well as health (mean = 3.4, SD = 0.46), were the strongest determinants (see Figure 2); while social and cultural (mean = 3.07, SD = 0.36), emotional (mean = 2.96, SD = 0.67), and economic and availability (mean = 2.86, SD = 0.51) motivations were less considered by respondents. Marketing and Commercial motivations were considered the least important drivers of food choices (mean = 2.46, SD = 0.53).

Twenty-three out of the 49 items had a median equal to 4 (median respondents agreed with the statements; see Table 3). It is worth noting that the non-inverted scores of statements M1.5, M1.9, M6.1, and M6.4 (negative statements, according to their global motivations) are shown here as well, as they were actually rated as 4 or above (i.e., agree). Respondents agreed about the social nature of meals ("Meals are a time of fellowship and pleasure"). They preferred to read food labels, instead of believing in marketing and commercial ("When I go shopping I prefer to read food labels instead of believing in advertising campaigns"). They also cared about the quality of their diet, in order to stay healthy ("It is important for me to eat food that keeps me healthy"), and about environmental sustainability ("When I cook I have in mind the quantities to avoid food waste", "It is important to me that the food I eat is prepared/packed in an environmental friendly way"). Overall, the respondents were very concerned about the environmental and health aspects of their food choices; nevertheless, they also considered emotional ("Food makes me feel good"), economic ("I usually choose food that has a good quality/price ratio"), and social ("I eat more than usual when I have company") aspects of food. Although the health aspect was crucial for them, they also regularly consumed some foods that may raise their cholesterol and blood glycemia ("There are some foods that I consume regularly, even if they may raise my cholesterol", "There are some foods that I consume regularly, even if they may raise my blood glycaemia").

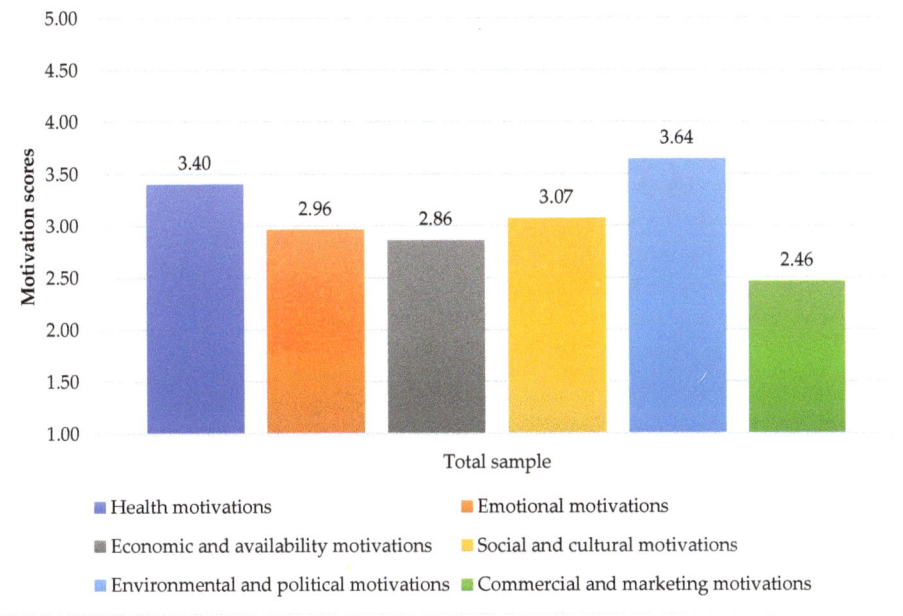

Figure 2. Average motivation scores of total sample (1 = strongly disagree, 2 = disagree, 3 = neither agree nor disagree, 4 = agree, 5 = strongly agree).

3.4. Consumer Segmentation

The items associated with the food choice motivations and results from the cluster analysis are shown in Figures 3 and 4. Two clusters were identified: Cluster 1 "Emotional eating consumers" and Cluster 2 "Health-driven consumers". Regarding the most and least important motivations, both clusters had the same idea: "Environmental and Policy motivations" were the most important, while "Marketing and Commercial motivations" were the least considered. Details of the scores of each item for each motivation, including the statistical difference between Clusters, are given in Appendix A.

Table 3. The most important food choice motivations for the total sample ($n = 531$).

	Statement	Mean	SD
M4.1	Meals are a time of fellowship and pleasure	4.34	0.68
M6.4	When I go shopping, I prefer to read food labels instead of believing in advertising campaigns	4.05	0.86
M1.8	It is important for me to eat food that keeps me healthy	4.02	0.76
M5.2	When I cook, I have in mind the quantities to avoid food waste	4.00	0.79
M5.1	It is important to me that the food I eat is prepared/packed in an environmentally friendly way	3.85	0.78
M4.6	I choose the foods I eat because it fits the season	3.82	0.83
M2.5	Food makes me feel good	3.81	0.85
M3.1	I usually choose food that has a good quality/price ratio	3.81	0.76
M5.4	I prefer to eat food that has been produced in a way that animals' rights have been respected	3.81	0.90
M4.2	I eat more than usual when I have company	3.79	0.90
M1.4	It is important for me that my daily diet contains a lot of vitamins and minerals	3.77	0.75
M4.8	I like to try new foods to which I am not accustomed	3.75	1.01
M5.5	I choose foods that have been produced in countries where human rights are not violated	3.71	0.92
M1.1	I am very concerned about the hygiene and safety of the food I eat	3.69	0.88
M3.4	I buy fresh vegetables to cook myself more often than frozen	3.66	1.10
M1.3	Usually, I follow a healthy and balanced diet	3.63	0.87
M1.10	I avoid foods with genetically modified organisms	3.60	1.11
M5.7	I prefer to buy foods that comply with policies of minimal usage of packaging	3.59	0.91
M5.3	It is important to me that the food I eat comes from my own country	3.56	1.03
M1.6	I try to eat foods that do not contain additives	3.50	0.96
M6.1	When I buy food, I usually do not care about the marketing campaigns happening in the shop	3.43	0.93
M1.5	There are some foods that I consume regularly, even if they may raise my cholesterol	3.35	0.95
M1.9	There are some foods that I consume regularly, even if they may raise my blood glycaemia	3.32	0.93

Note: Respondents were asked to indicate their opinion on the statements based on a 5-point semantic scale: 1 = strongly disagree, 2 = disagree, 3 = neither agree nor disagree, 4 = agree, 5 = strongly agree. Median scores of all items were equal to 4 (agree).

The first cluster accounted for 54.24% (288 persons) of the total sample and was described as "Emotional eating consumers" (Figure 3). Besides "Environmental and Policy motivations" (mean = 3.56, SD = 0.52), "Emotional motivations" (mean = 3.36, SD = 0.52) were very important for this cluster, as they scored most emotional items higher than the respondents in Cluster 2 ($t = 19.529$, $p < 0.001$). Food helped them to cope with stress, made them feel good, and served as their emotional consolation. In addition, they tended to emotionally eat, as they ate more when they felt lonely or had nothing to do, including craving sweets when they were depressed. They also consumed food to either keep them alert or relax. "Health motivations" (mean = 3.29, SD = 0.46) were the third most important for them; however, they scored most items in this category lower than respondents in Cluster 2, while they scored higher regarding consuming some foods regularly, even if they may raise their cholesterol or blood glycaemia (inverted scores). They also cared for "Social and cultural motivations" (mean = 3.15, SD = 0.37), "Economic and availability motivations" (mean = 3.09, SD = 0.44), and "Marketing and commercial motivations" (mean = 2.70, SD = 0.44) more than respondents in Cluster 2 ($t = 5.391$, $p < 0.001$; $t = 13.092$, $p < 0.001$; and $t = 12.998$, $p < 0.001$, respectively).

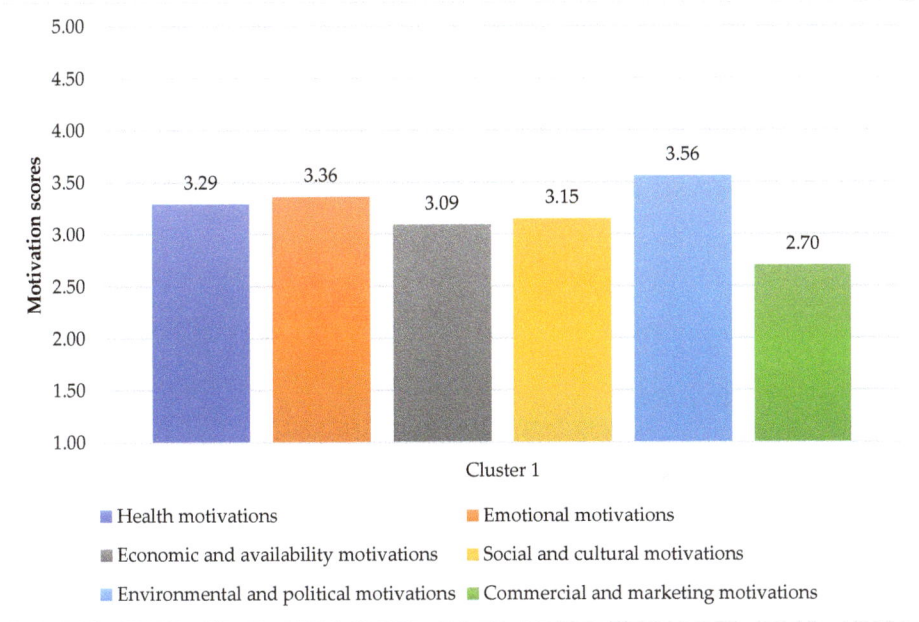

Figure 3. Average motivation scores of Cluster 1 (1 = strongly disagree, 2 = disagree, 3 = neither agree nor disagree, 4 = agree, 5 = strongly agree).

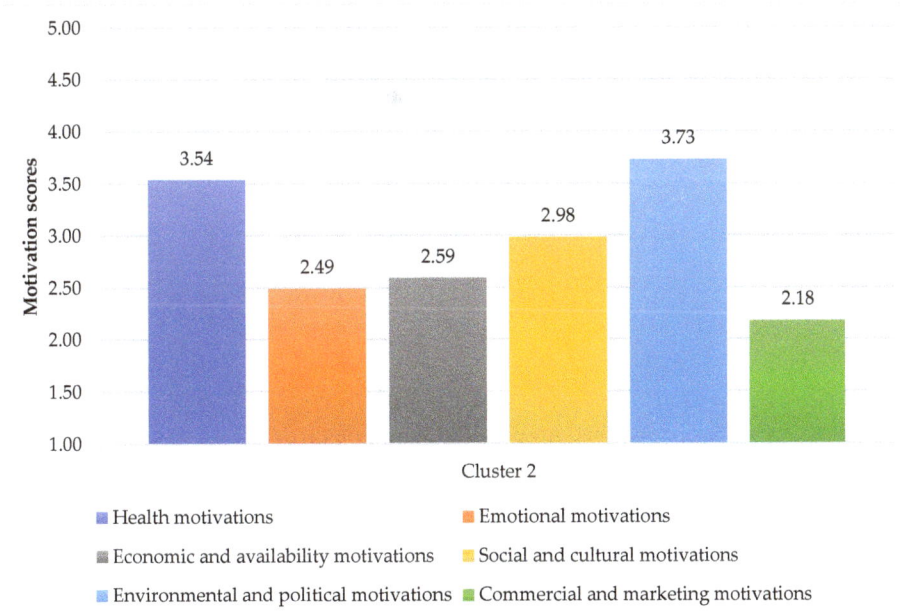

Figure 4. Average motivation scores of Cluster 2 (1 = strongly disagree, 2 = disagree, 3 = neither agree nor disagree, 4 = agree, 5 = strongly agree).

The second cluster was named "Health-Driven consumers", which accounted for 45.76% (243 persons) of the total sample. While "Environmental and Policy motivations" (mean = 3.73, SD = 0.61) were the most important drivers for them, "Health motivations" (mean = 3.54, SD = 0.43) were also highly considered. They agreed that they usually followed a healthy and balanced diet, it was important for them to eat foods that kept them healthy, and they tried to eat foods that did not contain additives. In addition, considering environmental motivations, they preferred to eat food that was prepared/packaged in an environmentally friendly way, and they were concerned about food waste and the reduction of food packages, differing from the respondents in Cluster 1. They cared for the environment more than the respondents in Cluster 1 ($t = -3.500$, $p = 0.001$). Besides those two motivations, "Social and cultural motivations" (mean = 2.98, SD = 0.34), "Economic and availability motivations" (mean = 2.59, SD = 0.44), "Emotional motivations" (mean = 2.49, SD = 0.50), and "Marketing and commercial motivations" (mean = 2.18, SD = 0.49) were less concerned by them.

3.5. Consumer Profiling

In order to understand the differences between the two segments, Pearson Chi-square, Student T-test, and Mann–Whitney U-test were performed on their demographic and anthropometric data and behavioral and health aspects. The results revealed that age, life environment, behavior, and health-related elements could significantly differentiate the segments (Table 4).

Table 4. Socio-demographic, anthropometric data, behavioral- and health-related elements of clusters.

Item	Frequency (%)			p-Value
	Total (n = 531)	Cluster 1 (n = 288)	Cluster 2 (n = 243)	
Age mean (SD)	42.09 (13.47)	40.30 (13.12)	44.21 (13.60)	0.001 [a]
Age range	35–44	35–44	35–44	<0.001 [b]
18–24	45 (8.5%)	29 (10.1%)	16 (6.6%)	
25–34	127 (23.9%)	78 (27.1%)	49 (20.2%)	
35–44	147 (27.7%)	88 (30.6%)	59 (24.3%)	
45–54	109 (20.5%)	48 (16.7%)	61 (25.1%)	
≥55	103 (19.4%)	45 (15.6%)	58 (23.9%)	
Gender	Female	Female	Female	0.180
Female	346 (65.2%)	195 (67.7%)	151 (62.1%)	
Male	185 (34.8%)	93 (32.3%)	92 (37.9%)	
Education (Highest level) (Median)	University	University	Secondary school	0.347
Primary school	26 (4.9%)	14 (4.9%)	12 (4.9%)	
Secondary school	238 (44.8%)	121 (42%)	117 (48.1%)	
University	267 (50.3%)	153 (53.1%)	114 (46.9%)	
Life environment (Median)	Urban	Urban	Urban	0.019
Rural	56 (10.5%)	31 (10.8%)	25 (10.3%)	
Urban	323 (60.8%)	189 (65.6%)	134 (55.1%)	
Suburban	152 (28.6%)	68 (23.6%)	84 (34.6%)	
Civil status (Median)	Married	Married	Married	0.278
Single	139 (26.2%)	82 (28.5%)	57 (23.5%)	
Married/Living together	351 (66.1%)	187 (64.9%)	164 (67.5%)	
Divorced/Separated	31 (5.8%)	16 (5.6%)	15 (6.2%)	
Widow	10 (1.9%)	3 (1.0%)	7 (2.9%)	

Table 4. Cont.

Item	Frequency (%)			p-Value
	Total (n = 531)	Cluster 1 (n = 288)	Cluster 2 (n = 243)	
Professional activity (Median)	Employed	Employed	Employed	0.106
Employed	299 (56.3%)	165 (57.3%)	134 (55.1%)	
Unemployed	30 (5.6%)	12 (4.2%)	18 (7.4%)	
Student	34 (6.4%)	24 (8.3%)	10 (4.1%)	
Retired	47 (8.9%)	20 (6.9%)	27 (11.1%)	
Student worker	20 (3.8%)	12 (4.2%)	8 (3.3%)	
Housewife	101 (19.0%)	55 (19.1%)	46 (18.9%)	
Responsible for food buying	Responsible	Responsible	Responsible	0.561
Responsible	451 (84.9%)	247 (85.8%)	204 (84%)	
Not responsible	80 (15.1%)	41 (14.2%)	39 (16%)	
BMI mean (SD)	23.65 (3.77)	23.88 (3.96)	23.36 (3.51)	0.110 [a]
BMI categories (Median)	Normal weight	Normal weight	Normal weight	0.066 [b]
Underweight (BMI < 18.50)	31 (5.8%)	16 (5.6%)	15 (6.2%)	
Normal weight (18.50 ≤ BMI ≤ 24.99)	339 (63.8%)	175 (60.8%)	164 (67.5%)	
Overweight (25.00 ≤ BMI ≤ 29.99)	130 (24.5%)	76 (26.4%)	54 (22.2%)	
Obese (BMI ≥ 30.00)	31 (5.8%)	21 (7.3%)	10 (4.1%)	
Physical exercise	Not enough	Not enough	Not enough	<0.001
Not enough physical exercise	331 (62.3%)	199 (69.1%)	132 (54.3%)	
Enough physical exercise	200 (37.7%)	89 (30.9%)	111 (45.7%)	
Healthy diet	Healthy diet	Unhealthy diet	Healthy diet	<0.001
Unhealthy diet	240 (45.2%)	164 (56.9%)	76 (31.3%)	
Healthy diet	291 (54.8%)	124 (43.1%)	167 (68.7%)	
Voluntary eating regimen	No	No	No	0.003
No voluntary regimen	401 (75.5%)	232 (80.6%)	169 (69.5%)	
Voluntary regimen	130 (24.5%)	56 (19.4%)	74 (30.5%)	
Chronic disease	No	No	No	0.089
No chronic disease	384 (72.3%)	217 (75.3%)	167 (68.7%)	
Chronic disease	147 (27.7%)	71 (24.7%)	76 (31.3%)	
Allergies/Intolerances	No	No	No	0.268
No allergies/intolerances	443 (83.4%)	245 (85.1%)	198 (81.5%)	
Allergies/intolerances	88 (16.6%)	43 (14.95%)	45 (18.5%)	
Have ever experienced eating disorder	No	No	No	0.053
No	482 (90.8%)	255 (88.5%)	227 (93.4%)	
Yes	49 (9.2%)	33 (11.5%)	16 (6.6%)	

Note: p-values were results from Pearson Chi-square, except [a], which resulted from a Student's T-test and [b], which resulted from a Mann–Whitney U-Test between the two Clusters.

The average age (44 years old) of respondents in Cluster 2 (or Health-Driven consumers) was significantly higher than that (40 years old) of Cluster 1 (or Emotional eating consumers; $t = -3.362$, $p = 0.001$). A significantly lower percentage of respondents in Cluster 2 (55%) lived in urban areas than those in Cluster 1 (66%; $\chi^2 = 7.936$, $p = 0.019$). Consistent with their scores for items in Health motivations, 69% of respondents in Cluster 2 stated that they followed a healthy diet. This was significantly higher than that in Cluster 1 (43%; $\chi^2 = 35.059$, $p < 0.001$). The respondents in Cluster 2 (46%) also physically exercised more than respondents in Cluster 1 (31%; $\chi^2 = 12.256$, $p < 0.001$). Respondents in Cluster 2 (30%) followed a voluntary food regimen more than those in Cluster 1 (24%; $\chi^2 = 8.639$, $p = 0.003$). The clusters were also differentiated—although with lower significance (statistically significant at 0.1 level)—in terms of the following issues: Based on BMI categories, a higher number of respondents in Cluster 2 (68%) had normal weight than in Cluster 1 (61%; $z = -1.839$, $p = 0.066$). However, more respondents in Cluster 2 (31%) had chronic diseases than in Cluster 1 (25%; $\chi^2 = 2.888$, $p = 0.089$), likely due to their higher average age. Additionally, the respondents in Cluster 1 (11%) had more experiences with eating disorders than those in Cluster 2 (7%; $\chi^2 = 3.738$, $p = 0.053$).

Regarding food motivations, respondents in Cluster 1 agreed with 19 out of 49 items (i.e., median respondents agreed with the statements; see Table 5). The non-inverted scores of statements M6.4, M4.5, M1.5, and M1.9 (negative statements, according to their global motivations) are shown here, as they were actually rated as agree. Respondents agreed that food had emotional value for them ("Food makes me feel good"). They also cared about the health ("It is important for me to eat food that keeps me healthy") and environmental ("When I cook I have in mind the quantities to avoid food waste") aspects of food. Although they were concerned about economics ("I usually choose food that has a good quality/price ratio"), they preferred to read food labels, instead of believing in advertisements ("When I go shopping I prefer to read food labels instead of believing in advertising campaigns"). Some preferred to eat alone ("I prefer to eat alone"). In general, the respondents in Cluster 1 concerned many aspects (motivations) of food, compared to respondents in Cluster 2. Emotional motivations seemed to be very important to them ("Food makes me feel good", "I eat more when I have nothing to do", "I have more cravings for sweets when I am depressed", and "Food helps me cope with stress").

Respondents in Cluster 2 agreed with 15 out of 49 items (i.e., median respondents agreed with the statements; see Table 6). The non-inverted scores of statements M6.1 and M6.4 (negative statements, according to their global motivations) are shown here as well. Respondents cared the most about health ("It is important for me to eat food that keeps me healthy") and environmental ("When I cook I have in mind the quantities to avoid food waste" and "It is important to me that the food I eat is prepared/packed in an environmental friendly way") aspects of food. They also agreed with social and cultural aspects ("I choose the foods I eat, because it fits the season"). Similar to the respondents in Cluster 1, they preferred to read labels, rather than believing in commercial advertisements ("When I go shopping I prefer to read food labels instead of believing in advertising campaigns"). Generally, the respondents in Cluster 2 were more concerned about health aspects than respondents in Cluster 1 ("It is important for me to eat food that keeps me healthy", "Usually I follow a healthy and balanced diet", "It is important for me that my daily diet contains a lot of vitamins and minerals", and "I try to eat foods that do not contain additives").

Regarding perceptions about healthy eating, there were also differences on perception about healthy diet between the two clusters (Table 7). Cluster 1 agreed significantly more than cluster 2 with the importance of eating everything (although in small quantities), with the role of tradition in a healthy diet, and that a healthy diet is not cheap. Differences between the clusters about totally avoiding sugary and fatty products were significant at the 0.10 level.

The frequency of finding information about eating a healthy diet from different sources of information is shown in Figure 5. Respondents in Cluster 2 used "specialized" sources, such as schools, health centers, hospitals, and family doctors (GP) more than respondents in Cluster 1. On the contrary, respondents in Cluster 1 used mass media—both traditional (radio and television) and internet—as well as books, magazines, and word-of-mouth between family and friends more than respondents in Cluster 2. All these sources, moreover, are cheaper than consulting experts (i.e., doctors).

Table 5. The most important food choice motivations for Cluster 1 (n = 288).

	Statement	Mean	SD
M2.5	Food makes me feel good	3.99	0.75
M1.8	It is important for me to eat food that keeps me healthy	3.92	0.79
M5.2	When I cook, I have in mind the quantities to avoid food waste	3.91	0.76
M6.4	When I go shopping, I prefer to read food labels instead of believing in advertising campaigns	3.89	0.84
M3.1	I usually choose food that has a good quality/price ratio	3.88	0.70
M4.5	I prefer to eat alone	3.85	0.99
M2.7	I eat more when I have nothing to do	3.76	0.97
M1.4	It is important for me that my daily diet contains a lot of vitamins and minerals	3.72	0.76
M4.6	I choose the foods I eat because it fits the season	3.69	0.81
M5.1	It is important to me that the food I eat is prepared/packed in an environmentally friendly way	3.67	0.75
M5.5	I choose foods that have been produced in countries where human rights are not violated	3.63	0.84
M1.5	There are some foods that I consume regularly, even if they may raise my cholesterol	3.58	0.79
M1.9	There are some foods that I consume regularly, even if they may raise my blood glycaemia	3.55	0.79
M1.10	I avoid foods with genetically modified organisms	3.54	1.05
M2.9	I have more cravings for sweets when I am depressed	3.54	1.08
M3.4	I buy fresh vegetables to cook myself more often than frozen	3.54	1.08
M3.5	I usually buy food that is easy to prepare	3.50	0.85
M2.1	Food helps me cope with stress	3.47	0.84
M1.3	Usually, I follow a healthy and balanced diet	3.44	0.90

Note: Respondents were asked to indicate their opinion on the statements, based on a 5-point semantic scale (1 = strongly disagree, 2 = disagree, 3 = neither agree nor disagree, 4 = agree, 5 = strongly agree). Median scores of all items were equal to 4 (agree).

Table 6. The most important food choice motivations for Cluster 2 (n = 243)

	Statement	Mean	SD
M1.8	It is important for me to eat food that keeps me healthy	4.14	0.70
M5.2	When I cook, I have in mind the quantities to avoid food waste	4.12	0.82
M5.1	It is important to me that the food I eat is prepared/packed in an environmentally friendly way	4.05	0.77
M4.6	I choose the foods I eat because it fits the season	3.97	0.83
M6.4	When I go shopping, I prefer to read food labels instead of believing in advertising campaigns	4.24	0.84
M1.3	Usually, I follow a healthy and balanced diet	3.86	0.76
M1.4	It is important for me that my daily diet contains a lot of vitamins and minerals	3.83	0.73
M3.4	I buy fresh vegetables to cook myself more often than frozen	3.81	1.11
M5.5	I choose foods that have been produced in countries where human rights are not violated	3.81	1.00
M5.7	I prefer to buy foods that comply with policies of minimal usage of packaging	3.76	0.92
M1.6	I try to eat foods that do not contain additives	3.73	0.89
M3.1	I usually choose food that has a good quality/price ratio	3.72	0.83

Table 6. Cont.

	Statement	Mean	SD
M1.10	I avoid foods with genetically modified organisms	3.68	1.17
M2.5	Food makes me feel good	3.60	0.91
M6.1	When I buy food, I usually do not care about the marketing campaigns happening in the shop	3.52	1.04

Note: Respondents were asked to indicate their opinion on the statements, based on a 5-point semantic scale (1 = strongly disagree, 2 = disagree, 3 = neither agree nor disagree, 4 = agree, 5 = strongly agree). Median scores of all items are equal to 4 (agree).

Table 7. Differences between clusters on perceptions about healthy eating.

Perception	Cluster 1 (n = 288)			Cluster 2 (n = 243)			p-Value
	Median	Mean	SD	Median	Mean	SD	
P.5 We can eat everything, as long as it is in small quantities	4	3.55	0.95	3	3.32	1.10	0.024
P.6 I believe that a healthy diet is not cheap	3	2.80	1.06	2	2.58	1.20	0.009
P.8 I believe that tradition is very important to a healthy diet	3	2.91	0.98	3	2.70	0.89	0.014
P.2 We should never consume sugary products	2	2.46	1.05	2	2.66	1.17	0.075
P.10 We should never consume fat products	2	2.43	0.92	2	2.32	1.03	0.099

Note: Respondents were asked to indicate their opinion on the statements based on a 5-semantic scale (1 = strongly disagree, 2 = disagree, 3 = neither agree nor disagree, 4 = agree, 5 = strongly agree). The p-values are the result of Mann–Whitney U-Test between two clusters.

In order to understand the differences between the information sources used by the two segments, a Mann–Whitney U-test was performed (Table 8). The results revealed that trust in TV and Radio significantly differentiated the segments. The respondents in Cluster 1 had more experience with using Radio and Television for information about healthy eating than those of Cluster 2.

Table 8. Difference in information sources about healthy diets between clusters.

Information Sources	Cluster 1 (n = 288)			Cluster 2 (n = 243)			p-Value
	Median	Mean	SD	Median	Mean	SD	
Radio	3	2.42	1.01	2	2.23	1.00	0.032
Television	3	2.93	0.98	3	2.74	1.09	0.041

Note: Respondents were asked to indicate the frequency at which they found information about eating a healthy diet, on the following scale: 1 = never, 2 = sporadically, 3 = sometimes, 4 = frequently, 5 = always. The p-values are the results of Mann–Whitney U-Test between two clusters.

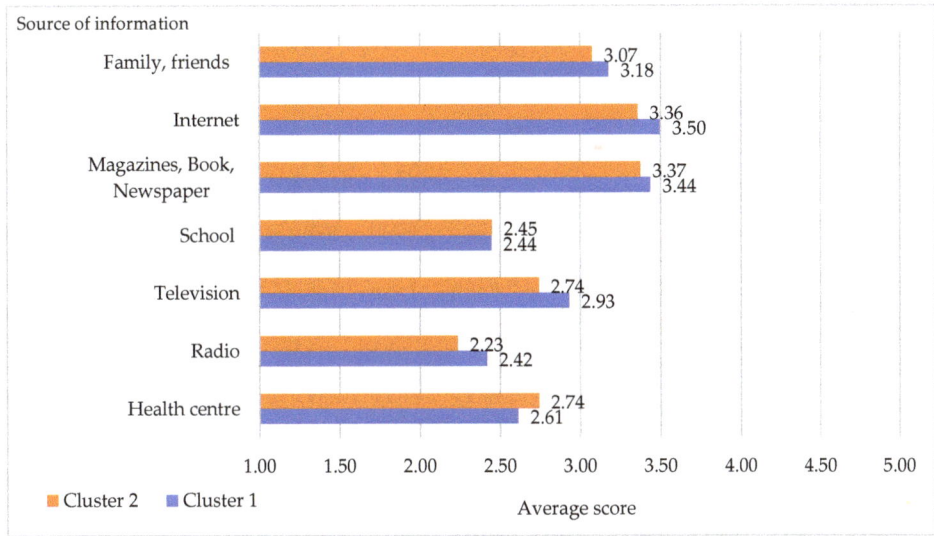

Figure 5. Average scores of information sources (1 = never, 2 = sporadically, 3 = sometimes, 4 = frequently, 5 = always).

4. Discussion

In this study, we investigated the motivations behind food choices in Italy and segmented the surveyed consumers to provide recommendations on effective tools to encourage healthy food choices. The main results indicated that some factors influenced consumer food choices more than others; for instance, in line with the previous literature [11,14,16–19], "Environmental and Political" and "Health" motivations were the most important determinants of food choices for Italian consumers, while "Marketing and Commercial" motivations were of the least concern [20].

When we looked at individual items, the highest rated items were as follows: Respondents mostly agreed that meals are linked to companionship and pleasure. This might be explained by the Italian tradition that meal time is a time to spend with family and friends [21]. They also stated that they preferred to read food labels when they shop for food, instead of believing in marketing campaigns. It was also highly important for them to eat food that keeps them healthy. Food waste was also highly considered by respondents when they prepare food, which was consistent with the results of Bravia et al. (2020): That Italian consumers tend to be proactive in planning their food purchases and checking 'use by' and 'best before' dates of food products, such that they can reduce their household food waste [22]. It has also been mentioned, in a report of the European Union, that trying to reduce waste was the number one action Italians carried out to address the issue of climate change [19].

Two consumer clusters were identified, according to the six analyzed food motivations: (1) "Emotional eating consumers", composed of respondents that were driven by their emotions; and (2) "Health-driven consumers" composed of those that based their choices on the health aspect of food. Although both clusters were primarily concerned with "Environmental and Political" motivations, when it came to food choice, their second-most important motivations differed; namely, "Emotional" and "Health", respectively.

The food choices of Emotional eating consumers were affected by psychological factors (e.g., mood). However, they also paid attention to health, food waste, food labels, and economic and availability factors of the product. Basically, they considered more aspects than Health-driven consumers. However, their choices could be highly affected by their mood or emotional state, as they mentioned that food made them feel good, that they ate more when they had nothing to do, that they had more cravings for sweets when they were depressed, and that food helped them to cope with stress. Their average age was lower than that of Health-driven consumers. Our results were in line with those of Cardoso et al. (2020), who stated that young adults had eating behaviors which were more conditioned by emotional motivations (e.g., to fight loneliness or boredom), compared to senior adults and elderly people [23]. Moreover, young adults have also been reported to link eating food with emotional consolation; for example, to help deal with stress and negative moods [24]. In addition, Emotional eating consumers had more experiences with eating disorders than Health-driven consumers, as they tended to exhibit emotional eating behaviors. Emotional eating consumers also agreed that there was some food that they consumed regularly, even if it may raise their cholesterol/blood glycaemia.

The food choices of Health-driven consumers were mainly driven by health-related aspects, seasonal availability, and label information. The relevance of sustainable consumption movements was also highlighted in this cluster. Besides avoiding creating food waste, similarly to Emotional eating consumers, they also believed that food should be prepared/packaged in an environmentally friendly manner, using minimal packaging. For them, it was also important that the foods they consume came from countries where human rights are not violated. When we looked at their profiles, the average age of Health-driven consumers was significantly higher than Emotional eating consumers. As a consequence, they had more chronic diseases than Emotional eating consumers. Health-driven consumers also stated that they followed a healthy diet and/or voluntary food regimen and exercised more than Emotional eating consumers. This is consistent with the fact that elderly individuals tend to eat more fruit and vegetables and are usually more adherent to healthy diets than young adults [25]. The fact that they have more chronic diseases may drive them to adhere to dietary recommendations and to be active. As a consequence, they tended to have a normal weight more than Emotional eating consumers.

Regarding perceptions related to healthy eating, most respondents perceived that a healthy diet should be balanced, varied, and complete and should include fruit and vegetables, which are aspects in accordance with suggestions for healthy eating by nutritionists [26–29]. This demonstrated that they were mostly aware about what healthy foods are. Nevertheless, only half of them stated that they followed a healthy diet. Hence, there existed a gap between declarative knowledge and behaviors. Several studies have confirmed that healthy eating knowledge is a significant predictor of both future knowledge and behavior [30–33]; however, knowledge alone is not sufficient to change the food behaviors of consumers, as such behaviors can also be influenced by personal, intra-individual, and environmental factors, including motivations [34–36]. The results of our cluster analysis underline that one such factor could be "Emotional" motivations; at least, for Emotional eating consumers. In addition, unconscious motivations and the link between nutritional knowledge, emotions, and food choice should be further investigated.

Most respondents also agreed that they could eat everything, as long as it is in a small quantity. In addition, they disagreed about the "total avoidance of sugary and fatty products". This may be because they believed that small quantities and variety are key to a healthy diet, as suggested by the Italian Food Dietary Guideline [37]. Moreover, they may have taken into account the emotional effect on food choice, as they generally agreed that having a craving for sweets is not unusual.

Respondents who had a normal body weight, declared to have healthy diet, and were active believed that a healthy diet should be balanced, varied, and complete. Overweight and obese respondents were more concerned about the consumption of fatty products than other groups (i.e., agreeing more that we should avoid consuming fatty products). Respondents who had a chronic disease perceived that they should avoid fatty and sweet products, as suggested in the various guidelines for the treatment of heart disease and for preventing dietary diseases in the general population (see, e.g., the Diet and Lifestyle Recommendations by the American Heart Association) [38].

In addition, following a voluntary food regimen led respondents to perceive healthy eating differently than those who did not follow any voluntary food regimen, with respect to fat and sugar consumption, the role of tradition, and the healthiness of organically produced foods. This might be because individuals who follow a particular diet are usually more attentive to their diet and are more informed about their diet, such that they are more aware of what should be limited (e.g., fat and sugar). They also considered that organic products are produced with more respect for the environment [39]. Especially in Italy, organic products are considered not only environmentally friendly but healthy; although, from a nutritional point of view, organic products are not considered to differ much from non-organic ones [39–41].

Concerning the sources of information used, our sample was well-informed and took information from various sources. The internet was the main source of information about healthy eating, followed by magazines, books, and newspapers. These answers were consistent with the emerging informative use of the Internet (i.e., reading online newspapers, documenting health, collecting information on products), although the Italian people are still in the last position in Europe, in terms of informative usage of the Internet, at present [42]. The internet also consists of the use of social networks. The use of social networks has been shown to change the way that consumers search for information and select products; they are becoming prominent sources of information, including for food choices (see [43,44], for example). From this perspective, social media can influence information strategies in two ways: Reducing the cost of releasing information, compared to that of traditional mass media (i.e., television or radio), and making specific consumer groups more easily targeted.

Offline and online word-of-mouth and social media, however, can be dangerous in transmitting misinformation; especially in the food sector [45,46]. Indeed, the recent study of Castellini et al. (2020) found that around half of Italians (48%) admitted that they had believed in a news story about the food sector that turned out to be false at least a few times in the last year, while a third of those (37%) had shared it on social media, thus contributing to the unstoppable spread of "food fake news" [46]. An even more interesting fact is that this phenomenon occurs in all social and educational classes. In particular, individuals who believe in such misinformation are psychologically different than consumers who are less persuaded by this kind of news. They are more driven by other motivations, related to familiarity with the product and the mood of the moment, rather than by the evaluation of healthiness of the food. They are more favorably oriented to experimentation with new products and are more predisposed to social influence, being less self-confident [46]. Hence, the Emotional eating consumers could be at risk of being more susceptible to such misinformation. This means that the role of institutions in educating the public is important, and that they should exploit different media forms, in order to aid citizens to be able to distinguish between reliable and non- reliable sources of information and enable them to make well-informed food choices.

For policy-makers, food labels could be promoted as a tool to assist consumers to make a conscious food choice. Information provision to promote sustainable and healthy diets could be carried out through educational campaigns (e.g., relating to the inclusion of sustainability in dietary guidelines) or improved sustainability labelling on packaging. Social media could be used to change social norms and food culture towards healthy diets and waste reduction, as recent studies have demonstrated that social media information also affects environmental awareness and consumer information and choices relating to sustainable food [44]. Further research is necessary to examine the role of the Internet in food information more closely, as well as the sources which are judged as most reliable by respondents. It will also be interesting, in future research, to deepen the multifaceted relationship between traditional and social media information and healthy or sustainable consumption, in terms of food choices for specific consumer segments.

For food marketers, there was a clear need, for both clusters, for food products that are healthy and sustainable. Environmentally friendly packaging and human rights in the producing countries were also emphasized by Health-driven consumers. Moreover, information regarding the environment and sustainability on these issues (e.g., product labelling) should be provided, in order to increase the purchase of such products [47].

The limitations of this research were as follows: There was a higher proportion of female participants and the sample had higher education, on average, than the Italian census. BMI values were calculated from self-reported height and weight and, therefore, the results should be interpreted with care. We also did not ask respondents about their dietary habits or their consumption of some food products, such that we could not compare their statements (e.g., following healthy diet) and (reported) consumption behavior. Future research should cover this aspect.

5. Conclusions

In conclusion, the respondents had a good awareness of what a healthy diet consists of. They mostly found information online or in newspapers and books, as well as through talking with friends and families. The strongest determinants for their food choice were Environmental and Health factors. The less influential reasons were those related to Marketing and Commercial. The clustering analysis resulted in two consumer segments: Emotional eating consumers and Health-driven consumers. Both segments considered Environmental and Political motivations as the most important issues. Nevertheless, their second-most important motivations divided them, as the Emotional eating consumers were more influenced by their emotions, while Health-driven consumers were more concerned with the health aspects of food. Emotional eating consumers were younger, while Health-driven consumers had more normal weight and stated that they followed a healthy diet and/or voluntary food regimen and exercised more than Emotional eating consumers. Food labels were used by respondents as an important tool when making food choices. Food waste and food packaging were issues also concerned by most respondents.

Author Contributions: Conceptualization, R.P.F.G., C.M., N.P. and E.V.; methodology, C.M. and R.W.; data collection: C.M., N.P., E.V. and E.C.; formal analysis, R.W.; writing—original draft preparation, R.W., C.M. and N.P.; writing—review and editing, R.P.F.G., G.S., N.P., E.C. and E.V. All authors have read and agreed to the published version of the manuscript.

Funding: The APC was funded by Parma University.

Institutional Review Board Statement: The study was conducted according to the guidelines of the Declaration of Helsinki, and approved by the Ethics Committee of Polytechnic Institute of Viseu (reference n° 04/2017).

Informed Consent Statement: Informed consent was obtained from all subjects involved in the study.

Data Availability Statement: The datasets generated for this study are available on request to the corresponding author.

Acknowledgments: This work was prepared in the ambit of the multinational project EATMOT from CI&DETS Research Centre [IPV—Viseu, Portugal] with reference PROJ/CI&DETS/CGD/0012. This work is supported by Portuguese National Funds through the FCT—Foundation for Science and Technology, I.P., within the scope of the project Ref^a UIDB/00681/2020. Furthermore, we would like to thank the CERNAS Research Centre and the Polytechnic Institute of Viseu for their support.

Conflicts of Interest: The authors declare no conflict of interest.

Appendix A

Food choice motivation of total sample, Cluster 1 and Cluster 2.

Table A1. Food choice motivation of total sample, Cluster 1 and Cluster 2.

Statement	Total (n = 531)			Cluster 1 (n = 288)			Cluster 2 (n = 243)			p-Value
	Median	Mean	SD	Median	Mean	SD	Median	Mean	SD	
M1. Healthy Motivations										
M1.1 I am very concerned about the hygiene and safety of the food I eat	4	3.69	0.88	4	3.66	0.85	4	3.71	0.93	0.347
M1.2 It is important for me that my diet is low in fat	3	3.26	0.88	3	3.28	0.85	3	3.23	0.91	0.422
M1.3 Usually I follow a healthy and balanced diet	4	3.63	0.87	4	3.44	0.90	4	3.86	0.76	<0.001
M1.4 It is important for me that my daily diet contains a lot of vitamins and minerals	4	3.77	0.75	4	3.72	0.76	4	3.83	0.73	0.047
M1.5 There are some foods that I consume regularly, even if they may raise my cholesterol [a]	2	2.65	0.95	2	2.42	0.79	3	2.93	1.05	<0.001
M1.6 I try to eat foods that do not contain additives	4	3.50	0.96	3	3.30	0.96	4	3.73	0.89	<0.001
M1.7 I avoid eating processed foods, because of their lower nutritional quality	3	3.23	0.98	3	3.14	0.95	3	3.33	1.01	0.024
M1.8 It is important for me to eat food that keeps me healthy	4	4.02	0.76	4	3.92	0.79	4	4.14	0.70	0.001
M1.9 There are some foods that I consume regularly, even if they may raise my blood glycaemia [a]	2	2.68	0.93	2	2.45	0.79	3	2.94	1.00	<0.001
M1.10 I avoid foods with genetically modified organisms	4	3.60	1.11	4	3.54	1.05	4	3.68	1.17	0.044
M2. Emotional Motivations										
M2.1 Food helps me cope with stress	3	2.98	1.05	4	3.47	0.84	2	2.40	0.98	<0.001
M2.2 I usually eat food that helps me control my weight	3	3.04	0.97	3	3.02	0.94	3	3.07	1.01	0.382
M2.3 I often consume foods that keep me awake and alert (such as coffee, coke, energy drinks)	2	2.67	1.20	3	3.05	1.20	2	2.22	1.04	<0.001
M2.4 I often consume foods that helps me relax (e.g., teas, red wine)	3	3.01	1.13	3	3.21	1.08	3	2.78	1.14	<0.001
M2.5 Food makes me feel good	4	3.81	0.85	4	3.99	0.75	4	3.60	0.91	<0.001
M2.6 When I feel lonely, I console myself by eating	2	2.47	1.07	3	3.05	0.98	2	1.70	0.73	<0.001
M2.7 I eat more when I have nothing to do	3	3.20	1.21	4	3.76	0.97	2	2.55	1.13	<0.001
M2.8 For me, food serves as an emotional consolation	2	2.56	1.16	3	3.18	1.03	2	1.82	0.82	<0.001
M2.9 I have more cravings for sweets when I am depressed	3	2.93	1.28	4	3.54	1.08	2	2.20	1.12	<0.001

Table A1. Cont.

Statement	Total (n = 531)			Cluster 1 (n = 288)			Cluster 2 (n = 243)			p-Value
	Median	Mean	SD	Median	Mean	SD	Median	Mean	SD	
M3. Economic and Availability Motivations										
M3.1 I usually choose food that has a good quality/price ratio	4	3.81	0.76	4	3.88	0.70	4	3.72	0.83	0.034
M3.2 The main reason for choosing a food is its low price	2	1.88	0.88	2	2.18	0.91	1	1.52	0.68	<0.001
M3.3 I choose the food I consume because it is convenient to purchase	2	2.54	1.00	3	1.86	0.94	2	2.17	0.94	<0.001
M3.4 I buy fresh vegetables to cook myself more often than frozen	4	3.66	1.10	4	3.54	1.08	4	3.81	1.11	0.001
M3.5 I usually buy food that is easy to prepare	3	3.11	1.04	4	3.50	0.85	3	2.66	1.06	<0.001
M3.6 I usually buy food that it is on sale	3	3.08	0.97	3	3.43	0.83	3	2.67	0.96	<0.001
M3.7 I prefer to buy food that is ready to eat or pre-cooked	2	1.94	0.94	2	2.24	0.99	1	1.57	0.73	<0.001
M4. Social and Cultural Motivations										
M4.1 Meals are a time of fellowship and pleasure	4	4.34	0.68	4	4.36	0.62	4	4.32	0.74	0.881
M4.2 I eat more than usual when I have company	4	3.79	0.90	4	3.82	0.90	4	3.76	0.91	0.482
M4.3 It is important to me that the food I eat is similar to the food I ate when I was a child	2	2.40	0.93	3	2.52	0.92	2	2.24	0.91	<0.001
M4.4 I eat certain foods because other people (my colleagues, friends, family) also eat it	2	2.15	0.93	2	2.43	0.94	2	1.81	0.80	<0.001
M4.5 I prefer to eat alone [a]	4	3.95	0.97	4	3.85	0.99	4	4.06	0.94	0.009
M4.6 I choose the foods I eat because it fits the season	4	3.82	0.83	4	3.69	0.81	4	3.97	0.83	<0.001
M4.7 I eat certain foods because I am expected to eat them	2	1.85	0.90	2	2.05	0.96	1	1.61	0.75	<0.001
M4.8 I like to try new foods to which I am not accustomed	4	3.75	1.01	4	3.75	1.02	4	3.75	0.99	0.925
M4.9 I usually eat food that is trendy	1	1.64	0.76	2	1.89	0.83	1	1.35	0.54	<0.001
M5. Environment and Political Motivations										
M5.1 It is important to me that the food I eat is prepared/packed in an environmentally friendly way	4	3.85	0.78	4	3.67	0.75	4	4.05	0.77	<0.001
M5.2 When I cook, I have in mind the quantities to avoid food waste	4	4.00	0.79	4	3.91	0.76	4	4.12	0.82	<0.001
M5.3 It is important to me that the food I eat comes from my own country	4	3.56	1.03	4	3.53	0.98	4	3.58	1.09	0.321
M5.4 I prefer to eat food that has been produced in a way that animals' rights have been respected	4	3.81	0.90	4	3.79	0.85	4	3.84	0.97	0.310

Table A1. *Cont.*

Statement	Total (*n* = 531)			Cluster 1 (*n* = 288)			Cluster 2 (*n* = 243)			*p*-Value
	Median	Mean	SD	Median	Mean	SD	Median	Mean	SD	
M5.5 I choose foods that have been produced in countries where human rights are not violated	4	3.71	0.92	4	3.63	0.84	4	3.81	1.00	0.009
M5.6 I avoid going to restaurants that do not have a recovery policy of food surplus	3	2.96	0.84	3	2.94	0.79	3	2.98	0.89	0.626
M5.7 I prefer to buy foods that comply with policies of minimal usage of packaging	4	3.59	0.91	3	3.45	0.87	4	3.76	0.92	<0.001
M6. Market and Commercials Motivations										
M6.1 When I buy food, I usually do not care about the marketing campaigns happening in the shop [a]	2	2.57	0.93	3	2.65	0.83	2	2.48	1.04	0.012
M6.2 I eat what I eat, because I recognize it from advertisements or have seen it on TV	2	1.85	0.81	2	2.09	0.81	1	1.57	0.73	<0.001
M6.3 I usually buy food that spontaneously appeals to me (e.g., situated at eye level, appealing colors, pleasant packaging)	2	2.27	0.97	3	2.63	0.90	2	1.85	0.87	<0.001
M6.4 When I go shopping, I prefer to read food labels instead of believing in advertising campaigns [a]	2	1.95	0.86	2	2.11	0.84	2	1.76	0.84	<0.001
M6.5 Food advertising campaigns increase my desire to eat certain foods	2	2.47	1.06	3	2.86	0.96	2	2.01	0.98	<0.001
M6.6 Brands are important to me when making food choices	3	2.96	1.10	3	3.14	0.99	3	2.75	1.18	<0.001
M6.7 I try to schedule my food shopping for when I know there are promotions or discounts	3	3.17	1.04	3	3.44	0.93	3	2.84	1.06	<0.001

Note: Respondents were asked to indicate their opinion on the statements based on a 5-point semantic scale (1 = strongly disagree, 2 = disagree, 3 = neither agree nor disagree, 4 = agree, 5 = strongly agree). [a] Inverted scale as they were negative questions (according to the motivations), *p*-values are results from Mann–Whitney U-Test between the two clusters.

References

1. Joint WHO/FAO Expert Consultation. *Diet, Nutrition and the Prevention of Chronic Diseases*; WHO technical report; WHO: Geneva, Switzerland, 2003; ISBN 92-4-120916-X.
2. GBD 2017 Diet Collaborators Health Effects of Dietary Risks in 195 Countries, 1990–2017: A Systematic Analysis for the Global Burden of Disease Study 2017. *Lancet* **2019**, *393*, 1958–1972. [CrossRef]
3. OECD/European Observatory on Health Systems and Policies. *Italy: Country Health Profile 2017, State of Health in the EU*; OECD Publishing: Brussels, Belgium, 2017; ISBN 978-92-64-28342-8.
4. OECD/European Observatory on Health Systems and Policies. *Italy: Country Health Profile 2019, State of Health in the EU*; OECD Publishing: Brussels, Belgium, 2019; ISBN 978-92-64-72593-5.
5. Bellisle, F. The Factors That Influence Our Food Choices. Available online: https://www.eufic.org/en/healthy-living/article/the-determinants-of-food-choice (accessed on 26 October 2020).
6. Steptoe, A.; Pollard, T.M.; Wardle, J. Development of a Measure of the Motives Underlying the Selection of Food: The Food Choice Questionnaire. *Appetite* **1995**, *25*, 267–284. [CrossRef]

7. Pollard, E.M.; Steptoe, A.; Wardle, J. Motives Underlying Healthy Eating: Using the Food Choice Questionnaire to Explain Variation in Dietary Intake. *J. Biosoc. Sci.* **1998**, *30*, 165–179. [CrossRef]
8. Appleton, K.M.; Dinnella, C.; Spinelli, S.; Morizet, D.; Saulais, L.; Hemingway, A.; Monteleone, E.; Depezay, L.; Perez-Cueto, F.J.A.; Hartwell, H. Consumption of a High Quantity and a Wide Variety of Vegetables Are Predicted by Different Food Choice Motives in Older Adults from France, Italy and the UK. *Nutrients* **2017**, *23*, 923. [CrossRef]
9. Renner, B.; Sproesser, G.; Strohbach, S.; Schupp, H.T. Why We Eat What We Eat. The Eating Motivation Survey (TEMS). *Appetite* **2012**, *59*, 117–128. [CrossRef] [PubMed]
10. Đorđević, Đ.; Buchtova, H. Factors Influencing Sushi Meal as Representative of Non-Traditional Meal: Consumption among Czech Consumers. *Acta Aliment.* **2017**, *46*, 76–83. [CrossRef]
11. Eertmans, A.; Victoir, A.; Notelaers, G.; Vansant, G.; Van den Bergh, O. The Food Choice Questionnaire: Factorial Invariant over Western Urban Populations? *Food Qual. Prefer.* **2006**, *17*, 344–352. [CrossRef]
12. Guiné, R.; Ferrão, A.C.; Ferreira, M.; Correia, P.; Cardoso, A.P.; Duarte, J.; Rumbak, I.; Shehata, A.M.; Vittadini, E.; Papageorgiou, M. The Motivations That Define Eating Patterns in Some Mediterranean Countries. *Nutr. Food Sci.* **2019**, *49*, 1126–1141. [CrossRef]
13. Ferrão, A.C.; Guiné, R.P.F.; Correia, P.; Ferreira, M.; Duarte, J.; Lima, J. Development of A Questionnaire To Assess People's Food Choices Determinants. *Curr. Nutr. Food Sci.* **2019**, *15*, 281–295. [CrossRef]
14. Guiné, R.P.F.; Bartkiene, E.; Szűcs, V.; Tarcea, M.; Ljubičić, M.; Černelič-Bizjak, M.; Isoldi, K.; EL-Kenawy, A.; Ferreira, V.; Straumite, E.; et al. Study about Food Choice Determinants According to Six Types of Conditioning Motivations in a Sample of 11,960 Participants. *Foods* **2020**, *9*, 888. [CrossRef]
15. World Health Organization. Global Dataset on Body Mass Index. Available online: http://apps.who.int/bmi/index.jsp?introPage=intro_3.html (accessed on 30 October 2020).
16. Banterle, A.; Ricci, E.C. Does the Sustainability of Food Products Influence Consumer Choices? The Case of Italy. *Int. J. Food Syst. Dyn.* **2013**, *4*, 149–158. [CrossRef]
17. Corallo, A.; Latino, M.E.; Menegoli, M.; Spennato, A. A Survey to Discover Current Food Choice Behaviors. *Sustainability* **2019**, *11*, 5041. [CrossRef]
18. Dinnella, C.; Spinelli, S.; Monteleone, E. Attitudes to Food in Italy: Evidence from the Italian Taste Project. In *Handbook of Eating and Drinking*; Springer: Cham, Switzerland, 2010; ISBN 978-3-030-14504-0.
19. European Union. *Climate Change Report: Italy*; Special Eurobarometer 490; European Commission: Brussels, Belgium, 2019.
20. Boyland, E.J.; Nolan, S.; Kelly, B.; Tudur-Smith, C.; Jone, A.; Halford, J.C.; Robinson, E. Advertising as a Cue to Consume: A Systematic Review and Meta-Analysis of the Effects of Acute Exposure to Unhealthy Food and Nonalcoholic Beverage Advertising on Intake in Children and Adults. *Am. J. Clin. Nutr.* **2016**, *103*, 519–533. [CrossRef] [PubMed]
21. Nuvoli, G. Family Meal Frequency, Weight Status and Healthy Management in Children, Young Adults and Seniors. A Study in Sardinia, Italy. *Appetite* **2015**, *89*, 160–166. [CrossRef] [PubMed]
22. Bravia, L.; Francioni, B.; Murmura, F.; Savelli, E. Factors Affecting Household Food Waste among Young Consumers and Actions to Prevent It. A Comparison among UK, Spain and Italy. *Resour. Conserv. Recycl.* **2020**, *153*, 104586. [CrossRef]
23. Cardoso, A.P.; Ferreira, V.; Leal, M.; Ferreira, M.; Campos, S.; Guiné, R.P.F. Perceptions about Healthy Eating and Emotional Factors Conditioning Eating Behaviour: A Study Involving Portugal, Brazil and Argentina. *Foods* **2020**, *9*, 1236. [CrossRef]
24. Sogari, G.; Velez-Argumedo, C.; Gómez, M.I.; Mora, C. College Students and Eating Habits: A Study Using an Ecological Model for Healthy Behavior. *Nutrients* **2018**, *10*, 1823. [CrossRef]
25. Leclercq, C.; Arcella, D.; Piccinelli, R.; Sette, S.; Le Donne, C.; Turrini, A. The Italian National Food Consumption Survey INRAN-SCAI 2005–06: Main Results in Terms of Food Consumption. *Public Health Nutr.* **2009**, *12*, 2504–2532. [CrossRef]
26. Aune, D.; Giovannucci, E.; Boffetta, P.; Fadnes, L.T.; Keum, N.; Norat, T.; Greenwood, D.C.; Riboli, E.; Vatten, L.J.; Tonstad, S. Fruit and Vegetable Intake and the Risk of Cardiovascular Disease, Total Cancer and All-Cause Mortality-a Systematic Review and Dose-Response Meta-Analysis of Prospective Studies. *Int. J. Epidemiol.* **2017**, *46*, 1029–1056. [CrossRef]
27. Slavin, J.L.; Lloyd, B. Health Benefits of Fruits and Vegetables. *Adv. Nutr.* **2012**, *3*, 506–516. [CrossRef]
28. Drescher, L.S.; Thiele, S.; Mensink, G.B.M. A New Index to Measure Healthy Food Diversity Better Reflects a Healthy Diet Than Traditional Measures. *J. Nutr.* **2007**, *137*, 647–651. [CrossRef] [PubMed]
29. World Health Organization. Healthy Diet. Available online: https://apps.who.int/iris/bitstream/handle/10665/325828/EMROPUB_2019_en_23536.pdf?sequence=1&isAllowed=y (accessed on 13 November 2020).
30. Spronk, I.; Kullen, C.; Burdon, C.; O'Connor, H. Relationship between Nutrition Knowledge and Dietary Intake. *Br. J. Nutr.* **2014**, *111*, 1713–1726. [CrossRef]
31. Chung, L.M.Y.; Chung, J.W.Y.; Chan, A.P.C. Building Healthy Eating Knowledge and Behavior: An Evaluation of Nutrition Education in a Skill Training Course for Construction Apprentices. *Int. J. Environ. Res. Public Health* **2019**, *16*, 4852. [CrossRef] [PubMed]
32. Kulik, N.L.; Moore, E.W.; Centeio, E.E.; Garn, A.C.; Martin, J.J.; Shen, B.; Somers, C.L.; Mc Caughtry, N. Knowledge, Attitudes, Self-Efficacy, and Healthy Eating Behavior Among Children: Results From the Building Healthy Communities Trial. *Health Educ. Behav.* **2019**, *46*, 602–611. [CrossRef] [PubMed]
33. Melesse, M.B.; van den Berg, M. Consumer Nutrition Knowledge and Dietary Behavior in Urban Ethiopia: A Comprehensive Study. *Ecol. Food Nutr.* **2020**. [CrossRef]

34. Worsley, A. Nutrition Knowledge and Food Consumption: Can Nutrition Knowledge Change Food Behaviour? *Asia Pac. J. Clin. Nutr.* **2002**, *11*, 579–585. [CrossRef]
35. Menozzi, D.; Sogari, G.; Mora, C. Understanding and Modelling Vegetables Consumption among Young Adults. *LWT Food Sci. Technol.* **2017**, *85*, 327–333. [CrossRef]
36. Nagy-Pénzes, G.; Vincze, F.; Sándor, J.; Bíró, É. Does Better Health-Related Knowledge Predict Favorable Health Behavior in Adolescents? *Int. J. Environ. Res. Public Health* **2020**, *17*, 1680. [CrossRef]
37. CREA Linee Guida per Una Sana Alimentazione. 2018. Available online: https://www.crea.gov.it/web/alimenti-e-nutrizione/-/linee-guida-per-una-sana-alimentazione-2018 (accessed on 12 October 2020).
38. Van Horn, L.; Carson, J.A.S.; Appel, L.J.; Burke, L.E.; Economos, C.; Karmally, W.; Lancaster, K.; Lichtenstein, A.H.; Johnson, R.K.; Thomas, R.J.; et al. Recommended Dietary Pattern to Achieve Adherence to the American Heart Association/American College of Cardiology (AHA/ACC) Guidelines: A Scientific Statement From the American Heart Association. *Circulation* **2016**, *134*, e505–e529. [CrossRef]
39. Dall'Asta, M.; Angelino, D.; Pellegrini, N.; Martini, D. The Nutritional Quality of Organic and Conventional Food Products Sold in Italy: Results from the Food Labelling of Italian Products (FLIP) Study. *Nutrients* **2020**, *12*, 1273. [CrossRef]
40. Annunziata, A.; Vecchio, R. Organic Farming and Sustainability in Food Choices: An Analysis of Consumer Preference in Southern Italy. *Agric. Agric. Sci. Procedia* **2016**, *8*, 193–200. [CrossRef]
41. Capitello, R.; Sirieix, L. Consumers' Perceptions of Sustainable Wine: An Exploratory Study in France and Italy. *Economies* **2019**, *7*, 33. [CrossRef]
42. We Are Social. Report Digital 2020: I Dati Global. Available online: https://wearesocial.com/it/blog/2020/01/report-digital-2020-i-dati-global (accessed on 31 October 2020).
43. Murphy, G.; Corcoran, C.; Tatlow-Golden, M.; Boyland, E.; Rooney, B. See, Like, Share, Remember: Adolescents' Responses to Unhealthy-, Healthy- and Non-Food Advertising in Social Media. *Int. J. Environ. Res. Public Health* **2020**, *17*, 2181. [CrossRef] [PubMed]
44. Simeone, M.; Scarpato, D. Sustainable Consumption: How Does Social Media Affect Food Choices? *J. Clean. Prod.* **2020**, *277*, 124036. [CrossRef]
45. Demestichas, K.; Remoundou, K.; Adamopoulou, E. Food for Thought: Fighting Fake News and Online Disinformation. *IT Prof.* **2020**, *22*, 28–34. [CrossRef]
46. Castellini, G.; Savarese, M.; Graffigna, G. I Consumatori Preda Delle Fake News Agro-Alimentari: Un Identikit Psicologico. *Micro Macro Mark.* **2020**, *2*, 433–445. [CrossRef]
47. Menozzi, D.; Nguyen, T.T.; Sogari, G.; Taskov, D.; Lucas, S.; Castro-Rial, J.L.S.; Mora, C. Consumers' Preferences and Willingness to Pay for Fish Products with Health and Environmental Labels: Evidence from Five European Countries. *Nutrients* **2020**, *12*, 2650. [CrossRef]

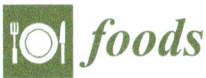

Article

Development and Validation of the Perceived Authenticity Scale for Cheese Specialties with Protected Designation of Origin

Katia Laura Sidali [1,*], Roberta Capitello [1] and Akhsa Joanne Taridaasi Manurung [2]

1 Department of Business Administration, University of Verona, via Cantarane, 24 1, 37129 Verona, Italy; roberta.capitello@univr.it
2 Marketing of Food and Agricultural Products Faculty of Agricultural Economics, G-A University of Goettingen, Platz der Goettinger Sieben 5, 37073 Goettingen, Germany; akhsamanurung@yahoo.de
* Correspondence: katialaura.sidali@univr.it; Tel.: +39-0458028592

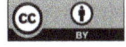

Citation: Sidali, K.L.; Capitello, R.; Manurung, A.J.T. Development and Validation of the Perceived Authenticity Scale for Cheese Specialties with Protected Designation of Origin. *Foods* **2021**, *10*, 248. https://doi.org/10.3390/foods10020248

Received: 31 December 2020
Accepted: 21 January 2021
Published: 26 January 2021

Publisher's Note: MDPI stays neutral with regard to jurisdictional claims in published maps and institutional affiliations.

Copyright: © 2021 by the authors. Licensee MDPI, Basel, Switzerland. This article is an open access article distributed under the terms and conditions of the Creative Commons Attribution (CC BY) license (https://creativecommons.org/licenses/by/4.0/).

Abstract: Authenticity has become increasingly important in the modern market as consumers seek products more resonant of tradition and originality. This study aimed to develop and validate a perceived authenticity scale for food specialties. Furthermore, this work exposed the causal relationship between authenticity and consumer behaviour, by quantitatively analysing the effects of perception of authenticity and identification with a product on consumers' willingness to consume the cheese Algovian Emmentaler, an iconic dairy product produced in southern Germany and protected with the designation of origin. Three surveys were conducted over two different timeframes. One served as a pre-test in Germany with a representative sample for the second two in Germany and Italy with a gourmet sample. Both objective authenticity and subjective authenticity were considered, with the former comprising concepts such as whether the respondent was sure of the cheese's origin and the latter what the cheese embodied. Identification with Algovian Emmentaler was also surveyed. Exploratory factor analysis and confirmatory factor analysis were conducted on the survey data in order to construct an authenticity scale. Based on this scale, structural equation models were constructed. Objective authenticity was found to positively contribute to stated willingness to consume, as well as mediate subjective authenticity, which itself mediated the effects of identification. Subjective authenticity was a large contributing factor to willingness to consume among German consumers, whereas the effects of objective authenticity were higher in Italy compared with the former. Expectedly, identification with Algovian Emmentaler also had a high direct effect on willingness to consume in Germany.

Keywords: authenticity scale; genuine; cheese specialty; country-of-origin labels; product identification; stated willingness to consume

1. Introduction

The increasing appeal of traditional, less sophisticated products among consumers on the marketplace has led to an increase in the significance of authenticity [1]. Many studies focusing explicitly on authenticity have been conducted across various domains, including tourism [2–4] wines, brands [5–9], business organization [10], advertising [5–11] and culture [12,13]. In the agrifood sector, worldwide interest in food-related issues is growing, making determining the origin of food of paramount importance [14,15]. According to Kuznesof et al. [16], the perceived authenticity of a product attributes by consumers applies above all to regional food. Moreover, Verbeke et al. [17] state that the perception of better product quality is one of the reasons for the consumption of specialty food that is often branded via quality labels or geographical indications (GIs) such as protected designation of origin (PDO) and protected geographical indication (PGI).

Furthermore, food safety issues, such as bovine spongiform encephalopathy (BSE), foot-and-mouth disease and malpractice among food producers have intensified public sensitivity regarding the origin of food. This has led to a surge in demand for high-quality products and desire for cultural identification [18]. There is, however, a gap in knowledge in various areas of research. Despite the number of studies on authenticity, very few focus on food marketing. This is particularly true for quantitative studies. To the best of our knowledge only a single study, conducted by Sidali and Hemmerling [19], has attempted to measure consumers' perceived authenticity of a specialty food, which was found to have a positive influence on stated consumption. No study to date has used a similar approach in a cross-country context. Therefore, this study attempts to fill this gap by quantitatively measuring customers' perceived authenticity of a German traditional specialty cheese in relation to their consumption of it. To achieve this, a perceived authenticity scale was developed using data from online surveys of gourmet consumers that were conducted during two different timeframes and in two different countries, namely Germany, where this cheese originates, and Italy, where lower knowledge of the product is compensated by a higher general culinary awareness. After the validity of the authenticity scale was verified, its effect on German and Italian respondents' stated willingness to consume the cheese was analysed.

Product authenticity is a keystone of modern marketing [19]. Spiggle et al. [7] observed that an authentic product comprehends the meaning and essence of the tradition it embodies. Authenticity can be treated as a unidimensional, bi-dimensional, or multidimensional construct, with consumers' desiring uniqueness [5,20,21], naturalness [15,20], country-specific origin [22] or credibility [5,23]. Liao and Ma [22] found that respondents with a high need for authenticity tend to associate it with six characteristics: (1) originality, (2) quality commitment and credibility, (3) heritage and style persistence, (4) scarceness, (5) sacredness and (6) purity. In her study on food authenticity and tourism, Sims [24] claims that consumers' demand for traditional and local food can also be viewed as linked to a quest for authenticity. Especially on holiday, the consumption of local food and drink products is a way of restoring a more meaningful sense of connection between the consumers and the people and places that produce their food [24]. Sidali and Hemmerling [25] suggest that the best way of surveying authenticity systematically is the multidimensional method. As such, a large number of studies distinguish between subjective authenticity and objective authenticity. The former depends on a consumer's personal experience with a product, to which a set of values is attached [16,21,23,26,27], as well as the social and environmental issues associated with sustainability, which includes supporting the local economy, fairly compensating local farmers and maintaining biodiversity [28]. Onozaka et al. [29] reported that purchasing behaviours were affected by the perceived availability of local food and perceived effectiveness of their actions, wherein customers believed that they made a difference in public outcomes, such as supporting the local economy. Contrary to subjective authenticity, perceived objective authenticity regards the physical attributes of the product and the production method, whether it is the traditionality of the recipe, the provenance of the ingredients, or the combination of soil and climatic conditions that are peculiar to the production area. Grayson and Martinec [30] recognized physical attributes as indexical authenticity. Moreover, Carcea et al. [15] stated that the perception of food authenticity is important at the emotional level because of the involvement of trust in the buying decision. Tradition and identity also play an important role in how food authenticity is perceived, as part of what makes it authentic is the traditional methods used. Research on perceived authenticity has largely succeeded in matching the challenges presented by consumer demand for original products. The tourism sector, for example, has benefited significantly. Unfortunately, there is little empirical evidence to support the bi-dimensionality of (subjective and objective) authenticity in the food sector. Thus, in contrast to what happened in the study of other topics or in other economic sectors, there exists no psychometrically validated measurement scales that is consistent with the theory of authenticity as a bi-dimensional construct. Therefore, the purpose of this study is to address this issue by developing and validating a measurement of consumers' views of authenticity of traditional cheese specialties and to analyse both its antecedent, i.e., identification with the product, and its consequence, namely how it affects stated-willingness to consume.

2. Research Framework

The central role of identification with a product is often espoused in marketing literature. Lunardo and Guerinet [6] suggest that the relevance of a product depends on whether it is able to trigger its consumption by projecting the consumer's personality. Furthermore, identity refers to upbringing, beliefs, stories, cultural ways of living and conceptions of what the product is to be [26]. Based on these factors, we postulate that (Figure 1):

Hypothesis 1 (H1). *The higher the identification with a product, the higher the subjective authenticity.*

Hypothesis 2 (H2). *The higher the identification with a product, the higher the objective authenticity.*

Hypothesis 3 (H3). *The higher the identification with a product, the higher the stated willingness to consume.*

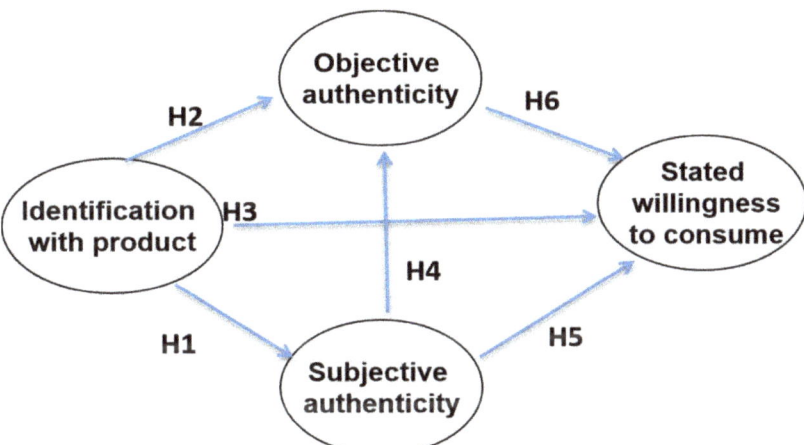

Figure 1. Research hypotheses.

Based on Marsden [30], we also state that food is not simply a commodity, but a social construct, as well. As a consequence, this social construct reinforces the mental images of the perceived product's setting, such as place, method of production, quality and time, among consumers. Thus, our fourth hypothesis is:

Hypothesis 4 (H4). *The higher the subjective authenticity elicited by a product, the higher the perceived objective authenticity.*

According to Bemporad and Baranowski [31], consumers reward producers of authentic products by displaying a preference for these products. Moreover, Langen [27] proposes that social and environmental issues related to sustainably produced food can affect consumers' decision-making. Therefore, we assume that authenticity has a positive impact on stated consumption behaviour. This leads us to hypotheses five and six:

Hypothesis 5 (H5). *The higher the subjective authenticity elicited by a product, the higher the stated willingness to consume.*

Hypothesis 6 (H6). *The higher the objective authenticity elicited by a product, the higher the stated willingness to consume.*

3. Methodology

3.1. The Research Steps

The scale construction and assessment techniques employed in this study follow those advocated by Gerbing and Anderson [32], Byrne [33], Homburg and Giering [34] and Brunsø et al. [35]. A seven-step procedure was implemented. The first step involved a review of the literature which led to the generation of a pool of items. The second step involved expert validation and the subsequent cleansing of some statements. A group of three experts in food marketing was asked to evaluate the accuracy of the items. They needed to reflect the factors of subjective and objective authenticity, identification with a traditional food specialty and stated willingness to consume. As a result of this step, the number of items included in the initial version of the measurement instrument was reduced. In the third step, the reduced measurement instrument was pre-tested. The survey was conducted in Germany in December 2012 with 136 German consumers. A private marketing research panel provider recruited the participants using three quotas in order to achieve a sample which was representative of the German population in the following aspects: age, gender and income. In the fourth step, we conducted an exploratory factor analysis (EFA) for assessing and optimizing the measurement model. This led to the further cleansing of some items and the introduction of new ones. In the fifth step, the cross-country study took place in Germany and in Italy. Since we strived for samples of consumers of traditional specialty foods, we applied the following filtering questions: (1) only respondents who consume cheese at least once a month were chosen and (2) we selected those respondents that declared, on a scale from 1 (never) to 5 (very often), to at least sometimes buy food from a specialty store, such as organic and farm shops, or delicatessens. Both the pre-test, as well as the 2013 questionnaire, were designed in German. The Italian version of the questionnaire was checked against the German version by translation and back translation by Italian and German native speaking researchers. As far as data collection is concerned, this step computed 220 complete responses, with a completion rate of 90.16% in Germany and 273 complete responses with a completion rate 90.75% in Italy. However, the total number of valid replies was 208 for the German survey and 200 for the Italian study, as survey responses finished in less than four minutes were cut off as untrustworthy. In the sixth step, we conducted an exploratory factor analysis for both the German and the Italian sample and compared the factor solutions across and within the samples. Finally, in the seventh step, we ran the final model, by means of confirmatory factor analysis (CFA), and we compared results across the German and the Italian sample by testing for cross-cultural validity of the scale measurement (Figure 2).

In all three surveys, respondents were asked to evaluate the two dimensions (subjective and objective) of authenticity concerning the PDO cheese Algovian Emmentaler (AE). AE is a well-known cheese made from the raw milk of cows that have been fed with grass and hay from the Algovian region in southern Germany. The decision to choose a traditional cheese as the object of our research is manifold: firstly, cheese belongs to the category Dairy Products, and dairy plays a fundamental role in the nutritional habits of Europeans [36]. Secondly, cheeses are the most represented traditional food speciality protected with the PDO label in Europe (http://ec.europa.eu/agriculture/quality/door/list.html?locale=de). Finally, this cheese specialty had almost disappeared during the 1990s due to the rapid increase in availability of the industrialized Emmentaler cheese, which is made with pasteurized milk [37,38]. Consequently, the production of Algovian Emmentaler is more expensive, due to the extra costs implicit in the artisanal mode of production. The PDO certification scheme helped Algovian Emmentaler producers to sell at a premium price and, in this way, to keep on producing it.

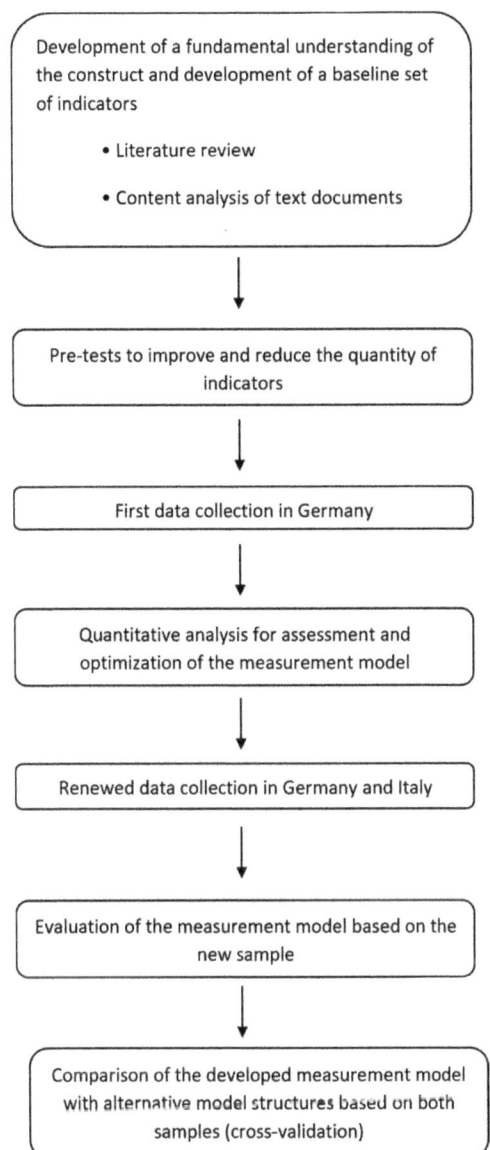

Figure 2. The research steps.

3.2. The Questionnaire

The questionnaire used in the surveys had four components: (a) perceived objective authenticity (methods of production, ingredients and origin of ingredients), (b) perceived subjective authenticity (idealization of agrarian life, solidarity with farmers and respect for natural biodiversity), (c) identification with the product (the potential of the product to elicit projective attributes in the consumer's personality) and d) overall stated willingness to buy the cheese or to purchase it again (only one item). The questions were supplemented with a picture of the AE cheese. Being an artisanal product, the cheese was shown without packaging, as it is usually sold in delicatessen stores. However, the picture of the cheese was complemented by the red label of the PDO as is mandated by European regulation regarding geographical indications which obliges retailers to expose the labelling next to the products [39].

4. Results

4.1. Sample Description

Three online surveys were conducted, with the first taking place in December 2012 and comprising a panel of 136 German consumers. Three quotas were used to achieve a representative sample (Table 1): age, gender and income. Respondent ages ranged from 18 to 82, with an average of 49 years of age. In terms of gender, 48% of the respondents were male while 52% were female. Meanwhile, respondent incomes ranged from ca. €900 a month to over €4501. Using a 5-point scale ranging from 1 (never) to 5 (very often), mean cheese consumption was 3.06, showing a modest consumption of Algovian Emmentaler. However, after reading a description of Algovian Emmentaler, mean interest in purchasing it ("I'm going to buy this cheese in the future") was higher, 3.96 with 1 meaning "strongly disagree", 3 meaning "neither" and 5 meaning "fully agree to". This survey served as a pre-test for the next cross-country survey that took place in Germany and Italy with samples of gourmet consumers. The two surveys were executed by a provider of survey panellists from 3 September 2013 to 9 September 2013. The total number of valid responses was 208 in the German sample and 200 in the Italian sample. The demographics of these German and Italian respondents are presented in Table 1.

Table 1. Socio-demographics of the pre-test (n = 136), German (n = 208), and Italian (n = 200) samples.

Variable	Survey Response	Pre-Test Survey (% unless Otherwise Stated)	German Survey (%)	Italian Survey (%)
Gender	Female	52	47.6	46.4
	Male	48	52.4	53.6
Age	<50	47.5	46.2	48.8
	51–70	42.6	45.2	47.4
	71 or older	9.6	8.6	3.8
	Average age, years	49	53	50.6
Household composition	1 member	30.1	21.2	10.5
	2 members	41.9	44.7	28.7
	3 members	15.4	16.8	29.7
	4 or more members	12.5	17.3	31.1
Monthly income per household	Less than €900	13.9	3.4	7.2
	€900–€1500	25.5	15.4	18.2
	€1501–€2000	16.1	15.9	22.5
	€2001–€3200	24.5	33.2	26.8
	€3201–€4500	12.0	23.1	17.2
	€4501 or more	8.0	9.1	8.1

The majority of German respondents (14.4%) were located in the German state of Baden-Württemberg, followed by 12% located in the German state of Bavaria and 7.7% in Berlin (data not shown). In contrast to the pre-test, in the German gourmet sample 47.8% were female and 52.4% were male. Similarly, in the Italian sample, 46.4% of the respondents were female while 53.6% were male. The majority of them (24.9%) were located in the region of Lombardy, followed by 11% who were located in the region of Campania and 7.2% in the region of Lazio. Average ages were also similar between the two countries; 53 years old in the German sample and 50.6 years old in the Italian one, with the youngest respondent being 30 and the oldest being 81 years old. In terms of monthly household income, in both samples dominated the income ranges between ca. €2001 and €3200.

4.2. Scale Construction: Exploratory and Confirmatory Factor Analyses

4.2.1. Exploratory Factor Analyses

Separate exploratory factor analyses (EFA) with principal component analyses and Varimax rotations were carried out for each sample. The aim of this procedure was to check whether items would tend to group together in similar factors across the three samples, which then led to the rejection of some items. Appendix A presents the items obtained through the EFA and how they loaded on the respective factor in each of the three samples, showing in bold which items were used in the confirmatory factor analysis (CFA) that followed. Regarding objective authenticity, items 1–4 showed constantly loading values higher than five both across time (in the pre-test of 2012 and German survey of 2013) and across countries (Germany and Italy). The item "Algovian Emmentaler comes from the best-known country in the world for the production of this type of cheese" was introduced after the pre-test, so its loading was only calculated for the cross-country surveys, while another item was loaded in a different factor. Interestingly, items 5–11 displayed consistent patterns only in the pre-test but not in the second pair of surveys with gourmet consumers. Therefore, they were not kept for further analysis. Concerning subjective authenticity, items 1–5 also showed consistent loading values higher than five across time, while items 6–9 displayed no clear pattern and were thus not further considered for the CFA. In terms of identification, items 1–4 were used for the following CFA, whereas items 5–8 were excluded. However, two items in the identification factor were only introduced after the pre-test: "The consumption of this product contributes to the improvement of my wellbeing" and "This cheese is the pride of a culture with which I can identify myself." All in all, three factors were identified that appeared to be constant across the three samples: objective authenticity, subjective authenticity and identification. As shown in the next section, those items with loadings consistently high in all three samples were combined into scales.

4.2.2. Confirmatory Factor Analyses

Originally, there were 33 indicators spread over five factors. Following the EFA, this number was narrowed down to 13 indicators in three factors (Table 2).

The objective authenticity factor contained four items, two of which referred to the traditional method of production and the region of production. The latter is particularly important, as it indicates not only the origin of the specialty's ingredients but its reputation, as well, which is a fundamental requisite when obtaining protected labels of designation of origin.

Subjective authenticity contained five items highlighting the social and economic sustainability values attached to the product, such as feeling close to the producers, allowing the producer to express themselves, and supporting the region economically. Another item revealed consumers' idealization of niche products originating from rural areas, through their "moral purity" versus mass-produced products.

Finally, the identification factor consisted of four items disclosing how the consumer identifies with the product personally, symbolically, culturally and in terms of their wellbeing. Factors related to objective and subjective authenticity were found to share similar tendencies across all three samples. Both gourmet samples identified more with Algovian Emmentaler than the pre-test sample. Expectedly, the identification factor's values also scored higher among the German respondents, as the Italian respondents identified less with Algovian Emmentaler.

Table 2. Confirmatory factor analysis.

Factor	Item	Factor Loadings/Item Reliability		
		Pre-Test	Germany	Italy
Objective Authenticity	I can trust the name AE.	0.909/0.827	0.830/0.689	0.829/0.688
	AE cheese-makers are very oriented toward respect for tradition.	0.754/0.569	0.783/0.614	0.811/0.658
	AE comes from the best-known country in the world for the production of this type of cheese.	*	0.706/0.499	0.770/0.593
	I am sure that all the ingredients of this product come from the Algovian region.	0.716/0.512	-	0.723/0.523
Subjective Authenticity	AE makes me feel close to the producer.	0.756/0.571	0.789/0.622	0.841/0.708
	AE allows producers to charge fair prices.	0.742/0.550	0.763/0.582	0.758/0.575
	AE is the embodiment of moral purity.	0.790/0.624	0.813/0.660	0.749/0.560
	AE allows the cheese-makers to express themselves and be creative.	0.760/0.577	0.731/0.534	0.766/0.587
	AE supports the region economically.	0.773/0.598	0.722/0.521	0.654/0.428
Identification	This cheese fits my lifestyle and the way I shop.	0.902/0.814	0.884/0.782	0.808/0.653
	The consumption of this product contributes to the improvement of my wellbeing.	*	0.793/0.629	0.873/0.763
	This cheese is the pride of a culture with which I can identify myself.	*	0.842/0.709	0.779/0.607
	I can identify with this cheese.	0.758/0.575	0.879/0.773	0.816/0.666
Intention to consume	I will definitely (continue to) eat Algovian Emmentaler in the future.	-/0.59	-/0.35	-/0.47

AE = Algovian Emmentaler cheese * = Item was not given in the pre-test; - = Item did not load on the same factor. Sources of items: Objective authenticity, 1. based on Liao and Ma [22], 2. based on Beverland [5], 3. based on Camus [40], 4. own item; subjective authenticity, 1. and 2. own item, 3. based on Liao and Ma [22], 4. and 5. own item; identification, 1. based on Grunert et al. [41], 2. based on Davis [42], 3. based on Carstensen [43], 4. based on Camus [40]; intention to consume: own item (for one-item statements only item reliabilities are calculated).

Confirmatory factor analysis was conducted using the software AMOS 21. CFA indicates a special case of the general model of causal analysis, which is identified in more precise formulation as covariance structure analysis [34]. A complete causal analysis model consists of two components:

- The measurement model:

Through confirmatory factor analysis, it shows how the indicators explain the latent variables (factors).

- The structural model:

With the help of structural equation analysis, it shows the explanation of the exogenous variables by the endogenous latent variables (factors).

Furthermore, Ref. [41] demonstrated that CFA can be used to determine whether a set of data is compatible with a pre-specified factor structure. It can also be applied to multiple samples, and then used to confirm whether the factor structure in each sample is the same. This allows the reliability of a factor to be examined, as well as how well it is measured together with its associated indicators [34]. In the present case, all the factors had good factor reliability (FR), i.e., composite reliability, and average variance extracted (AVE) values (FR: > 0.6 and AVE: > 0.5), as is found in Table 3.

Table 3. Composite reliability.

Factor	Factor Reliability/AVE		
	Pre-Test	Germany	Italy
Objective Authenticity	0.84/0.64	0.83/0.56	0.86/0.62
Subjective Authenticity	0.88/0.58	0.88/0.58	0.87/0.57
Identification	0.82/0.69	0.91/0.72	0.89/0.67

In covariance-based structural equation modelling the adequacy of the model is measured by a range of goodness-of-fit criteria (see Table 4). Using different indices is considered by many scholars the best strategy to overcome the limitations of each index [33,34].

Table 4. Model fit (measurement and structural equation models).

Survey	Model Fit					
	Cmin/DF	CFI	RMSEA	GFI	NFI	TLI
Pre-Test	1.036	0.998	0.016	0.946	0.953	0.998
Germany	2.353	0.941	0.081	0.883	0.902	0.927
Italy	1.420	0.980	0.046	0.929	0.936	0.976
Cut-off criteria	1–3	0.90–0.95	≤0.05 very good ≤0.08 good	0.90–0.95	0.90–0.95	0.90–0.95

Legend: Cmin/DF = Chi-Squared/Degrees of Freedom; CFI = Comparative Fit Index; RMSEA = Root Mean Square Error of Approximation; GFI = Goodness-of-Fit Index; NFI = Normed Fit Index; TLI = Tucker–Lewis Index.

The overall fit met the conventional cutoff-criteria in all three samples [34]. Furthermore, the best scores in terms of Root Mean Square Error of Approximation (RMSEA) and Goodness-of-Fit Index (GFI) were those displayed in the pre-test and the Italian samples. On the contrary, the German sample scored best with regards to the Comparative Fit Index (CFI) and the Tucker–Lewis Index (TLI).

4.2.3. Structural Equation Model

Using the validated authenticity scale produced by the confirmatory analysis and the identification factor, evidence was found of the influence of consumers' perceptions of authenticity and identification with a specialty product on their purchasing intentions. Furthermore, using the software AMOS 21, identical models were built based on the two samples obtained by the cross-country surveys (Germany and Italy). The robustness of the theoretical framework was tested with covariance-based structural equation modelling (SEM). According to Byrne [33], the RMSEA is one of the most informative criteria in assessing the fit of the structural equation model. As already shown in Table 4, both the Italian and the German sample had adequate RMSEA scores (0.046 vs. 0.081, respectively) when judged based on the recommended cut-off criteria (values less than 0.05 indicate good fit, and values as high as 0.08 represent reasonable errors of approximation in the population. Whilst RMSEA values ranging from 0.08 to 0.10 are still acceptable, those greater than 0.10 indicate poor fit).

Both German and Italian models comprised one exogenous latent variable (identification with the product) and three endogenous latent variables (subjective and objective authenticity, as well as stated willingness to consume).

4.2.4. Outlook

Identification with Algovian Emmentaler directly accounted for 26% of the explained variance of the subjective authenticity in Germany and 62% in Italy (Figure 3). Subjective authenticity was directly responsible for the majority of objective authenticity's variation in both samples, albeit more so in the German sample's case (60%) than in the Italian sample (29%). Finally, objective authenticity-together with identification-explained 47% of the variation of the stated willingness to consume in the Italian sample, followed by 35% in the German one.

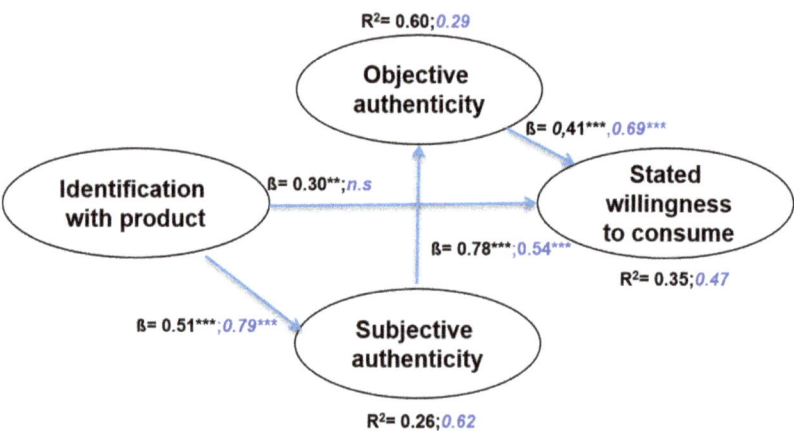

Figure 3. Results of the two structural equation models; *** = $p < 0.001$, ** = $p < 0.01$, n.s. = non statistically significant.

The hypotheses were tested by examining the sign, size and statistical significance of the structural coefficients. The hypotheses regarding the relationship among the constructs tested in the final model were partially accepted in both models. In the following, only direct effects are taken into consideration. The parameter estimates for the relationship between identification and subjective authenticity were statistically significant and consistent with the proposed direction of our first hypothesis (H1) in both the German and Italian samples (ß = 0.51 *** and ß = 0.79 ***, respectively). However, this does not hold true for the effect of identification on objective authenticity—H2 was rejected in both samples.

In terms of the relationship between subjective authenticity and objective authenticity, the path coefficient was statistically significant and consistent with the proposed direction of our fourth hypothesis. H4 was accepted in both samples, with ß = 0.78 *** in the German sample and ß = 0.54 in the Italian sample. Contrarily, the effect of subjective authenticity on the stated willingness to consume (H5) was not statistically significant in either of the two samples, and thus not accepted. Objective authenticity's effect on stated willingness to consume was relatively strong and statistically significant in both Germany and Italy (ß = 0.41 *** and ß = 0.69 ***, respectively; H6 was accepted). Finally, the expected effect of identification on the stated willingness to consume was significant and positive in Germany (ß = 0.30 **), but not in Italy; therefore, H3 was accepted in the German sample and not accepted in the Italian sample. The latter's rejection is expected considering Algovian Emmentaler's origin is outside of Italy.

Overall, the subjective dimensions of authenticity were found to be consistently higher in Germany than in Italy. This, along with the high direct effect of identification, could be interpreted as a higher emotional anchorage of consumers in Germany with "their" food specialty compared with the Italian sample. Conversely, the effects of the objective dimensions of authenticity on stated willingness to consume were higher in Italy, which may be caused by the country's more developed culinary culture and the generally higher knowledge of GIs. In a nutshell, both models explained significant amounts of the variation in the endogenous variables.

5. Discussion

The objective of this research was to build an authenticity scale of traditional cheese specialties and we tested it in two regions that are positioning themselves as food destinations in Germany and in Italy. Another goal of this work was to explore the effect of customers' perception of authenticity—whether it is perceived subjective authenticity or objective authenticity—and their identification with a product on their stated willingness to consume it, as well as how this effect varies across countries. Using a sample of consumers of specialty foods from the above-mentioned countries, the findings of our model generally showed that objective and subjective authenticity as well as identification with a product affected stated willingness to consume. Objective authenticity had a direct influence on stated willingness to consume in both countries. This was also a mediator of subjective authenticity, while the latter was a mediator of the effect of identification on objective authenticity. Unsurprisingly, only in the German sample did respondents' identification with Algovian Emmentaler have a direct effect on their stated willingness to consume it.

This finding confirms previous literature. For instance, several studies showed that consumers prefer products that reflect their actual or desired personality [44–46]. Niinimaki [47] affirmed that consumers continuously construct their identity through the consumption of products that reflect their personality. In this sense, a person's identification with the profile of green consumers positively influences his/her intention to purchase environmentally friendly products [48,49]. As such, being a German specialty, the sample of German consumers could identify with this cheese, but not the Italian one, although both samples considered the cheese specialty to be authentic. Furthermore, being held across two different timeframes and with a cross-country design, our scale seems to suggest that a bi-dimensional construct might be a suitable means to measure authenticity".

While the proposed model shows that subjective authenticity is clearly linked to consumers' ethical and sustainability-related attributes (Table 2), objective authenticity displays a direct and measurable effect on the stated intention to consume the food specialty. As mentioned before, the construct of objective-authenticity consists of items that range from respect for the tradition, to the unique connection of the product with the place of origin (Table 2). Thus, this dimension reflects the rationale of country-of-origin labels such as PDO, Slow Food, etc., which identify a food with its origin and link food quality with its geographical environment, including natural and human factors [39]. In line with the results of Sidali and Hemmerling [25], this finding shows once again the reassuring importance of food claims on credence attributes of food.

Modern consumers purchase foods from certified sources in order to access high-quality foods and to contribute to environmental and society-friendly agriculture. However, as remarked by De Haen and Réquillart [50], an important precondition for consumers to express their preferences for food from sustainable production is availability of objective information about the product and about process quality. Hence, policy intervention is called for to find a balance between the right of consumers to be adequately informed, and in this way reduce their food illiteracy, and the right of the different stakeholders along the food supply chain to run their businesses with the right amount of 'entrepreneurial freedom' [50]. In other words, on the one hand, farmers and/or processors are already overtasked by burdensome rules and standards, to the extent that it appears unrealistic to expect them to accept further rules or certification schemes [50], but on the other hand, many scholars agree on the necessity of investing in equity and sustainability in modern agricultural systems as a moral societal task [51].

It is the opinion of the authors that country-of-origin such as PDO and PGI seem to be effective means of conveying and reinforcing ethical and sustainability-related values, as well as promoting best practices among agricultural food systems. GIs stem from the necessity of reducing moral hazards in the way food is produced and consumed when traded in the international marketplace, thus protecting both producers and consumers from counterfeiting and fraud. As mentioned earlier in our study, governmental support towards such specific certification schemes was successful in the past in helping those producers who could not, or did not want to, opt for a product reformulation (pasteurized milk instead of raw milk; forage instead of hay)—a recognized business practice of the food industry, [51]—and enabled the emergence of long-term societal benefits with regard to both product quality and consumer empowerment.

Furthermore, governmental support towards such schemes helps counterbalance the downstream shift in the drivers of product differentiation, to the benefit of upstream producers, as is shown in the case of wine production by [50]. A targeted and exemplary policy to increase GI schemes has been offered through a piece of legislation in Italy. In order to boost regional gastronomy, farms offering agrotourism are called upon to offer mostly locally produced food products to their guests. Furthermore, to promote Italian regional gastronomic traditions, the law recommends the provision of foods with protected quality names such as PDO and PGI. In order to obtain 'new relationships between agriculture and society' [52], policy-makers need to facilitate the promotion of alternative food supply chains, even if this means a rethinking of those food policies of Western governments that have aimed to keep food prices low at all costs. The cost of tracking food specialties is higher compared to the cost of producing a "placeless" product [53]. However, the statistically significant effect of perceived authenticity on stated willingness to consume displayed in our model indicates that consumers of traditional food specialties are ready to pay a higher cost, if they perceive these products as authentic. This is also reflected in the literature: on average consumers honour producers' higher costs by paying a higher premium that can range from an average of 21% [54] to up to 300% [53], for a specialty with a country-of-origin label. At an aggregated level, this means an empowerment of consumers who are less distant from the locus of food production, as well as a redistribution of profits along the food chain from those who sell on a large scale to those who grow the food [51].

6. Conclusions

Prior studies have documented the importance of analysing the potential perception of food products and have called for more work to analyse the communication of food distinctiveness in both qualitative and quantitative ways [55]. In this article, the authors have built an authenticity scale of food specialties using a cross-country design and have tested the scale in two different timeframes in order to facilitate the comparison of results. The findings of this study will be helpful for producers of certified foods by helping them to improve their understanding of consumers' specific views on authenticity, along with which dimensions of authenticity—subjective or objective authenticity—most strongly affect their stated willingness to consume specialty products. These findings also provide a basis for marketing strategies that emphasize the origins of products and can help policy-makers to develop national food policies. As an avenue for future research, it would be interesting to analyse whether the proposed scale of perceived authenticity also holds true for other categories of traditional food specialties such as fresh fruits and vegetables or meat products. This study does contain limitations as well. Although traditional food specialties are at the heart of European Union initiatives in the food sector, rural areas host even richer homemade, local and varied produce, which has been neglected by the authors in this current study. To survey consumer understanding of such embedded, often artisanal food, the current work could have integrated the authenticity scale with qualitative research designed to unearth different levels of awareness of such products among consumers. This would have provided the reader with a more complete picture of consumers' cognitive and affective dimensions of territorialized food. All in all, the proposed scale is a departure point for further research. The authors are aware that the validity of the current work remains in the hands of the research community who may replicate this instrument and further define the extent of appropriateness of this measure for future studies on authenticity in the food sector.

Author Contributions: All three authors conceived and designed the article; K.L.S. is responsible for the introduction, study case, data analysis and conclusion; R.C. contributed to the overall structure of the study and data analysis; A.J.T.M. is responsible for the overall conception and the data analysis. All authors have read and agreed to the published version of the manuscript.

Funding: The authors are covering the costs to publish in open access.

Conflicts of Interest: The authors declare no conflict of interest. "The funding sponsors had no role in the design of the study; in the collection, analyses, or interpretation of data; in the writing of the manuscript, and in the decision to publish the results".

Abbreviations

The following abbreviations are used in this manuscript:

SEM	Structural Equation Modelling
PDO	Protected Denomination of Origin
PGI	Protected Geographical Indication
GIs	Geographical Indications
Cmin/DF	Chi-Squared/Degrees of Freedom
CFI	Comparative Fit Index
RMSEA	Root Mean Square Error of Approximation
GFI	Goodness-of-Fit Index
NFI	Normed Fit Index
TLI	Tucker–Lewis Index
PDO	Protected Designation of Origin

Appendix A

Exploratory factor analysis. Items in bold were used in the confirmatory factor analysis described in the article, while the others were excluded.

Factor	Item	Pre-Test	Germany	Italy
Objective Authenticity	I can trust the name AE.	-	0.733	0.775
	AE cheese-makers are very oriented toward respect for tradition.	0.581	0.701	0.799
	AE comes from the best-known country in the world for the production of this type of cheese.	*	0.696	0.765
	I am sure that all the ingredients of this product come from the Algovian region.	0.775	0.656	0.738

Factor	Item	Pre-Test	Germany	Italy
	AE cheese-makers are not mass-production companies.	-	0.625	0.574
	I can imagine where this cheese was produced.	0.742	-	-
	I can imagine how this cheese is produced.	0.712	-	#
	I am certain that this cheese is produced using traditional methods.	0.720	#	#
	I am certain that the quality of this product is above average.	0.702	#	-
	This cheese does not seem to contain artificial additives.	0.588	#	-
	I am certain of the origin of this product.	0.578	#	-
	AE makes me feel close to the producer.	0.616	0.805	0.836
	AE allows producers to charge fair prices.	0.622	0.713	0.784
	AE is the embodiment of moral purity.	0.646	0.677	0.745
	AE allows the cheese-makers to express themselves and be creative.	0.512	0.588	0.743
Subjective Authenticity	AE supports the region economically.	0.775	0.767	0.576
	AE is trustworthy	0.720	0.774	#
	AE tastes like all of the "earlier" products and is certainly better than conventional products	#	0.734	#
	AE is traditionally hand-made.	0.722	0.714	#
	This cheese protects the biodiversity of the Algovian region	0.660	#	-
	This cheese fits my lifestyle and the way I shop.	0.788	0.840	#
	The consumption of this product contributes to the improvement of my wellbeing.	*	0.839	#
Identification	This cheese is the pride of a culture with which I can identify myself.	*	0.782	#
	I can identify with this cheese.	0.750	0.811	#

Factor	Item	Pre-Test	Germany	Italy
	AE makes me smile because it is a product from my childhood.	#	0.709	#
	It doesn't bother me that the taste of this cheese can vary from day to day like any other product made by hand.	0.605	0.590	-
	I find this cheese particularly attractive because you cannot find it in any store.	0.750	#	0.824
	This cheese expresses who I am.	-	#	-

Legend: Allgäuer Emmentaler = Algovian Emmentaler. * Item was not given in the pre-test. - Item did not load on same factor. # Item loaded to more than one factor or displayed loading < 0.5. Stated intention to consume Algovian Cheese was measured by the following statement: I will definitely (continue to) eat Allgäuer Emmentaler in the future.

References

1. Carroll, G.R.; O'Connor, K. Socially constructed authenticity and consumer choice: Empirical tests of an organizational theory. In Proceedings of the Annual Meeting of the Academy of Management, Boston, MA, USA, 3–7 August 2012.
2. Cohen, E. Authenticity and commoditization in tourism. *Ann. Tour. Res.* **1988**, *15*, 371–386. [CrossRef]
3. Wang, N. Rethinking Authenticity in Tourism Experience. *Ann. Tour. Res.* **1999**, *26*, 349–370. [CrossRef]
4. Olsen, S.O. Comparative evaluation and the relationship between quality, satisfaction, and repurchase loyalty. *J. Acad. Mark. Sci.* **2002**, *30*, 240–249. [CrossRef]
5. Beverland, M.B. Crafting brand authenticity: The case of luxury wines. *J. Manag. Stud.* **2005**, *42*, 1003–1029. [CrossRef]
6. Lunardo, R.; Guerinet, R. The Influence of Label on Wine Consumption: Its Effects on Young Consumers' Perception of Authenticity and Purchasing Behavior. In Proceedings of the EAAE Seminar "International Marketing and International Trade of Quality Food Products", Bologna, Italy, 8–10 March 2007. Available online: http://ageconsearch.umn.edu/bitstream/7847/1/cp070005.pdf (accessed on 23 January 2017).
7. Spiggle, S.; Nguyen, H.T.; Caravella, M. More than Fit: Brand Extension Authenticity. *J. Mark. Res.* **2012**, *49*, 967–983. [CrossRef]
8. Newman, G.E.; Dhar, R. Authenticity is contagious: Brand essence and the original source of production. *J. Mark. Res.* **2014**, *51*, 371–386. [CrossRef]
9. Schallehn, M.; Burmann, C.; Riley, N. Brand authenticity: Model development and empirical testing. *J. Prod. Brand Manag.* **2014**, *23*, 192–199. [CrossRef]
10. Skilton, P.F.; Purdy, J.M. Authenticity, power, and pluralism: A framework for understanding stakeholder evaluations of corporate social responsibility activities. *Bus. Ethics Q.* **2017**, *27*, 99–123. [CrossRef]
11. Stern, B. Authenticity and the textual persona: Postmodern paradoxes in advertising narrative. *Int. J. Res. Mark.* **1994**, *11*, 387–400. [CrossRef]
12. Leigh, T.W.; Peters, C.; Shelton, J. The consumer quest for authenticity: The multiplicity of meanings within the MG subculture of consumption. *Acad. Mark. Sci. J.* **2006**, *34*, 481–493. [CrossRef]
13. Neff, K.D.; Suizzo, M.-A. Culture, power, authenticity and psychological well-being within romantic relationships: A comparison of European American and Mexican Americans. *Cogn. Dev.* **2006**, *21*, 441–457. [CrossRef]
14. Kelly, S.; Heaton, K.; Hoogewerff, J. Tracing the geographical origin of food: The application of multi-element and multi_isotope analysis. *Trends Food Sci. Technol.* **2005**, *16*, 555–567. [CrossRef]
15. Carcea, M.; Brereton, P.; Hsu, R.; Kelly, S.; Marmiroli, N.; Melini, F.; Soukoulis, C.; Wenping, D. Food authenticity assessment: Ensuring compliance with food legislation and traceability requirements. *Qual. Assur. Saf. Crop. Foods* **2009**, *1*, 93–100. [CrossRef]
16. Kuznesof, S.; Tregear, A.; Moxey, A. Regional foods: A consumer perspective. *Br. Food J.* **1997**, *99*, 199–206. [CrossRef]
17. Verbeke, W.; Pieniak, Z.; Guerrero, L.; Hersleth, M. Consumers' Awareness and Attitudinal Determinants of European Union Quality Label Use on Traditional Foods". *Bio-Based Appl. Econ.* **2012**, *1*, 213–229.
18. McCluskey, J.J.; Loureiro, M.L. Consumer preferences and willingness to pay for food labelling: A discussion of empirical studies. *J. Food Distrib. Res.* **2003**, *34*, 95–102.
19. Brown, S.; Kozinets, R.V.; Sherry, J.F., Jr. Teaching old brands new tricks: Retro branding and the revival of brand meaning. *J. Mark.* **2003**, *67*, 19–33. [CrossRef]
20. Gilmore, J.H.; Pine, J.B. *Authenticity. What Consumers Really Want*; Harvard Business School Press: Boston, MA, USA, 2007.
21. Molleda, J.-C. Authenticity and the construct's dimensions in public relations and communication research. *J. Commun. Manag.* **2010**, *14*, 223–236. [CrossRef]
22. Liao, S.; Ma, Y.Y. Conceptualizing Consumer Need for Product Authenticity. *Int. J. Bus. Inf.* **2009**, *4*, 89–114.
23. Tregear, A.; Kuznesof, S.; Moxey, A. Policy initiatives for regional foods: Some insights from consumer research. *Food Policy* **1998**, *23*, 383–394. [CrossRef]

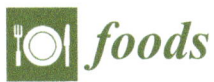

Article

Study of the Influence of Sociodemographic and Lifestyle Factors on Consumption of Dairy Products: Preliminary Study in Portugal and Brazil

Raquel P. F. Guiné [1], Sofia G. Florença [2,*], Solange Carpes [3] and Ofélia Anjos [4,5]

1. CERNAS Research Centre, Polytechnic Institute of Viseu, 3504-510 Viseu, Portugal; raquelguine@esav.ipv.pt
2. Faculty of Food and Nutrition Sciences, University of Porto, 4200-465 Porto, Portugal
3. Department of Chemistry, Federal University of Technology—Paraná (UTFPR), 85503-390 Pato Branco, Brazil; carpes@utfpr.edu.br
4. Polytechnic Institute of Castelo Branco, 6001-909 Castelo Branco, Portugal; ofelia@ipcb.pt
5. Forest Research Centre, School of Agriculture, University of Lisbon, 1349-017 Lisbon, Portugal
* Correspondence: sofiaguine@gmail.com

Received: 27 October 2020; Accepted: 26 November 2020; Published: 30 November 2020

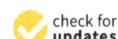

Abstract: Sociodemographic characteristics, including regional variations, have been associated with different food consumption patterns. Behavioral factors and lifestyle variables may also contribute to different food dietary trends. In this way, the present study intended to investigate the consumption habits of the most relevant types of dairy products around the world and relate them to sociodemographic factors, for example, age, sex, education and country as well as with some anthropometric and behavioral aspects, for example, body mass index, satisfaction with body weight and exercise or sedentary lifestyles. One other objective of the study was to categorize the lifestyles of the participants, according to measured variables linked with hours of inactivity or exercise, in order to use these as possible differentiating variables for the consumption of dairy products. The study involved a questionnaire survey undertaken on a non-probabilistic convenience sample of participants from Portugal (PT) and Brazil (BR), and participation was voluntary and anonymous. The data analysis involved different statistical techniques: basic statistics, chi-square tests, factor analysis, cluster analysis and tree classification analysis. The results showed that semi skimmed milk is never consumed by about half of the participants (47.4% for PT and 46.7 for BR), and those numbers increase for skimmed (64.8% for PT and 50.9% for BR), chocolate flavored milk (82.6% for PT and 65.6% for BR) and enriched milks (94.8% for PT and 85.3% for BR). Cheeses are also consumed in the two countries by small numbers of people. The number of participants consuming imported cheeses in both countries was particularly low (only 4.0% consume these more than once a week in both countries), suggesting national products may be preferred. It was further observed that those who consume cheese do it seldom (once a week) or sometimes (2–3 times per week). Butter is also consumed by only about half of the adult population (43.8% for PT and 49.5% for BR), but the percentage of those who never consume butter increases for skimmed butter (66.0% for PT and 82.6% for BR) and unsalted butter (70.2% for PT and 69.1% for BR). The consumption of yogurts also follows similar low consumption patterns. The most frequently consumed yogurt types in Portugal are liquid (30.5% consume regularly) and natural yogurts (34.8% consume regularly), while in Brazil the most frequent are creamy fruit pulp yogurt (14.4% consume regularly), liquid (13.7% consume regularly) and Greek type yogurt (10.2% consume regularly). A factor analysis and a cluster analysis established groups according to lifestyles, as follows: 1—Screeners, 2—Exercisers, 3—Travelers and 4—Others. These lifestyles were found to be influential in the consumption of dairy products for all classes of dairy tested: milk, cheese, yogurt and butter. For example, the screeners were found to consume more milk, more butter, more cheese and more yogurt. Additionally, other influential factors were age, sex, education, BMI and satisfaction with body weight. Nevertheless, country was not a meaningfully discriminant variable in relation to the other variables included in the classification analysis. The results concluded that, despite some small differences in the patterns of consumption of dairy products in both countries, the levels of consumption of dairy products are extremely low, for all classes studied (milk, cheese, yogurt or butter). Additionally, it was concluded that some factors are influential on the level of consumption of dairy products, and therefore decision makers can plan their interventions according to the characteristics of the targeted segments of the population, according to lifestyle, age, sex, education, BMI and satisfaction with body weight.

Keywords: milk; cheese; butter; yogurt; questionnaire survey

1. Introduction

Dairy products are one of the basic food categories in human diets all over the world. These food products include milk and its derivatives, for example, butter, cheese, fermented milk and yoghurts. According to the Milk Market Observatory of the European Commission in October 2020 [1], in the European Union in the last 12 months there was an increase of 1.6% in the collection of cow's milk, a small decrease in the production of fermented milk by 0.6%, an increase of 1.4% in the production of cheese and an increase of 2.2% in the production of butter. The highest increase was observed for powdered whole milk at 5.6%. Regarding yogurt production in the 28 countries of the European Union, in 2019 8163 thousand tons of acidified milk products were produced, including yogurts and others [2]. Data reporting to the World production of the main dairy products issued by the Milk Market Observatory of the European Commission released in May 2020 [3] show that in the United States in 2019 5959 thousand tons of cheese and 904 thousand tons of butter were produced. The data further shows that the primary milk producer in 2019 was India (194,200 thousand tons), followed by the European Union (160,000 thousand tons) and the United States (99,155 thousand tons).

The consumption of dairy products is recommended by many organizations around the world due to their nutritional richness, and for that reason they are indicated for consumption throughout the entire life cycle, from infants to elderly [4,5].

Dairy products can contain high amounts of protein of high biological value, as well as vitamins (particularly the fat-soluble vitamins A and D and the B complex vitamins B_2—riboflavin and B_{12}—cobalamin) [6–9] and dietary minerals (such as calcium, phosphorus, sodium, magnesium, potassium and iodine) [10–12]. They also contain carbohydrates, especially in the form of lactose, which might be problematic for some consumers with lactose intolerance. However, people suffering from this pathology, which causes gastrointestinal malfunctioning, do not derive their symptoms exclusively form the consumption of dairy products, contrarily to popular belief, as discussed by Jansson-Knodell et al. [13]. Usual gastrointestinal symptoms that can appear after lactose ingestion in individuals with lactose intolerance include abdominal pain, diarrhea, flatulence and bloating [14]. Some people believe they have lactose intolerance when they in fact have not been diagnosed by a physician, and their gastrointestinal problems are derived from something other than lactose [13,15]. Nevertheless, those individuals who believe themselves to be lactose intolerant or who follow fashionable dietary trends tend to avoid milk and other related dairy products [15–17]. By avoiding the consumption of dairy products these individuals may suffer from insufficient basic nutrients, increasing the risk of certain health problems, for example, poor bone health, in turn increasing the risk for osteoporosis [14,18]. Besides, dairy products contain fat, part of which is saturated, a type of fat that has been associated with some health problems. However, this is not consensual because there are a large number of studies which have proven the contrary, i.e., that limiting dietary saturated fatty acid intake showed no benefits on cardiovascular disease and total mortality, while showing protective effects against stroke and high blood pressure [19,20]. Finally, dairy products also contain substances with physiologically active properties, such as antioxidants, oligosaccharides, probiotic bacteria, butyric acid, immunoglobulins and active peptides, which have been investigated for their beneficial roles in the human body [21–25].

Sociodemographic characteristics are usually associated with different food consumption patterns. Additionally, behavioral factors and lifestyle variables also contribute to different food dietary trends. For example, Khandpur et al. [26] found differences in the consumption of ultra-processed foods according to age, socioeconomic status, area of residence and geographical region but not gender. Riedeiger et al. [27] reported that female gender, household education and high income had a positive impact on fruit and vegetable consumption among adolescents. Nayga [28] reported sociodemographic influences on consumer concern about irradiated foods, or foods containing antibiotics, hormones and pesticides.

In the case of dairy products, Richter and Sanders [29] evaluated sociodemographic influences on the consumption of dairy products in Switzerland and concluded that age and income were important influencers for consumption of organically produced dairy products. Miftari et al. [30] investigated the role of demographic and socioeconomic factors on dairy product consumption in Kosovo and found that age, education, income, household size and number of children influenced consumption patterns. Shi et al. [31] reported that socio-economic status was strongly associated with consumption of milk in Chinese adolescents. Baek and Chitekwe [32] observed differences in the consumption of diverse foods, including dairy products, according to geographic location and income.

The consumption of dairy products may have a preventive role in some diseases that affect people all over the world, and therefore in Portugal and Brazil. One of the most recognized health benefits associated with the consumption of dairy products is the prevention of osteoporosis [33–35]. The study by Rodrigues et al. [36] aimed at characterizing the state of osteoporosis in post-menopausal women in Portugal and showed that 43% of them suffered from osteoporosis, leading to important healthcare consumption and treatment costs. In Brazil, according to Radominski et al. [37], the guidelines issued by the Osteoporosis and Osteo-metabolic Diseases Committee of the Brazilian Society of Rheumatology, in conjunction with the Brazilian Medical Association and other Societies, dictate that women over 50 should ingest up to 1200 mg of calcium per day, preferably in their diet, by consuming milk and dairy products. As far as we know, the consumption of dairy products in Portugal and Brazil have not been investigated, and therefore, this study was carried out to investigate people's consumption of dairy products and to what extent sociodemographic, anthropometric and behavioral factors associated with lifestyle influence the consumption of dairy products. Additionally, and because the study was carried out in two countries, differences between the countries were investigated. One other objective of the study was to categorize the lifestyles of the participants, according to measured variables linked with hours of inactivity or exercise, for example, in order to use these as possible differentiating variables for the consumption of dairy products.

2. Materials and Methods

2.1. Data Collection and Sample Characterization

This work was based on the application of a questionnaire, which was developed purposely for this research, in order to investigate consumption habits regarding dairy products, such as milk, yogurt, cheese or butter. The questionnaire was validated and approved for the study. The questionnaire included different parts, as follows: Part I: Sociodemographic data (5 questions); Part II: Anthropometric and behavioral aspects (10 questions); Part III: Consumption habits regarding dairy products (21 questions distributed as follows—4 for milk products, 7 for cheeses, 3 for butter, 7 for yogurt). The complete questionnaire is attached in Appendix A. The data collected was based on the participants' self-responses for frequencies of consumption on the scale provided: Never, Seldom (Once/week), Sometimes (2–3 times/week), Frequently (once/day) and Always (+ 1 time/day).

To undertake this descriptive cross-sectional study a non-probabilistic convenience sample was used, consisting of adult citizens from Brazil and Portugal. Hence only participants aged 18 years or older were included in the study, and these had to provide consent to participate. One other inclusion criteria, derived from the mode of survey delivery, was to have access to a computer and internet as well as to have the necessary knowledge to be able to use the technology and the platform through which the questionnaire was presented. These two countries were selected due to being connected through language and culture, since Brazil was once a colony of Portugal, and also because nowadays they receive different influences related to geographical location: one in the South American continent and the other in Western Europe. The choice of a convenience sample was owing to facility of recruitment and place of residence, and it was intended to have a similar sample size in each of the countries. One important advantage of convenience samples is precisely the ease of recruitment, despite not allowing generalization according to estimates of sociodemographic differences. Still, they represent an adequate tool for exploratory research, as is the present case [38–42]. The survey took place through an internet questionnaire platform and 914 answers were obtained. The data collection took place between November 2019 and April 2020. The answers were obtained only from adult citizens (aged 18 or over), and after informed consent. Extreme care was taken to verify all ethical guidelines when formulating and applying the questionnaire. Finally, confidentiality of the individual answers was guaranteed to comply with ethical principles. The survey was registered and approved by the Ethics Committee of the Polytechnic Institute of Viseu before application.

2.2. Data Analysis

Body mass index (BMI) was calculated from self-reported values of height and weight, according to the equation:

$$BMI\ (kg/m^2) = \frac{Weight\ (kg)}{[Height\ (m)]^2} \qquad (1)$$

Participants were then classified according to the World Health Organization (WHO) classification for BMI as: underweight: BMI < 18.5; normal weight: $18.5 \leq BMI < 25$; overweight: $25 \leq BMI < 30$; obesity: $BMI \geq 30$. There are other classes of obesity, differentiating the degree of obesity, but for the present study these four classes were considered sufficient [43,44].

Sociodemographic information was also collected and age was classified into categories according to: young adults (aged between 18 and 30 years), middle aged adults (between 31 and 50 years), senior adults (between 51 and 65 years), and the elderly (aged 66 years or over).

For the analysis of the data different basic descriptive statistical tools were used, such as frequencies and descriptives, including minimum, maximum, mean value and standard deviation. The crosstabs and the chi square test were used to access the relations between some of the categorical variables under study. Moreover, the Cramer's V coefficient was used to analyze the strength of the significant relations found between some of the variables. This coefficient ranges from 0 to 1 and can be interpreted as follows: $V \approx 0.1$, the association is considered weak, $V \approx 0.3$, the association is moderate, and $V \approx 0.5$ or over, the association is strong [45].

Factor analysis (FA) and cluster analysis (CA) were used to treat data obtained for lifestyle variables: •Practice of physical exercise; ·Daily hours traveling walking or riding a bike; •Daily hours watching TV; •Daily hours playing with computer or mobile phone or on social networks; •Daily hours working on computer; •Daily hours traveling inactively (in car, motorbike, bus, train, etc.). The correlation matrix, the Kaiser-Meyer-Olkin measure of adequacy of the sample (KMO) and Bartlett's test were all used to confirm the adequacy of data for FA [46]. The FA was applied with extraction by principal component analysis (PCA) method and Varimax rotation with Kaiser Normalization, being the number of components determined by the Kaiser criterion (eigenvalues $\geq$1) and also by the scree plot. Communalities were calculated to show the percentage of variance explained by the factors extracted [46]. Only factor loadings with absolute of 0.4 or higher were used [47,48].

Cluster analysis (CA) of the factors resulting from FA started with four hierarchical methods to find the most adequate number of clusters, based on the agglomeration schedule: average linkage—between groups (AL-BG), average linkage—within groups (AL-WG), centroid and Ward. This procedure allowed fixing the number of clusters at four and then applying the k-means, which is particularly recommended and frequently used in cluster analysis [49]. The application of k-means was made using the initial solutions obtained with the four hierarchical methods.

To treat the data obtained for the frequency of consumption of certain dairy products, a mean value was computed for each of the dairy product categories: milk, cheese, butter and yogurt. The measurement scale for the individual consumption variables was: 1—Never, 2—Seldom (once/week), 3—Sometimes (2–3 times/week), 4—Frequently (once/day) and 5—Always (more than once/day). However, the variables accounting for the average consumption for each category were real numbers varying from 1 to 5, and their interpretation was made according to the following defined scale: low consumption—value $\in$ (1.0, 2.5), moderate consumption—value $\in$ (2.5, 3.5), high consumption—value $\in$ (3.5, 5).

The variables accounting for the average level of consumption of the four categories of dairy products were submitted to a tree classification analysis for evaluation of the relative importance of each of the possible influential variables considered: country, sex, age class, education, BMI class, satisfaction with body weight, balanced diet, and lifestyle clusters. The analysis followed the CRT (Classification and Regression Trees) algorithm with cross validation and with minimum change in improvement of 0.0001, considering a limit of 5 levels and the minimum number of cases for parent or child nodes equal to 30 and 20, respectively.

The data were processed using the SPSS program, version 26 from IBM, Inc, and the level of significance used was 5%.

3. Results and Discussion

3.1. Sociodemographic Characterization of the Sample

From the 914 participations obtained, 64 were rejected because the questionnaires were incomplete or not properly filled out, resulting in a sample of 850 valid responses, 430 from Brazil and 420 from Portugal. Table 1 shows the sociodemographic characteristics of the 850 participants included in the sample studied. The number of participants from both countries was similar, corresponding to 50.6% from Brazil and 49.4% from Portugal, but the distribution according to sex was not equal, having more women (65.1%) than men (34.9%).

Table 1. Sociodemographic characteristics of the participants.

Variable	Class	N	%
Country	Brazil	430	50.6
	Portugal	420	49.4
Sex	Female	553	65.1
	Male	297	34.9
Age Class	Young adults (18 ≤ age ≤ 25 years)	231	27.2
	Middle aged adults (26 ≤ age ≤ 50 years)	403	47.5
	Senior adults (51 ≤ age ≤ 65 years)	203	23.9
	Elderly (age ≥ 66 years)	12	1.4
Marital status	Single	372	43.8
	Married or living together	412	48.5
	Divorced or separated	53	6.2
	Widowed	13	1.5
Education level	Primary school (4 years)	5	0.6
	Basic school (9 years)	7	0.8
	Secondary school (12 years)	101	11.9
	University degree	737	86.7

The participants were aged between 18 and 82, most of them, 47.5%, were middle aged adults (26 ≤ age ≤ 50 years), and those less represented, only 1.4%, were the elderly (age ≥ 66 years). The distribution of the participants according to their marital status shows that most of them were married (48.5%) or single (43.8%). Regarding the level of education, the large majority of the participants had completed a university degree (86.7%).

3.2. Anthropometric Measures

Table 2 presents the anthropometric measures of the participants. The average height was 1.68 ± 0.09 m for the whole sample, with men showing higher values (1.76 ± 0.07) as compared with women (1.63 ± 0.06), as usually happens. The average weight was 70.06 ± 15.80 kg, and the difference between men and women was considerable for this sample: 63.71 ± 11.96 and 81.87 ± 15.28 kg, respectively. The calculated BMI was 24.73 ± 4.50 kg/m^2 for the whole sample, being also higher for the men (26.34 ± 4.40 kg/m^2) as compared to women (23.86 ± 4.31 kg/m^2). It is important to notice that these measures were self-reported and, therefore, some inaccuracy might be present, this being a limitation of this kind of assessment of anthropometric measures.

Table 2. Anthropometric measures of the participants.

Sex	Measure [a]	N [b]	Minimum	Maximum	M ± SD [c]
Women	Height (m)	552	1.38	1.80	1.63 ± 0.06
	Weight (kg)	552	40.00	120.00	63.71 ± 11.96
	BMI (kg/m^2)	552	15.43	43.03	23.86 ± 4.31
Men	Height (m)	297	1.54	2.00	1.76 ± 0.07
	Weight (kg)	297	44.0	140.0	81.87 ± 15.28
	BMI (kg/m^2)	297	15.94	41.67	26.34 ± 4.40
Global	Height (m)	849	1.38	2.00	1.68 ± 0.09
	Weight (kg)	849	40.0	140.00	70.06 ± 15.80
	BMI (kg/m^2)	849	15.43	43.03	24.73 ± 4.50

[a] BMI = body mass index = (weight/height^2). [b] N = number of values used in the calculations. [c] Mean values (M) and standard deviation (SD).

The participants' BMI was classified according to the World Health Organization into the four principal classes as shown in Table 3. Most participants have a normal weight (56.5% for the whole sample), but mostly in women (65.0%) when compared with men (40.4%). However, the incidence of overweight is worrying (26.0% for the whole sample), particularly in men (39.1%), while in women the percentage is lower (19.0%), but still important. Even raising more concern is the percentage of obese participants (13.4%, 18.5% and 10.7%, respectively for global, men and women), considering the risks that this brings to health, associated with diabetes and heart related diseases [50–53].

Table 3. Classification of the participants' Body Mass Index (BMI = weight/height^2).

BMI [1] Classification:	Women N	Women %	Men N	Men %	Global N	Global %
Underweight: BMI < 18.5	29	5.3	6	2.0	35	4.1
Normal weight: 18.5 ≤ BMI < 25	359	65.0	120	40.4	479	56.5
Overweight: 25 ≤ BMI < 30	105	19.0	116	39.1	221	26.0
Obese: BMI ≥ 30	59	10.7	55	18.5	114	13.4

[1] BMI = body mass index = (weight/height^2).

3.3. Lifestyle

One aspect investigated related to the participant's self-perception about the practice of a balanced diet. Unbalanced diets lead to malnutrition, referring either to under-nutrition or to over nutrition. Nevertheless, very often malnutrition is associated with excessive calories in relation to requirements, coupled with low intake of micronutrient-rich foods [54]. Food security entails aspects such as availability, utilization and access, but these may not necessarily cover nutritional aspects. In fact, easily accessed and available food products may not necessarily provide a healthy and balanced diet. The Family Nutrition Guide of the FAO (Food and Agriculture Organization of the United Nations) [55] states that a balanced diet should be able to provide the right amount of food, energy and nutrients needed during the day to cover the dietary requirements of a particular person. Additionally, a balanced diet must include a variety of foods from different food groups to ensure the supply of all the nutrients needed for adequate body functioning, thus significantly contributing to a healthy life, while at the same time lowering mortality incidences related to malnutrition. Because a healthy diet needs to be balanced, the participants were asked about the frequency with which they practiced a balanced diet.

Table 4 shows the results obtained for this question, considering the possible effect of some sociodemographic variables, assessed through chi-square tests. When considering the global sample, it was found that nearly half of the participants (46.9%) believed they frequently practice a balanced diet, while 16.5% responded that they always have a balanced diet. A considerable fraction (30.0%) responded to eating a balanced diet only sometimes.

Additionally, Table 4 also shows that no significant differences were found between sexes ($p = 0.060$), but considering the two countries involved significant differences were encountered ($p < 0.0005$), with participants from Portugal reporting a higher frequency of balanced diet as compared with Brazilians, although the association between these two variables (balanced diet and country) was weak ($V = 0.198$). The results in Table 4 also show that high percentages of underweight and obese participants admitted to practicing a balanced diet only sometimes (45.7% and 37.7%, respectively), and people who are overweight believed they frequently consume a balanced diet (50.7%). These differences were significant ($p = 0.001$), but with a low association ($V = 0.116$). Considering age classes, an significant number of young adults state that they have a balanced diet only sometimes (41.6%), but the care for a balanced diet increases for the elderly, with 58.3% saying that they always have a balanced diet. These differences were significant ($p < 0.0005$). Older people tend to have more health problems, sometimes suffering from non-communicable and age related diseases, thus making it more important to have a healthier food intake, either because they want to remain healthy or to diminish the morbidity associated with their diseases. Results from countless studies have revealed that healthy dietary patterns are associated with a reduced risk of developing several chronic diseases or having a better control of these, such as obesity, dyslipidemia, hypertension and diabetes mellitus. Hence, for the elderly, nutrition assumes a particular role in the maintenance of acceptable health standards and functional capacity [56,57]. As for marital status, the widowed showed a higher frequency of balanced diet as compared with the other groups (single, married or divorced), with 61.5% having a balanced diet frequently and 15.4% always. These results are in line with those of age class, since most often the widowed consisted of older people, who had already lost their spouses. The differences are significant ($p = 0.009$), although the association between balanced diet and marital status is weak ($V = 0.102$). Finally, the results showed that higher education levels are associated with higher frequency of practicing a balanced diet, with the percentages of participants who report this frequently increasing systematically from 20.0% for people with the lowest level of education completed, up to 47.8% for participants with a university degree. Again, these differences were significant ($p < 0.0005$). These results clearly indicate that more educated people are better aware of the importance given to a proper diet to benefit from a globally healthier status [58].

Table 4. Practice of a balanced diet.

Variable/Group		Never	Seldom	Sometimes	Frequently	Always
Global (%)		0.9	5.6	30.0	46.9	16.5
Sex	Women (%)	0.4	5.1	28.9	47.9	17.7
	Men (%)	2.0	6.8	32.0	45.1	14.1
	χ^2 test *		N = 850; p-value = 0.060			
Country	Brazil (%)	1.2	8.4	35.8	41.6	13.0
	Portugal (%)	0.7	2.9	24.0	52.4	20.0
	χ^2 test *		N = 850; p-value < 0.0005; Cramer´s V = 0.198			
BMI class	Underweight	0.0	5.7	45.7	37.1	11.5
	Normal weight	0.4	4.2	27.3	47.8	20.3
	Overweight	0.9	6.8	29.4	50.7	12.2
	Obese	3.5	9.6	37.7	38.6	10.6
	χ^2 test *		N = 849; p-value = 0.001; Cramer´s V = 0.116			
Age class	Young adults	1.7	8.7	41.6	35.0	13.0
	Middle aged adults	0.7	5.5	25.3	53.8	14.9
	Senior adults	0.5	3.0	26.6	48.3	21.6
	Elderly	0.0	0.0	25.0	16.7	58.3
	χ^2 test *		N = 849; p-value < 0.0005; Cramer´s V = 0.148			
Marital status	Single	1.3	7.0	36.3	43.8	11.6
	Married	0.5	5.1	24.5	49.3	20.6
	Divorced	1.9	1.9	30.2	47.2	18.8
	Widowed	0.0	0.0	23.1	61.5	15.4
	χ^2 test *		N = 850; p-value = 0.009; Cramer´s V = 0.102			
Education	Primary	20.0	0.0	60.0	20.0	0.0
	Basic	0.0	14.3	57.1	14.3	14.3
	Secondary	0.0	11.9	32.7	44.6	10.8
	University	0.9	4.7	29.2	47.8	17.3
	χ^2 test *		N = 850; p-value < 0.0005; Cramer´s V = 0.123			

* Chi-square test, level of significance of 5% ($p < 0.05$). The Cramer´s V was only indicated for cases where significant differences were observed.

Another aspect investigated in this research was the satisfaction with body weight, and the results are shown in Table 5 for the global sample and also according to BMI classes and to the practice of a balanced diet. Most participants (40.1%) believed they are of normal weight but would still like to lose 2 to 5 kg.

Considering the underweight participants, 42.9% are aware of their condition, and stated they would like to gain a few kilos (Table 5). Of the participants with normal weight, an important part (39.5%) is satisfied with their body weight and wish to maintain it, while 46.4% would like to lose 2 to 5 kg, even though they know their weight is normal. For those participants who are overweight, a high percentage (48.9%) wrongly think they have normal weight but would still like to lose 2 to 5 kg, and 32.1% are conscientious about being overweight. From the obese participants, 75.4% know about their condition and would like to lose a few kilos, but say they have tried and not succeeded. These results are interesting, because they reveal that, in general, the participants were aware of their bodyweight status.

The results in Table 6 refer to the practice of physical exercise and also the level of activity related to active daily traveling, by walking or riding a bike, for example. Most participants (38.8%) practiced exercise occasionally, i.e., once a week, but a considerable part (33.9%) does 2 to 3 times a week, which is the frequency recommended for most cases. Nevertheless, 17.4% of participants never do physical exercise, which can have a very negative impact on health at so many levels [59–62]. Regarding active traveling, for example to and from work, most participants (52.2%) do not or do less than half an hour per day, but 33.8% spend between 30 min and 1 h daily in these activities.

Table 5. Satisfaction with body weight.

Satisfaction	Global	BMI Class			
		Underweight	Normal weight	Overweight	Obese
I am satisfied with my body weight and I want to keep it (%)	25.5	22.9	39.5	7.2	3.5
I have normal weight, but would like to lose 2 to 5 kg (%)	40.1	5.7	46.4	48.9	7.0
I am underweight, but I feel good like this (%)	2.5	25.7	2.5	0.0	0.0
I am underweight and would like to gain 2 to 5 kg (%)	4.2	42.9	4.2	0.0	0.0
I am overweight and I would like to lose a few kilos, but I have tried and I cannot (%)	20.9	2.8	4.2	32.1	75.4
I am overweight and do nothing to change this (%)	0.0	0.0	0.0	0.0	0.0
Other (%)	6.8	0.0	3.2	11.8	14.1
χ^2 test * (for BMI Class)		N = 849; p-value < 0.0005; Cramer's V = 0.500			

Satisfaction	Balanced diet				
	Never	Seldom	Sometimes	Frequently	Always
I am satisfied with my body weight and I want to keep it (%)	12.5	14.6	17.6	26.6	41.4
I have normal weight, but would like to lose 2 to 5 kg (%)	12.5	29.2	37.3	45.4	35.7
I am underweight, but I feel good like this (%)	12.5	6.3	4.7	1.0	0.7
I am underweight and would like to gain 2 to 5 kg (%)	0.0	4.2	6.7	3.3	2.1
I am overweight and I would like to lose a few kilos, but I have tried and I cannot (%)	25.0	45.7	26.7	16.5	14.4
I am overweight and do nothing to change this (%)	0.0	0.0	0.0	0.0	0.0
Other (%)	37.5	0.0	7.1	7.2	5.7
χ^2 test * (for balanced diet)	N = 850; p-value < 0.0005; Cramer's V = 0.165				

* Chi-square test, level of significance of 5% ($p < 0.05$). The Cramer's V was only indicated for cases where significant differences were observed.

Table 6. Physical activity.

Intensity of Physical Activity		N	%
Physical exercise	Never	148	17.4
	Occasionally (1 time/week)	330	38.8
	Moderate (2–3 times/week)	288	33.9
	Intense (>3 times/week)	84	9.9
Daily time walking or riding a bike	0:00–0:30 h	444	52.2
	0:30–1:00 h	287	33.8
	1:00–2:00 h	85	10.0
	2:00–5:00 h	26	3.1
	>5:00 h	8	0.9

Table 7 presents the results obtained for the hours spent daily on sedentary activities. The results indicated that a high percentage (32.4%) spend between 1 and 2 h watching TV, and 13.8% spend up to 5 h watching TV. The participants do not engage much in activities like playing with computers or mobile phones or on social networks, i.e., screen entertainment, with 39.9% spending less than 30 min per day in those activities. On the other hand, the use of computers for professional purposes is a reality for the great majority of the participants, with 30.4% spending between 2 to 5 h, and 39.6% spending more than 5 h daily working on the computer. Finally, the daily hours of inactive traveling, for example in a car, motorbike, bus or train, are low, less than 30 min for 54.2% of participants, or between 30 min and 1 h for 30.4% of participants.

Table 7. Sedentary lifestyle.

Inactivity		Hours per day				
		0:00–0:30	0:30–1:00	1:00–2:00	2:00–5:00	>5:00
Watching TV	N	193	246	275	117	19
	%	22.7	28.9	32.4	13.8	2.2
Screen entertaining [1]	N	339	189	194	98	30
	%	39.9	22.2	22.8	11.5	3.6
Working on computer	N	65	70	121	258	336
	%	7.6	8.2	14.2	30.4	39.6
Traveling inactive [2]	N	461	258	104	19	8
	%	54.2	30.4	12.2	2.2	1.0

[1] Playing with computer or mobile phone or on social networks. [2] In car, motorbike, bus, train, etc.

3.3.1. Factor Analysis for Lifestyle

Some variables related to lifestyle were subjected to exploratory FA, starting with Principal Component Analysis (PCA), to identify a possible grouping structure between the variables used to evaluate aspects related to physical activity or sedentary lifestyle of the participants.

The correlation matrix showed some correlations between the variables, although they were relatively weak. The value of KMO was low (0.496), but the results of the Bartlett's test of sphericity indicated adequacy for applying FA ($p < 0.0005$), thus leading to the rejection of the null hypothesis that the correlation matrix was equal to the identity matrix. Analysis of the anti-image matrix revealed that values of MSA (Measure of Sampling Adequacy) were close or above 0.5, meaning that in general the variables could be included in the analysis. The solution obtained by rotation of FA with PCA originated three components, explaining 59.7% of total variance, distributed by the three factors as: F1—22.4%, F2—19.3% and F3—18.0%. All variables had communalities higher than 0.4: the variable practice of physical exercise had the highest value (0.827, indicating that this variable had 82.7% of its variance explained by the solution), while the variable with lowest communality was daily hours working on computer (0.509). Rotation converged in five iterations and extracted three factors, grouping the variables as shown in Table 8.

Table 8. Component matrix obtained by factor analysis to variables related with active or sedentary lifestyles.

Factors	Variable	Component
F1: Screens	TV = daily hours watching TV	0.675
	LC = daily hours leisure: playing with computer or mobile phone or on social networks	0.722
	WC = daily hours working on computer	−0.558
F2: Travelling	TI = daily hours traveling inactive (in car, motorbike, bus, train, etc.)	0.727
	WR = daily hours traveling walking or riding a bike	0.739
F3: Exercise	PE = practice of physical exercise	0.904

Considering the components in Table 8, F1 was clearly linked to activities related to screens, where watching TV and playing on screen devices have positive high loads, while the use of computer for work has a considerable load, but negative, indicating that these variables contribute strongly to the definition of the factor. Factor F2 is strongly linked with variables related to daily hours of traveling, either active or inactive, and finally F3 is very strongly related with only one variable, which is physical exercise.

3.3.2. Cluster Analysis for Lifestyle

The factors identified though FA were subject to CA in order to perceive if there was a cluster structure among the people surveyed. Cluster analysis was based on the three factors resulting from FA and started with four hierarchical methods that indicated that four clusters was the most suitable grouping structure for this set of data. Following that, the k-means method was applied using as initial solutions those obtained with the hierarchical methods. In all cases, the k-means cluster analysis produced clustering variables with means that differ significantly, as indicated by ANOVA since p-value < 0.0005 for the three input variables, i.e., factors F1 to f3. The results obtained for the cluster centers and number of members are presented in Table 9 and show that the four initial solutions tested converged to a similar final solution. Because the final solutions obtained from WARD and AL-BW methods converged to the exact same one, this was then considered as the final solution, which is characterized by:

- Cluster 1: individuals with strong focus on F1 and negative input for F2 and F3, i.e., those whose lifestyle is very much dominated by screens. These were named screeners;
- Custer 2: individuals with strong focus on F3 and negative input for F1 and F2, i.e., those whose lifestyle is very influenced by physical exercise. There were named exercisers;
- Cluster 3: individuals with strong focus on F2 and negative input for F1 and F3, i.e., those whose lifestyle is very strongly dominated by daily travelling hours. There were named travelers;
- Cluster 4: individuals with negative input for all three factors, i.e., those whose lifestyle is inversely associated with screens, travelling and exercise. Because these participants did not present a specific feature, this group was named others.

Table 9. Final cluster centers and number of members.

Cluster	Hierarchical Initial Solution	Number of Members	Final Cluster Centers		
			Factor F1	Factor F2	Factor F3
Cluster C1	Ward	179	1.390	−0.167	−0.451
	AL-WG	179	1.390	−0.167	−0.451
	AL-BG	177	1.351	−0.229	−0.465
	Centroid	178	1.364	−0.211	−0.440
Cluster C2	Ward	272	−0.168	−0.285	1.009
	AL-WG	272	−0.168	−0.285	1.009
	AL-BG	284	−0.238	−0.386	0.922
	Centroid	281	−0.202	−0.321	0.964
Cluster C3	Ward	132	−0.261	1.697	−0.083
	AL-WG	132	−0.261	1.697	−0.083
	AL-BG	140	−0.048	1.681	0.114
	Centroid	135	−0.156	1.720	−0.033
Cluster C4	Ward	267	−0.632	−0.437	−0.685
	AL-WG	267	−0.632	−0.437	−0.685
	AL-BG	249	−0.662	−0.342	−0.785
	Centroid	256	−0.645	−0.407	−0.735

3.3.3. Cluster Characterization

To better understand the type of people who fall into each of the four categories that cluster analysis indicated, cross tabulation between cluster membership and the sociodemographic and behavioral variables was undertaken (Table 10).

Table 10. Cluster membership according to sociodemographic variables.

Variable	Group	Cluster 1 Screeners	Cluster 2 Exercisers	Cluster 3 Travelers	Cluster 4 Others
Country	Brazil (%)	30.0	22.8	32.8	14.4
	Portugal (%)	11.9	40.2	31.2	16.7
Sex	Women (%)	20.8	34.2	30.4	14.6
	Men (%)	21.5	26.3	35.0	17.2
Age	Young adults (%)	44.2	19.9	24.2	11.7
	Middle aged adults (%)	11.4	36.5	33.5	18.6
	Senior adults (%)	12.8	35.0	38.4	13.8
	Elderly (%)	33.3	25.0	25.0	16.7
Education level	Primary (%)	60.0	0.0	0.0	40.0
	Basic (%)	42.9	28.6	0.0	28.6
	Secondary (%)	36.6	22.8	27.7	12.9
	University (%)	18.5	32.8	33.1	15.6
Marital status	Single (%)	31.7	24.5	28.5	15.3
	Married (%)	12.9	37.4	34.2	15.5
	Divorced (%)	11.3	32.1	37.7	18.9
	Widowed (%)	15.4	38.5	38.5	7.7

The results in Table 10 show that Portuguese participants are essentially exercisers (40.2%) while Brazilians were travelers (32.8%). While a major part of the women surveyed were exercisers (30.4%), men were mostly travelers (35.0%). Regarding the age class, young adults and the elderly were mostly screeners (44.2% and 33.3%, respectively), while middle aged adults were exercisers (36.5%), and senior adults were travelers (38.4%). While participants with a university degree were exercisers and travelers (32.8 and 33.1%, respectively) those with lower levels of education were mostly screeners (60.0% for primary school, 42.9% for basic school and 36.6% for secondary school). As for marital status, most single participants were screeners (31.7%), while those married, divorced and widowed were exercisers and travelers, in relatively similar percentages.

Table 11 shows the cross tabulation between cluster membership and some anthropometric and lifestyle variables, specifically BMI and frequency of practicing a balanced diet. Results showed that underweight people are essentially screeners (37.1%) and travelers (34.3%), those with normal weight are exercisers (31.7%) and travelers (32.4%) and so are the overweight (34.4% exercisers and 32.6% travelers). The obese are equally distributed by clusters 1 (screeners: 28.1%), 2 (exercisers: 27.2%) and 3 (travelers: 28.9%). Regarding the practice of a balanced diet, those who practice it frequently or always are exercisers and travelers, while those who never or seldom have a balanced diet are screeners or exercisers.

Table 11. Cluster membership according to some anthropometric and lifestyle variables.

Variable	Group	Cluster 1 Screeners	Cluster 2 Exercisers	Cluster 3 Travelers	Cluster 4 Others
IMC class	Underweight (%)	37.1	20.0	34.3	8.6
	Normal weight (%)	20.9	31.7	32.4	15.0
	Overweight (%)	15.4	34.4	32.6	17.6
	Obese (%)	28.1	27.2	28.9	15.8
Balanced diet	Never (%)	37.5	37.5	0.0	25.0
	Seldom (%)	37.5	37.5	12.5	12.5
	Sometimes (%)	32.9	29.4	20.0	17.6
	Frequently (%)	14.8	32.1	40.9	12.3
	Always (%)	10.7	30.7	37.1	21.4

3.4. Consumption Habits Regarding Dairy Products

Table 12 shows the consumption habits of dairy products in Portugal and Brazil. Concerning milk consumption, for both countries the percentage of participants who never consume milk products is high, ranging between 46.7% (Brazil: never consume semi skimmed milk) to 94.8% (Portugal: never consume enriched milk). For those who consume milk, it was observed that 52.6% of Portuguese and 53.3% of Brazilians consume semi skimmed milk revealing a similar trend in both countries, although with variability according to the frequency of consumption. In Portugal, a higher frequency was observed for consumption of semi skimmed milk once a day (20.2%) and for Brazil for once a week (24.2%). On the other hand, the consumption of skimmed milk presents bigger differences between countries: 49.1% of Brazilians and 35.2% of Portuguese consume it, and in both countries a higher percentage of participants consume it rarely (13.8% and 27.9%, respectively, for Portugal and Brazil). This survey shows that the consumption of chocolate flavored and enriched milks is very low in these two countries, particularly in Portugal. Brazilians consume more chocolate flavored milk (34.4%) than the Portuguese (17.4%), but in both countries this is consumed with a very low frequency (seldom). In Portugal there is a slightly higher percentage of people who never consume enriched milk (94.8%) as compared with Brazil (85.3%). However, because portion and serving sizes were not specified in the questionnaires, the obtained responses may not be fully indicative, given that different participants may have interpreted the questions differently.

Milk and dairy products are considered by the FAO as important in the human diet, given their high quality protein and micronutrients in an easily absorbed form [63]. However, it has been reported in several sources that milk intake has gradually declined over the past decades [64–66], maybe due to the aforementioned gastrointestinal problems that can appear after lactose ingestion [14]. There are considerable studies related to the health benefits of milk consumption e.g., for bone strength [33,67–69], risk factor of osteoporosis [70] and protective effects against asthma, current wheeze, hay fever or allergic rhinitis, and atopic sensitization [71]. Concerning this point of view, some controversial studies can be found, like that of Wang et al. [72], which concluded that the risk associated with the consumption of milk depends on the quantities, so that moderate milk consumption diminished the risk of mortality associated with cardiovascular diseases and a high milk consumption showed an increased risk of cancer mortality. Specifically, in the two countries under study, some studies have addressed the problem of osteoporosis in Portugal and in Brazil [36,37], a recent investigation evaluated the sleep patterns in Brazilian children and the consumption of dairy products [73] and one study shows arterial hypertension management strategies according to some factors, such as dietary management, including milk and dairy product recommendations [74].

More recently a variety of enriched milks have appeared in the market, mainly with calcium and vitamin D. Calcium is critical for children's development and is necessary for skeletal consolidation and preventing fractures and osteoporosis in old age [75,76]. According to the Dietary Guidelines Advisory Committee [77], lower calcium consumptions are linked with adverse health outcomes. The importance of vitamin D is well known owing to its importance in helping with the fixation of calcium in the bones, among other roles in the human body, namely regulating the brain, liver, lungs, heart, kidneys, skeletal, immune and reproductive systems. This vitamin also has significant anti-inflammatory, anti-aging, anti-stress, anti-arthritic, anti-osteoporosis, anti-apoptotic, wound healing, anti-cancer, anti-psychotic and anti-fibrotic actions [78–83].

Table 12. Frequency of consumption of dairy products in Portugal and Brazil.

Product	Country [1]	Frequency of Responses [2] (%)				
		Never	Seldom	Sometimes	Frequently	Always
Category: Milk						
Semi skimmed	Portugal	47.4	17.4	11.0	20.2	4.0
	Brazil	46.7	24.2	14.2	9.1	5.8
Skimmed milk	Portugal	64.8	13.8	7.1	9.5	4.8
	Brazil	50.9	27.9	9.3	6.7	5.1
Chocolate flavored	Portugal	82.6	11.2	4.3	0.7	1.2
	Brazil	65.6	24.0	6.7	3.3	0.5
Enriched milk	Portugal	94.8	2.9	1.7	0.7	0.0
	Brazil	85.3	10.7	2.8	0.7	0.5
Category: Cheese						
Soft paste cheese	Portugal	43.3	44.0	9.8	2.6	0.2
	Brazil	70.7	21.2	6.0	1.4	0.7
Cured hard paste cheese	Portugal	45.2	38.3	12.9	3.3	0.2
	Brazil	57.7	29.3	10.2	2.1	0.7
Fresh cheese	Portugal	28.8	46.4	18.3	5.7	0.7
	Brazil	41.4	38.8	14.0	4.4	1.4
Whey cheese	Portugal	46.9	42.9	7.1	2.9	0.2
	Brazil	37.2	39.1	15.6	6.3	1.9
Semi skimmed sliced cheese	Portugal	35.0	31.0	24.0	8.1	1.9
	Brazil	39.3	30.7	21.2	6.5	2.3
Skimmed sliced cheese	Portugal	35.0	31.0	24.0	8.1	1.9
	Brazil	39.3	30.7	21.2	6.5	2.3
Imported cheeses	Portugal	67.9	28.1	3.8	0.2	0.0
	Brazil	77.0	19.1	3.3	0.5	0.2
Category: Butter						
Milk butter	Portugal	43.8	22.9	17.1	11.0	5.2
	Brazil	49.5	24.0	14.7	6.3	5.6
Skimmed butter	Portugal	66.0	19.5	8.3	5.0	1.2
	Brazil	82.6	14.0	3.5	0.0	0.0
Butter without salt	Portugal	70.2	20.5	4.8	3.1	1.4
	Brazil	69.1	20.0	6.7	3.5	0.7
Category: Yogurt						
Natural yogurt	Portugal	40.2	29.3	19.3	8.8	2.4
	Brazil	57.7	30.9	7.9	2.3	1.2
Aromatized yogurt	Portugal	42.1	33.3	20.0	3.3	1.2
	Brazil	62.1	25.6	8.6	2.6	1.2
Creamy fruit pulp yogurt	Portugal	60.5	25.7	11.0	2.1	0.7
	Brazil	55.6	30.0	9.8	3.7	0.9
Yogurt with fruit pieces	Portugal	61.4	23.8	11.4	2.1	1.2
	Brazil	65.1	26.5	5.3	2.3	0.7
Liquid yogurt	Portugal	33.1	32.1	20.5	11.2	3.1
	Brazil	52.3	34.0	9.5	3.5	0.7
With separated flavors	Portugal	73.3	20.5	4.3	1.7	0.2
	Brazil	74.2	18.4	5.1	2.1	0.2
Greek type yogurt	Portugal	50.0	33.3	11.7	4.0	1.0
	Brazil	59.8	30.0	5.8	3.5	0.9

[1] Number of participants: N(Portugal) = 420, N(Brazil) = 430. [2] Frequency: Seldom = once/week, Sometimes = 2 to 3 times/week, Frequently = once/day, Always = more than once/day.

As observed previously for milk consumption, a high number of participants in both countries never eat cheese (Table 12). However, this percentage is higher for Brazilians compared with the Portuguese for most types of cheese, except only for whey cheese. In fact, Portugal has a long history of eating traditional cheeses that are presently recognized with PDO (Protected Designation of Origin) [84]. The highest percentage of Portuguese who never eat a certain type of cheese is verified for imported cheeses (67.9%) and the lowest for fresh cheeses (28.8%), while for Brazilians, those who never eat cheese are, also, predominantly for imported cheeses (77.0%) and with least expression for whey cheeses (37.2%). For all categories of cheese and in both countries, the more usual consumption frequency is once a week. The differences observed in the cheese consumption patterns in both countries could be attributed to the different habits and production modes. The Brazilian cheese market has been reported to vary according to place of origin, type of milk (cow, buffalo, goat), manufacturing procedures, texture, and maturation time, among other factors [85]. For Portugal, with good pastures and a tradition in pastoralism, there are several types of cheese, made with cow, goat, sheep or mixtures of different milks, which have different tastes and consistencies. According to Guiné et al. [84], the traditional Portuguese cheeses can be classified according to the type of milk used for the cheese production, the fat content, ripening and paste consistency.

Whey is a dilute liquid resulting from cheese manufacture that contains lactose, proteins, minerals, such as calcium, and traces of fat and organic acids [84]. An important difference was observed in the consumption of whey cheese. Brazilians eat whey cheese in higher percentages (62.8%) compared to the Portuguese (54.1%), but in both cases the frequency of consumption is mostly once/week (42.9% of Portuguese and 39.1% of Brazilians).

According to Ferrão & Guiné [84], cheese is a good source of calcium, fat, protein, and some vitamins (A, B_2 and B_{12}), as well as other dietary minerals such as zinc or phosphorus. Cheese is not only consumed in its original form, and during the last decade, it has become one of the most widely used food ingredients, leading to the development of several types of low-fat cheeses that have health-promoting benefits beyond their nutritional value [86,87].

Butter is one of the most ancient and popular dairy products. This dairy product contains valuable fatty acids, as well as fat-soluble vitamins (A, D, E, K), tocopherols and carotenoids, among its important nutrients. However, the consumption of butter must be moderate because it has been linked to high cholesterol, atherosclerosis, and heart disease [88,89]. Consumer acceptance of butter is influenced by its sensory properties, which are dependent on milk raw material quality that influence the final flavor, aroma, appearance, and rheological properties [90]. Table 12 also presents the results for butter consumption in Portugal and Brazil. Around 50% of Brazilians never consume butter and the observed percentage is 43.8% for the Portuguese who also never consume butter. These percentages increase for the consumption of skimmed butter (Brazil: 82.6% never consume it; Portugal: 66.0% never consume it) and unsalted butter (Brazil: 69.1%; Portugal: 70.2%). For those who consume butter, the highest percentage of people consume it seldom, only once/week.

Yogurts are obtained from milk fermented by lactic acid bacteria such as *Lactobacillus*, *Lactococcus*, and *Leuconostoc* which allows for an extension of the product shelf life and improves its taste compared to milk, giving way to differentiated products in the market. Fermented dairy products' consumption has been increasing widely around the world and different companies encourage new product development to satisfy the consumers with new tastes and flavors. Some of these products have demonstrated nutritional value and health benefits. For example, it has been shown that intestinal bacterial microbiota contributes to a healthy life and increases life expectancy [91–94]. This kind of product contains a high amount of live bacteria, which has benefits for human health, contributing to the maintenance and balance of the intestinal flora, facilitating digestion and preventing constipation and other gastrointestinal disorders [94,95]. Several studies state that yogurt presents antimutagenic and anticarcinogenic effects and provides protection against colorectal adenomas [95–98].

The results regarding yogurt consumption (Table 12) reveal that a high percentage of participants never consume yogurt and, on average, this value is higher for Brazilians (52.3% to 74.2% depending on the type of yogurt) when compared with the Portuguese (33.1% to 73.3%). Regarding the results in Table 12, it is observed that the classes of yogurts which are consumed by a lower percentage of participants are the ones with separated flavors (only by 26.7% of Portuguese and by 25.8% of Brazilians). Natural yogurt is consumed more frequently by the Portuguese (59.8%): 29.3% once a week and 19.3% 2–3 times/week, while the Brazilians consume 42.3% of this kind of yogurt: 30.9% once a week and 7.9% 2–3 times/week. A relatively similar trend is also observed for the aromatized yogurt. For the other classes of yogurt, the differences between Portuguese consumers and Brazilian are small.

From the collected data it was further possible to determine those participants who never consumed certain classes of dairy products or those who never consumed any of the investigated dairy products at all, and these results are shown in Table 13 for the global sample and separated by country. The results indicate that butter is the class which a highest percentage of participants never consume, 30.0%, with a higher expression in Brazil as compared to Portugal. The second class corresponds to milk products, which are never consumed by 22.8% of people, but in this case it is in Portugal that the percentage in higher. Following comes the yogurt category, never consumed by 21.1% of Brazilians and by 7.6% of Portuguese. Last appears the cheese category, with the lowest percentage of people who never consume this type of dairy product. Finally, one can see that a residual number of participants identified as never consuming any of the dairy products considered, and this result might not correspond to the reality in both countries, since this was a questionnaire survey in which the volunteers participated knowing from the start that it was about the consumption of dairy products (this information was provided before the participants gave their informed consent). Therefore, it is possible that people who never consume dairy products did not even respond to the questionnaire, by considering that their participation was not useful, or because they did not want to spend time with a subject that was not important for them.

Table 13. Participants who "never" consume dairy products in Portugal and Brazil.

	Portugal (N = 420)		Brazil (N = 430)		Global (N = 850)	
	N	%	N	%	N	%
Participants who "never" eat dairy products in the category Milk	121	28.8	73	17.0	194	22.8
Participants who "never" eat dairy products in the category Cheese	36	8.6	26	6.0	62	7.3
Participants who "never" eat dairy products in the category Butter	100	23.8	155	36.0	255	30.0
Participants who "never" eat dairy products in the category Yogurt	32	7.6	91	21.1	123	14.4
Participants who "never" eat dairy products in any of the categories	5	1.2	5	1.2	10	1.2

3.5. Variables Influencing Dairy Product Consumption

As explained in the section Materials and Methods, the variables accounting for the average level of consumption of the four categories of dairy products (milk, cheese, butter and yogurt) were submitted to a tree classification analysis for evaluation of the relative importance of each of the possible influential variables considered: country, sex, age class, education, BMI class, satisfaction with body weight, balanced diet and lifestyle clusters. Figures 1–4 show the obtained classification trees, and they reveal that some of the variables considered in the analysis were not influential, for example, variables such as country and balanced diet never appeared in any of the diagrams, meaning that they do not determine the consumption of any of the dairy products evaluated.

The tree in Figure 1, for consumption of milk products, contains 4 levels and 17 nodes, of which 9 are terminal. The risk estimate for re-substitution was 0.062 with standard error 0.008 and the risk estimate for cross-validation was 0.061 with standard error 0.008. These values indicate goodness of fit to the model. The results in Figure 1 reveal that, for the whole sample (node 0), a huge majority of participants have a low milk consumption (93.8%) and that the first discriminant variable was age, so that younger people (from 18 to 30 years) tend to have a slightly higher consumption of milk than older people (moderate consumption: 11.2% and 4.2%, respectively, for people up to 30 years and older). For young people, the second discriminating factor was sex, with men showing higher consumption of milk as compared with women. For young men, the next discriminant variable was body weight satisfaction and the final differentiating factor was lifestyle cluster. Regarding older people, the next discriminating factor after age was education, with lower milk consumption for people with university degrees or higher levels of education. Following in the order of appearance the discriminating variables were sex, lifestyle cluster and age class again, differentiating in the last level middle aged adults (93.5% low and 6.5% moderate consumption) from senior adults and elderly (100% low consumption).

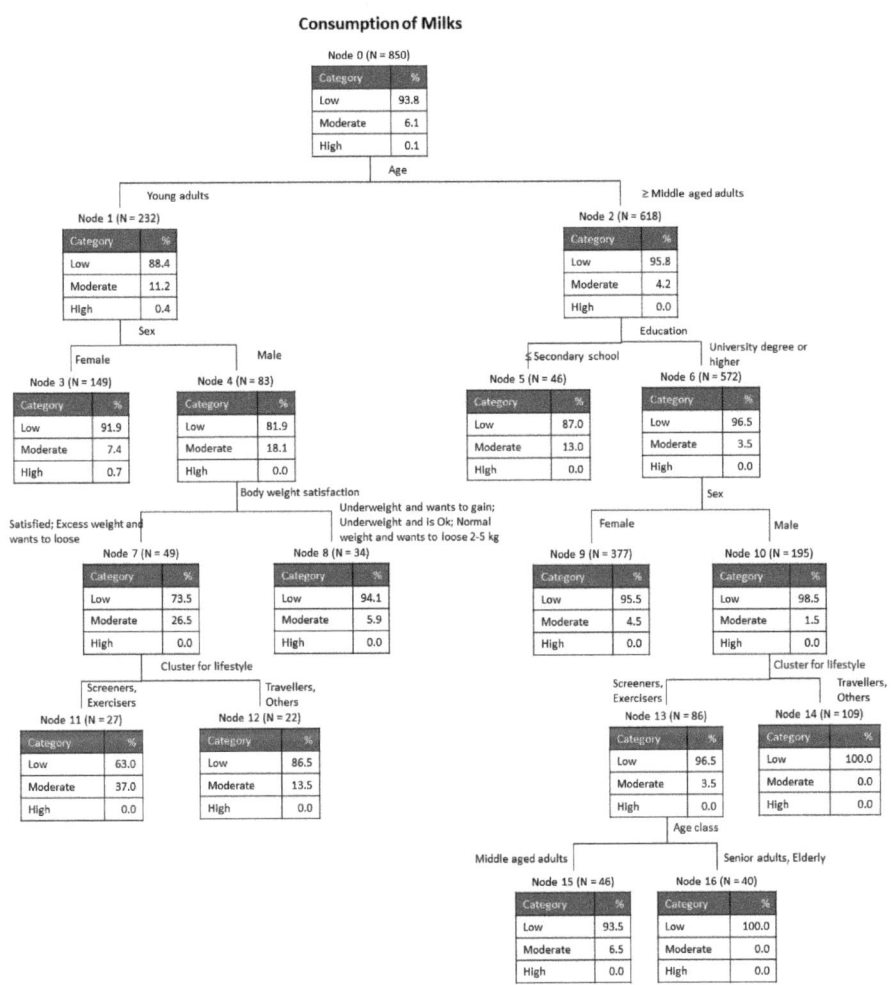

Figure 1. Tree classification for consumption of milks.

The tree in Figure 2 for the consumption of cheese has 5 levels with 17 nodes, including 9 terminals. The risk estimates for re-substitution and for cross-validation were in both cases 0.062 with standard error 0.008. The results for the whole set of participants (node 0) indicate that, similarly to milk consumption, cheese consumption is also very low (93.8% low, and only 5.9% moderate). The discriminant variable in the first level was BMI class, separating the overweight and obese participants as having slightly higher consumption of cheese (8.6% moderate and 91.1% low). For these, the next discriminant variable was education and in this case those with higher levels of education tend to have a higher consumption of cheese (8.6% moderate against 0% for those with lower education). For the branch of underweight and normal weight, BMI class was again the differentiating factor, with lower consumption for normal weight participants (3.5% moderate against 11.4% moderate for the underweight). The following discriminant variables were body weight satisfaction (level 3), sex and age class (level 4) and lifestyle cluster (level 5).

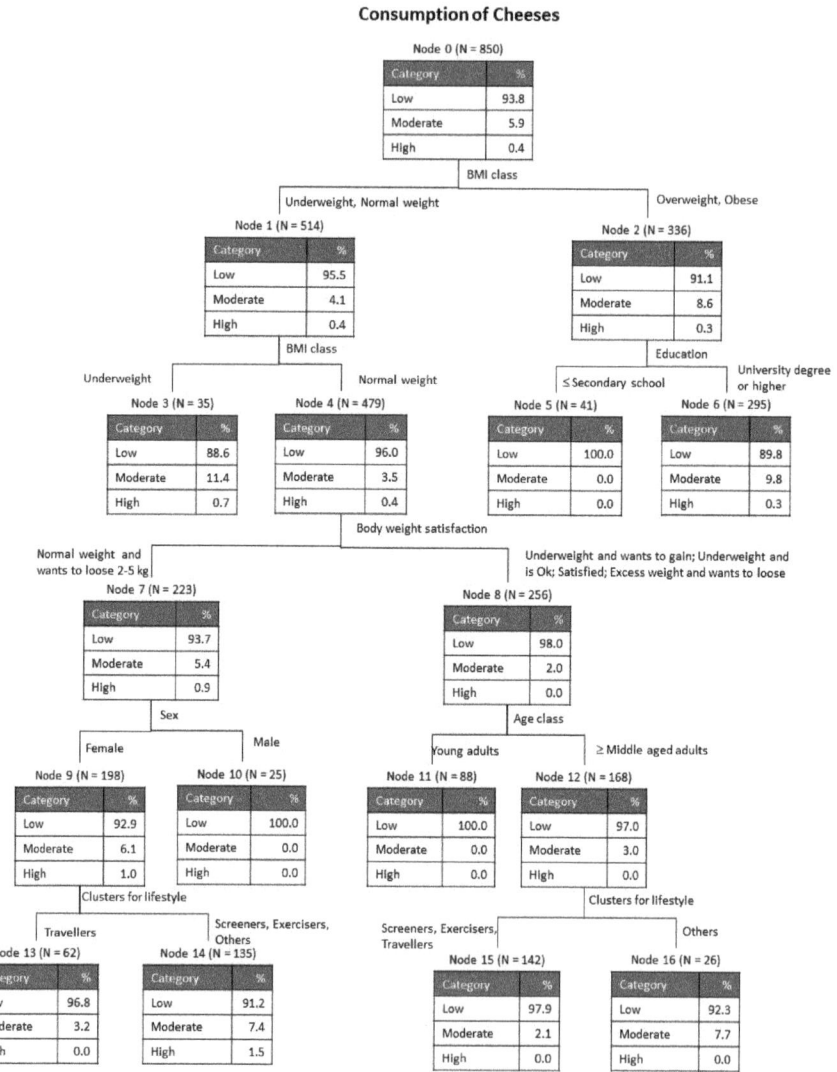

Figure 2. Tree classification for consumption of cheeses.

Figure 3 presents the results of the tree obtained for butter consumption. This has only 3 levels, representing 7 nodes, of which 4 were terminal. The risk parameters were equal for re-substitution and cross-validation: risk estimate = 0.076, standard error = 0.009. In the case of butter, the values for the whole sample are low (92.4% low, 6.6% for moderate and 1.1% for high consumption), being in line with the trends previously observed for milk and for cheese. The first discriminant was sex, differentiating men as having lower consumption than women (94.9% and 91.0%, respectively). For women the node was terminal, while for the men, the following discriminant was lifestyle cluster, separating the screeners and exercisers as showing a slightly higher butter consumption (6.3% moderate as compared with 1.9% moderate for travelers and others). Finally, at level 3 the discriminating variable was age class, separating people over 50 years, which presented a higher butter consumption (4.7% moderate).

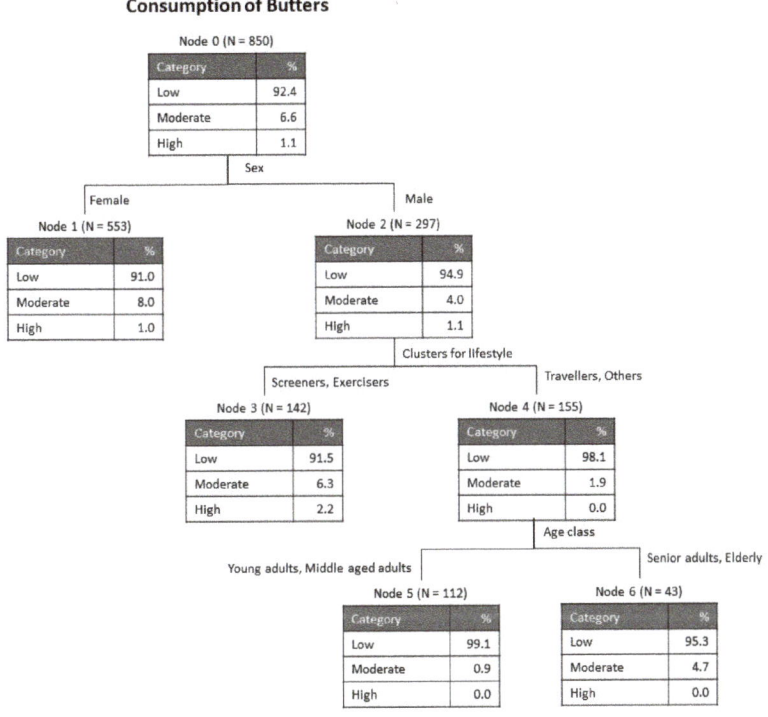

Figure 3. Tree classification for consumption of butters.

Figure 4 shows the tree for yogurt consumption, with 4 levels and 11 nodes (six of which are terminal). The risk estimate for re-substitution was 0.085 with standard error 0.010 and equal values were obtained for cross-validation. The consumption of yogurts is again low (91.5% at node 0). The first discriminant was BMI, as was observed for cheese, and the discriminant at level 2 was body weight satisfaction, regardless of the BMI class (i.e., on both branches). For the overweigh and obese (i.e., BMI of 25 or over) who are satisfied with their body weight, 25% have a moderate yogurt consumption. For these, the next level was separated according to their age class, and for the participants aged up to 50 years the last discriminant was lifestyle cluster.

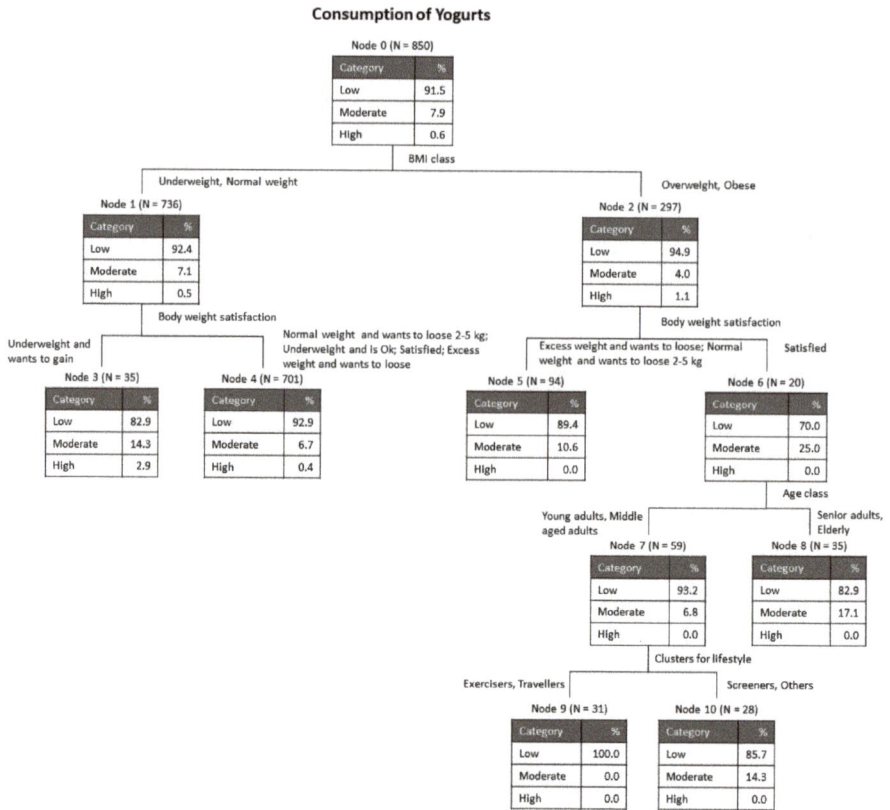

Figure 4. Tree classification for consumption of yogurts.

Overall, these results seem to indicate that the most relevant discriminant factors for dairy consumption were age, BMI, sex, education, satisfaction with body weight and lifestyle cluster, following more or less the same order regardless of the type of dairy product. On the contrary, factors such as country or balanced diet were found to have no discriminant capacity for the variables under study, i.e., the consumption of dairy products is not influenced significantly by these two variables.

According to Wolf et al. [99,100] age is a factor determining milk consumption in the United States, with people born in the 1990s consuming milk less often than earlier generations, and this trend is expected to continue with the replacement of older generations by younger ones. Nevertheless, the consumption of other dairy products seems to be increasing in the US, in the case of cheese mostly because it is widely used in pizzas and in the case of butter because there has been a setback regarding health views of butterfat [101]. The study by Xu et al. [4] highlighted also differences in dairy consumption according to sex and BMI. On the other hand, lifestyle behaviors have been proven to influence dairy consumption according to the recent study by Santaliestra-Pasías et al. [102]. Their results suggest that European children with healthier lifestyles, specifically regarding aspects such as physical activity and sedentary behaviors, tend to consume higher quantities of milk and yogurt.

4. Limitations of the Study

Although providing important insights into the consumption habits of the Portuguese and Brazilian citizens, this study has some limitations, that are worth mentioning. One of these limitations is related to the sample sizes. Although it was possible to recruit a similar number of participants from the two countries involved, the size of Portugal and Brazil are unequal, and therefore it could be beneficial to have samples proportional to the population of each of the countries. Also, the group sizes for the sociodemographic variables considered are not equal, for example there were more women than men and a lower number of older participants or with lower levels of education. However, due to financial restrictions it was not possible to organize another type of data collection. One other limitation can be associated with the period of data collection. Although the data collection was mostly done in the period pre covid-19 outbreak, in Portugal the outbreak was felt after mid-March, but in Brazil the most critical period was later and therefore this outbreak may have had some influence only on data collected in Portugal in the last month. Still, in Portugal during the confinement period, no shortage whatsoever in the food supply was observed, and people were always allowed to go out for food shopping, so the possible influences are expected to be very mild. Another factor is related to possible loss of jobs and consequent reduction in the available monthly budget, which could influence people's food purchases. However, in the early days of the confinement the social measures implemented prevented a mass loss of jobs and therefore this problem could have had a higher importance if the data collection was extended beyond April, which it was not.

Other limitations relate to some additional aspects of the research that could in future studies be addressed, such as for example the motivations that drive consumers in relation to the consumption or non-consumption of dairy products. This would also be an interesting aspect to explore in the future, to better understand the reasons why people consume or avoid different dairy products. Finally, it would also be interesting to replicate this investigation in other countries to see if the observed low influence of the country on the dairy products' pattern of consumption would still be maintained, or if these similarities observed are because the two countries involved share a common culture and history due to the colonization of Brazil by the Portuguese.

5. Conclusions

The present work established some relevant facts about the consumption of dairy products in two counties, one situated in Europe and the other in Latin America. Although some small differences were observed in the consumption patterns in both countries, a worrying fact is that the levels of consumption for all dairy products studied were frankly low. Regarding milk consumption, semi skimmed milk is never consumed by about half of the participants, those who never consume skimmed milk are even more in number, and these numbers increase again for chocolate flavored and enriched milks. Cheeses are also consumed by only small parts of the population in these two countries, with the least consumed being imported cheeses in both countries followed by soft paste cheeses in Brazil and Portugal and whey cheese in Portugal. For those who consume cheese, they do so with a low frequency: once a week or sometimes (2–3 times per week). Butter is also consumed by only about half of the adult population, but the percentage of those who never consume butter increases for skimmed butter and unsalted butter, these last being least preferred when compared to regular milk butter. Yogurt consumption follows the same low consumption trends of other dairy products. In order of preference, the most frequently consumed yogurt types are liquid yogurts and natural yogurts in Portugal and creamy fruit pulp yogurt, liquid yogurt and Greek type yogurt in Brazil.

This work further studied some anthropometric facts of the surveyed sample as well as behavioral aspects, allowing the establishment of groups according to lifestyles, as determined by cluster analysis. Four clusters were identified: 1—Screeners, 2—Exercisers, 3—Travelers and 4—Others. The screeners were mostly single young adults, with low education and from Brazil. The Exercisers were mostly women with ages comprised between 30 and 65 years, with a university degree and from Portugal. The Travelers were mostly men aged between 30 and 65 years, also with a university degree and divorced or widowed. These lifestyles were found to be influential to the consumption of dairy products for all classes of dairy tested: milk, cheese, yogurt and butter. Additionally, other influential factors found were age, sex, education, BMI and satisfaction with body weight. The influence of country was not a meaningful discriminant, in relation to the other variables included in the classification analysis. This might be due to the cultural similarity between the two countries studied, which, although being in different parts of the globe, have a historic and cultural common past. For these reasons it would be interesting to replicate this study in the future in other countries to evaluate the extension of possible country variability in the consumption of dairy products.

Author Contributions: Conceptualization, R.P.F.G. and O.A.; methodology, R.P.F.G. and O.A.; software, R.P.F.G.; validation, R.P.F.G.; formal analysis, R.P.F.G. and O.A.; investigation, R.P.F.G., S.G.F., S.C., O.A.; resources, R.P.F.G.; data curation, R.P.F.G.; writing—original draft preparation, R.P.F.G., S.G.F. and O.A.; writing—review and editing, all authors; visualization, R.P.F.G.; supervision, R.P.F.G.; project administration, R.P.F.G.; funding acquisition, R.P.F.G. and O.A. All authors have read and agreed to the published version of the manuscript.

Funding: The APC was funded by FCT—Foundation for Science and Technology (Portugal) project Reference UIDB/00681/2020.

Acknowledgments: This work was supported by National Funds through the FCT—Foundation for Science and Technology, I.P., within the scope of the project Reference UIDB/00681/2020. Furthermore, we would like to thank the CERNAS Research Centre and the Polytechnic Institute of Viseu for their support. We would also like to thank Isabel Lavado for proofreading and revising the English in the article.

Conflicts of Interest: The authors declare no conflict of interest.

Appendix A

The questions included in the questionnaire were distributed by tree different sections as follows:

Part 1—Sociodemographic data

Country: Portugal $\square_1$ Brazil $\square_2$
1. Age: _____ years
2. Sex: Female $\square_1$ Male $\square_2$
3. Level of education:
Primary (4 school years) $\square_1$ Basic school (9 years) $\square_2$ Secondary school (12 years) $\square_3$
University degree or higher $\square_4$
4. Marital status:
Single $\square_1$ Married $\square_2$ Divorced $\square_3$ Widowed $\square_4$
5. Profession:
Student $\square_1$ Employee for the government $\square_2$ Employee for private companies $\square_3$
Self-employed freelance $\square_4$ Businessmen $\square_5$ Unemployed $\square_6$ Other $\square_7$

Part 2—Anthropometric data and behavioural aspects

6. Height: _____ meters
7. Weight: _____ kg
8. Do you practice physical exercise?
Never $\square_1$ Occasional (once/week) $\square_2$ Moderate (2–3 times/week) $\square_3$ Intense (+ 3 times/week) $\square_4$
9. Daily hours watching TV:
0–30 min $\square_1$ 30 min–1 hour $\square_2$ 1–2 hour $\square_3$ 2–5 hours $\square_4$ More than 5 hours $\square_5$
10. Daily time playing on computer or mobile phone or on social networks:
0–30 min $\square_1$ 30 min–1 hour $\square_2$ 1–2 hour $\square_3$ 2–5 hours $\square_4$ More than 5 hours $\square_5$
11. Daily time working on the computer:
0–30 min $\square_1$ 30 min–1 hour $\square_2$ 1–2 hour $\square_3$ 2–5 hours $\square_4$ More than 5 hours $\square_5$
12. Daily time traveling sedentary (car, motorcycle, train, bus, etc ...):
0–30 min $\square_1$ 30 min–1 hour $\square_2$ 1–2 hour $\square_3$ 2–5 hours $\square_4$ More than 5 hours $\square_5$
13. Daily walking time (on foot, by bicycle, ...):
0–30 min $\square_1$ 30 min–1 hour $\square_2$ 1–2 hour $\square_3$ 2–5 hours $\square_4$ More than 5 hours $\square_5$
14. Do you believe that you have a balanced diet?
Never $\square_1$ Seldom $\square_2$ Sometimes $\square_3$ Several times/week $\square_4$ Always $\square_5$
15. Are you satisfied with your bodyweight?

I am satisfied with my weight and wish to keep it ☐$_1$
I am of normal weight, but I would like to lose 2 to 5 kg ☐$_2$
I am underweight, but I feel good ☐$_3$
I am underweight and would like to gain 2 to 5 kg ☐$_4$
I am overweight and I would like to lose a few pounds, but I have tried and I cannot ☐$_5$
I am overweight and do nothing to change ☐$_6$
Other ☐$_7$

Part 3—Consumption habits regarding dairy products

16. How often do you consume the following dairy products?

Product	Never	Seldom *Once/week*	Sometimes *2–3 x/week*	Frequently *once/day*	Always *+ 1 x/day*
Category: Milk					
(1) Semi skimmed milk					
(2) Skimmed milk					
(3) Chocolate flavored milk					
(4) Enriched milk					
Category: Cheese					
(5) Soft paste cheese					
(6) Cured hard paste cheese					
(7) Fresh cheese					
(8) Whey cheese					
(9) Semi skimmed sliced cheese					
(10) Skimmed sliced cheese					
(11) Imported cheeses					
Category: Butter					
(12) Milk butter (not vegetable spreads)					
(13) Skimmed butter					
(14) Butter without salt					
Category: Yogurt					
(15) Natural yogurt					
(16) Aromatized yogurt					
(17) Creamy fruit pulp yogurt					
(18) Yogurt with fruit pieces					
(19) Liquid yogurt					
(20) Yogurt with separated flavors (cereals, jam, chocolate chips, etc.)					
(21) Greek type yogurt					

References

1. EC. *Milk Market Observatory: EU Production of Main Dairy Products*; European Commission: Brussels, Belgium, 2020; pp. 1–3.
2. CLAL EU-28: Yogurt Production. Available online: https://www.clal.it/en/?section=consegne_eu&p=D4100_THS_T (accessed on 10 October 2020).
3. EC. *Milk Market Observatory: World Production of Main Dairy Products*; European Commission: Brussels, Belgium, 2020; pp. 1–11.

4. Xu, P.P.; Yang, T.T.; Xu, J.; Li, L.; Cao, W.; Gan, Q.; Hu, X.Q.; Pan, H.; Zhao, W.H.; Zhang, Q. Dairy Consumption and Associations with Nutritional Status of Chinese Children and Adolescents. *Biomed. Environ. Sci.* **2019**, *32*, 393–405. [CrossRef]
5. Yousefi, M.; Jafari, S.M. Recent advances in application of different hydrocolloids in dairy products to improve their techno-functional properties. *Trends Food Sci. Technol.* **2019**, *88*, 468–483. [CrossRef]
6. Girard, C.L.; Graulet, B. Methods and approaches to estimate B vitamin status in dairy cows: Knowledge, gaps and advances. *Methods* **2020**. [CrossRef] [PubMed]
7. Wisnieski, L.; Brown, J.L.; Holcombe, S.J.; Gandy, J.C.; Sordillo, L.M. Serum vitamin D concentrations at dry-off and close-up predict increased postpartum urine ketone concentrations in dairy cattle. *J. Dairy Sci.* **2020**, *103*, 1795–1806. [CrossRef] [PubMed]
8. Zahedirad, M.; Asadzadeh, S.; Nikooyeh, B.; Neyestani, T.R.; Khorshidian, N.; Yousefi, M.; Mortazavian, A.M. Fortification aspects of vitamin D in dairy products: A review study. *Int. Dairy J.* **2019**, *94*, 53–64. [CrossRef]
9. Gutiérrez-Peña, R.; Fernández-Cabanás, V.M.; Mena, Y.; Delgado-Pertíñez, M. Fatty acid profile and vitamins A and E contents of milk in goat farms under Mediterranean wood pastures as affected by grazing conditions and seasons. *J. Food Compos. Anal.* **2018**, *72*, 122–131. [CrossRef]
10. Fadlalla, I.M.T.; Omer, S.A.; Atta, M. Determination of some serum macroelement minerals levels at different lactation stages of dairy cows and their correlations. *Sci. Afr.* **2020**, *8*, e00351. [CrossRef]
11. García, M.I.H.; Puerto, P.P.; Baquero, M.F.; Rodríguez, E.R.; Martín, J.D.; Romero, C.D. Mineral and trace element concentrations of dairy products from goats' milk produced in Tenerife (Canary Islands). *Int. Dairy J.* **2006**, *16*, 182–185. [CrossRef]
12. Reykdal, O.; Rabieh, S.; Steingrimsdottir, L.; Gunnlaugsdottir, H. Minerals and trace elements in Icelandic dairy products and meat. *J. Food Compos. Anal.* **2011**, *24*, 980–986. [CrossRef]
13. Jansson-Knodell, C.L.; Krajicek, E.J.; Savaiano, D.A.; Shin, A.S. Lactose Intolerance: A Concise Review to Skim the Surface. *Mayo Clin. Proc.* **2020**, *95*, 1499–1505. [CrossRef]
14. Rana, S.; Morya, R.K.; Malik, A.; Bhadada, S.K.; Sachdeva, N.; Sharma, G. A relationship between vitamin D, parathyroid hormone, calcium levels and lactose intolerance in type 2 diabetic patients and healthy subjects. *Clin. Chim. Acta* **2016**, *462*, 174–177. [CrossRef]
15. Nicklas, T.A.; Qu, H.; Hughes, S.O.; He, M.; Wagner, S.E.; Foushee, H.R.; Shewchuk, R.M. Self-perceived lactose intolerance results in lower intakes of calcium and dairy foods and is associated with hypertension and diabetes in adults. *Am. J. Clin. Nutr.* **2011**, *94*, 191–198. [CrossRef]
16. Vesa, T.H.; Marteau, P.; Korpela, R. Lactose intolerance. *J. Am. Coll. Nutr.* **2000**, *19*, 165S–175S. [CrossRef]
17. Bailey, R.K.; Fileti, C.P.; Keith, J.; Tropez-Sims, S.; Price, W.; Allison-Ottey, S.D. Lactose intolerance and health disparities among African Americans and Hispanic Americans: An updated consensus statement. *J. Natl. Med. Assoc.* **2013**, *105*, 112–127. [CrossRef]
18. Krela-Kaźmierczak, I.; Michalak, M.; Szymczak-Tomczak, A.; Czarnywojtek, A.; Wawrzyniak, A.; Łykowska-Szuber, L.; Stawczyk-Eder, K.; Dobrowolska, A.; Eder, P. Milk and dairy product consumption in patients with inflammatory bowel disease: Helpful or harmful to bone mineral density? *Nutrition* **2020**, *79–80*, 110830. [CrossRef]
19. Astrup, A.; Magkos, F.; Bier, D.M.; Brenna, J.T.; de Oliveira Otto, M.C.; Hill, J.O.; King, J.C.; Mente, A.; Ordovas, J.M.; Volek, J.S.; et al. Saturated Fats and Health: A Reassessment and Proposal for Food-Based Recommendations: JACC State-of-the-Art Review. *J. Am. Coll. Cardiol.* **2020**, *76*, 844–857. [CrossRef]
20. Roy, S.J.; Lapierre, S.S.; Baker, B.D.; Delfausse, L.A.; Machin, D.R.; Tanaka, H. High dietary intake of whole milk and full-fat dairy products does not exert hypotensive effects in adults with elevated blood pressure. *Nutr. Res.* **2019**, *64*, 72–81. [CrossRef]
21. Balthazar, C.F.; Silva, H.L.A.; Esmerino, E.A.; Rocha, R.S.; Moraes, J.; Carmo, M.A.V.; Azevedo, L.; Camps, I.; Abud, Y.K.D.; Sant'Anna, C.; et al. The addition of inulin and Lactobacillus casei 01 in sheep milk ice cream. *Food Chem.* **2018**, *246*, 464–472. [CrossRef]
22. Dantas, A.B.; Jesus, V.F.; Silva, R.; Almada, C.N.; Esmerino, E.A.; Cappato, L.P.; Silva, M.C.; Raices, R.S.L.; Cavalcanti, R.N.; Carvalho, C.C.; et al. Manufacture of probiotic Minas Frescal cheese with Lactobacillus casei Zhang. *J. Dairy Sci.* **2016**, *99*, 18–30. [CrossRef]
23. de Toledo Guimarães, J.; Silva, E.K.; de Freitas, M.Q.; de Almeida Meireles, M.A.; da Cruz, A.G. Non-thermal emerging technologies and their effects on the functional properties of dairy products. *Curr. Opin. Food Sci.* **2018**, *22*, 62–66. [CrossRef]

24. Martins, N.; Oliveira, M.B.P.P.; Ferreira, I.C.F.R. Development of Functional Dairy Foods. In *Bioactive Molecules in Food*; Mérillon, J.-M., Ramawat, K.G., Eds.; Reference Series in Phytochemistry; Springer International Publishing: Cham, Switzerland, 2017; pp. 1–19. ISBN 978-3-319-54528-8.
25. Rodríguez-Pérez, C.; Pimentel-Moral, S.; Ochando-Pulido, J. 4—New Trends and Perspectives in Functional Dairy-Based Beverages. In *Milk-Based Beverages*; Grumezescu, A.M., Holban, A.M., Eds.; Woodhead Publishing: Cambridge, UK, 2019; pp. 95–138. ISBN 978-0-12-815504-2.
26. Khandpur, N.; Cediel, G.; Obando, D.A.; Jaime, P.C.; Parra, D.C.; Khandpur, N.; Cediel, G.; Obando, D.A.; Jaime, P.C.; Parra, D.C. Sociodemographic factors associated with the consumption of ultra-processed foods in Colombia. *Rev. Saúde Pública* **2020**, *54*, 19. [CrossRef] [PubMed]
27. Riediger, N.D.; Shooshtari, S.; Moghadasian, M.H. The Influence of Sociodemographic Factors on Patterns of Fruit and Vegetable Consumption in Canadian Adolescents. *J. Am. Diet. Assoc.* **2007**, *107*, 1511–1518. [CrossRef] [PubMed]
28. Nayga, R.M. Sociodemographic Influences on Consumer Concern for Food Safety: The Case of Irradiation, Antibiotics, Hormones, and Pesticides. *Rev. Agric. Econ.* **1996**, *18*, 467–475. [CrossRef]
29. Richter, T.; Sanders, J. Impact of socio-demographic factors on consumption patterns and buying motives with respect to organic dairy products in Switzerland. In Proceedings of the 1st SAFO Workshop, Florence, Italy, 5–7 September 2003; pp. 211–217.
30. Miftari, I.; Ahmeti, S.; Gjonbalaj, M.; Shkodra, J. *The Role of Demographic and Socioeconomic Factors on Consumption Patterns and Demand for Dairy Products in Kosovo*; Social Science Research Network: Rochester, NY, USA, 2011.
31. Shi, Z.; Lien, N.; Kumar, B.N.; Holmboe-Ottesen, G. Socio-demographic differences in food habits and preferences of school adolescents in Jiangsu Province, China. *Eur. J. Clin. Nutr.* **2005**, *59*, 1439–1448. [CrossRef]
32. Baek, Y.; Chitekwe, S. Sociodemographic factors associated with inadequate food group consumption and dietary diversity among infants and young children in Nepal. *PLoS ONE* **2019**, *14*, e0213610. [CrossRef]
33. Yun, B.; Maburutse, B.E.; Kang, M.; Park, M.R.; Park, D.J.; Kim, Y.; Oh, S. Short communication: Dietary bovine milk–derived exosomes improve bone health in an osteoporosis-induced mouse model. *J. Dairy Sci.* **2020**, *103*, 7752–7760. [CrossRef]
34. Lee, C.S.; Kim, B.K.; Lee, I.O.; Park, N.H.; Kim, S.H. Prevention of bone loss by using Lactobacillus-fermented milk products in a rat model of glucocorticoid-induced secondary osteoporosis. *Int. Dairy J.* **2020**, *109*, 104788. [CrossRef]
35. Fardellone, P.; Séjourné, A.; Blain, H.; Cortet, B.; Thomas, T. Osteoporosis: Is milk a kindness or a curse? *Jt. Bone Spine* **2017**, *84*, 275–281. [CrossRef]
36. Rodrigues, A.; Laires, P.; Gouveia, N.; Eusébio, M.; Canhão, H.; Branco, J. PMS18—Characterization of Osteoporosis in Portugal—Treatment Patterns and Reasons for Under-Treatment and Non-Persistence With Pharmacological Treatments. *Value Health* **2015**, *18*, A636–A637. [CrossRef]
37. Radominski, S.C.; Bernardo, W.; de Paula, A.P.; Albergaria, B.-H.; Moreira, C.; Fernandes, C.E.; Castro, C.H.M.; de Zerbini, C.A.F.; Domiciano, D.S.; Mendonça, L.M.C.; et al. Brazilian guidelines for the diagnosis and treatment of postmenopausal osteoporosis. *Rev. Bras. Reumatol. (Engl. Ed.)* **2017**, *57*, 452–466. [CrossRef]
38. Hill, M.M.; Hill, A. *Investigação por Questionário*, 2nd ed.; Sílabo: Lisboa, Portugal, 2008.
39. Marôco, J. *Análise Estatística com o SPSS Statistics*, 7th ed.; ReportNumber: Lisboa, Portugal, 2018.
40. Robinson, O.C. Sampling in Interview-Based Qualitative Research: A Theoretical and Practical Guide. *Qual. Res. Psychol.* **2014**, *11*, 25–41. [CrossRef]
41. Bornstein, M.H.; Jager, J.; Putnick, D.L. Sampling in developmental science: Situations, shortcomings, solutions, and standards. *Dev. Rev.* **2013**, *33*, 357–370. [CrossRef]
42. Guiné, R.P.F.; Florença, S.G.; Villalobos Moya, K.; Anjos, O. Edible Flowers, Old Tradition or New Gastronomic Trend: A First Look at Consumption in Portugal versus Costa Rica. *Foods* **2020**, *9*, 977. [CrossRef] [PubMed]
43. Weir, C.B.; Jan, A. BMI Classification Percentile and Cut Off Points. In *StatPearls*; StatPearls Publishing: Treasure Island, FL, USA, 2020.
44. WHO Body Mass Index—BMI. Available online: https://www.euro.who.int/en/health-topics/disease-prevention/nutrition/a-healthy-lifestyle/body-mass-index-bmi (accessed on 27 October 2020).
45. Witten, R.; Witte, J. *Statistics*, 9th ed.; Wiley: Hoboken, NJ, USA, 2009.

46. Broen, M.P.G.; Moonen, A.J.H.; Kuijf, M.L.; Dujardin, K.; Marsh, L.; Richard, I.H.; Starkstein, S.E.; Martinez–Martin, P.; Leentjens, A.F.G. Factor analysis of the Hamilton Depression Rating Scale in Parkinson's disease. *Parkinsonism Relat. Disord.* **2015**, *21*, 142–146. [CrossRef] [PubMed]
47. Stevens, J.P. *Applied Multivariate Statistics for the Social Sciences*, 5th ed.; Routledge: New York, NY, USA, 2009; ISBN 978-0-8058-5903-4.
48. Rohm, A.J.; Swaminathan, V. A typology of online shoppers based on shopping motivations. *J. Bus. Res.* **2004**, *57*, 748–757. [CrossRef]
49. Dolnicar, S. A Review of Data-Driven Market Segmentation in Tourism. *J. Travel Tour. Mark.* **2002**, *12*, 1–22. [CrossRef]
50. Bailey, R.R.; Serra, M.C.; McGrath, R.P. Obesity and diabetes are jointly associated with functional disability in stroke survivors. *Disabil. Health J.* **2020**, 100914. [CrossRef]
51. Carbone, S.; Lavie, C.J.; Elagizi, A.; Arena, R.; Ventura, H.O. The Impact of Obesity in Heart Failure. *Heart Fail. Clin.* **2020**, *16*, 71–80. [CrossRef]
52. Pearson, E.S. Goal setting as a health behavior change strategy in overweight and obese adults: A systematic literature review examining intervention components. *Patient Educ. Couns.* **2012**, *87*, 32–42. [CrossRef]
53. Saliba, L.J.; Maffett, S. Hypertensive Heart Disease and Obesity: A Review. *Heart Fail. Clin.* **2019**, *15*, 509–517. [CrossRef]
54. Bvenura, C.; Sivakumar, D. The role of wild fruits and vegetables in delivering a balanced and healthy diet. *Food Res. Int.* **2017**, *99*, 15–30. [CrossRef] [PubMed]
55. Burgess, A.; Glasauer, P. *Family Nutrition Guide*; FAO—Food and Agriculture Organization of the United Nations: Rome, Italy, 2004.
56. De Fernandes, D.P.S.; Duarte, M.S.L.; Pessoa, M.C.; do Franceschini, S.C.C.; Ribeiro, A.Q. Evaluation of diet quality of the elderly and associated factors. *Arch. Gerontol. Geriatr.* **2017**, *72*, 174–180. [CrossRef] [PubMed]
57. De Silva, N.A.; Pedraza, D.F.; de Menezes, T.N.; de Silva, N.A.; Pedraza, D.F.; de Menezes, T.N. Physical performance and its association with anthropometric and body composition variables in the elderly. *Ciência Amp Saúde Coletiva* **2015**, *20*, 3723–3732. [CrossRef]
58. Gebreslassie, M.; Sampaio, F.; Nystrand, C.; Ssegonja, R.; Feldman, I. Economic evaluations of public health interventions for physical activity and healthy diet: A systematic review. *Prev. Med.* **2020**, 106100. [CrossRef]
59. Kemmler, W.; von Stengel, S. Exercise Frequency, Health Risk Factors, and Diseases of the Elderly. *Arch. Phys. Med. Rehabil.* **2013**, *94*, 2046–2053. [CrossRef]
60. Kroencke, L.; Harari, G.M.; Katana, M.; Gosling, S.D. Personality trait predictors and mental well-being correlates of exercise frequency across the academic semester. *Soc. Sci. Med.* **2019**, *236*, 112400. [CrossRef]
61. Owusu, C.; Nock, N.L.; Hergenroeder, P.; Austin, K.; Bennet, E.; Cerne, S.; Moore, H.; Petkac, J.; Schluchter, M.; Schmitz, K.H.; et al. IMPROVE, a community-based exercise intervention versus support group to improve functional and health outcomes among older African American and non-Hispanic White breast cancer survivors from diverse socioeconomic backgrounds: Rationale, design and methods. *Contemp. Clin. Trials* **2020**, *92*, 106001. [CrossRef]
62. Watson, S.J.; Lewis, A.J.; Boyce, P.; Galbally, M. Exercise frequency and maternal mental health: Parallel process modelling across the perinatal period in an Australian pregnancy cohort. *J. Psychosom. Res.* **2018**, *111*, 91–99. [CrossRef]
63. Muehlhoff, E.; Bennett, A.; McMahon, D. *Milk and Dairy Products in Human Nutrition*; Food and Agriculture Organization of the United Nations: Rome, Italy, 2013; pp. 1–404.
64. Park, J.; Lee, H.S.; Lee, C.; Lee, H.-J. Milk consumption patterns and perceptions in Korean adolescents, adults, and the elderly. *Int. Dairy J.* **2019**, *95*, 78–85. [CrossRef]
65. Zingone, F.; Bucci, C.; Iovino, P.; Ciacci, C. Consumption of milk and dairy products: Facts and figures. *Nutrition* **2017**, *33*, 322–325. [CrossRef]
66. Pierre, M.S. *Changes in Canadians' Preferences for Milk and Dairy Products*; Canadian Minister of Industry: Ottawa, ON, Canada, 2017; pp. 1–9.
67. Batty, B.S.; Bionaz, M. Graduate Student Literature Review: The milk behind the mustache: A review of milk and bone biology. *J. Dairy Sci.* **2019**, *102*, 7608–7617. [CrossRef] [PubMed]
68. Cashman, K.D. Milk minerals (including trace elements) and bone health. *Int. Dairy J.* **2006**, *16*, 1389–1398. [CrossRef]

69. Kalkwarf, H.J. Childhood and adolescent milk intake and adult bone health. *Int. Congr. Ser.* **2007**, *1297*, 39–49. [CrossRef]
70. Bazarra-Fernandez, A. Children, milk, bone and osteoporosis in menopause. *Bone* **2009**, *45*, S102–S103. [CrossRef]
71. Brick, T.; Hettinga, K.; Kirchner, B.; Pfaffl, M.W.; Ege, M.J. The Beneficial Effect of Farm Milk Consumption on Asthma, Allergies, and Infections: From Meta-Analysis of Evidence to Clinical Trial. *J. Allergy Clin. Immunol. Pr.* **2020**, *8*, 878–889.e3. [CrossRef] [PubMed]
72. Wang, X.J.; Jiang, C.Q.; Zhang, W.S.; Zhu, F.; Jin, Y.L.; Woo, J.; Cheng, K.K.; Lam, T.H.; Xu, L. Milk consumption and risk of mortality from all-cause, cardiovascular disease and cancer in older people. *Clin. Nutr.* **2020**, *39*, 3442–3451. [CrossRef]
73. De Oliveira, M.T.; Lobo, A.S.; Kupek, E.; de Assis, M.A.A.; Cezimbra, V.G.; Pereira, L.J.; Silva, D.A.S.; Di Pietro, P.F.; de Hinnig, P.F. Association between sleep period time and dietary patterns in Brazilian schoolchildren aged 7–13 years. *Sleep Med.* **2020**, *74*, 179–188. [CrossRef]
74. de Oliveira, G.M.M.; Mendes, M.; Malachias, M.V.B.; Morais, J.; Filho, O.M.; Coelho, A.S.; Capingana, D.P.; Azevedo, V.; Soares, I.; Menete, A.; et al. 2017 Guidelines for the management of arterial hypertension in primary health care in Portuguese-speaking countries. *Rev. Port. Cardiol. (Engl. Ed.)* **2017**, *36*, 789–798. [CrossRef]
75. Muros, J.J.; Cabrera-Vique, C.; Briones, M.; Seiquer, I. Assessing the dietary intake of calcium, magnesium, iron, zinc and copper in institutionalised children and adolescents from Guatemala. Contribution of nutritional supplements. *J. Trace Elem. Med. Biol.* **2019**, *53*, 91–97. [CrossRef]
76. Mesías, M.; Seiquer, I.; Navarro, M.P. Calcium nutrition in adolescence. *Crit. Rev. Food Sci. Nutr.* **2011**, *51*, 195–209. [CrossRef]
77. DGAC. *Scientific Report of the 2015 Dietary Guidelines Advisory Committee*; U.S. Department of Agriculture: Washington, DC, USA, 2015; pp. 1–436.
78. Lee, A.C.; Trivedi, M.K.; Branton, A.; Trivedi, D.; Nayak, G.; Mondal, S.C.; Jana, S. The Potential Benefits of Biofield Energy Treated Vitamin D_3 on Bone Mineralization in Human Bone Osteosarcoma Cells (MG-63). *Int. J. Nutr. Food Sci.* **2018**, *7*, 30. [CrossRef]
79. Holick, M.F. Sunlight and vitamin D for bone health and prevention of autoimmune diseases, cancers, and cardiovascular disease. *Am. J. Clin. Nutr.* **2004**, *80*, 1678S–1688S. [CrossRef] [PubMed]
80. Asbaghi, O.; Sadeghian, M.; Mozaffari-Khosravi, H.; Maleki, V.; Shokri, A.; Hajizadeh-Sharafabad, F.; Alizadeh, M.; Sadeghi, O. The effect of vitamin d-calcium co-supplementation on inflammatory biomarkers: A systematic review and meta-analysis of randomized controlled trials. *Cytokine* **2020**, *129*, 155050. [CrossRef]
81. Erfanian, A.; Rasti, B.; Manap, Y. Comparing the calcium bioavailability from two types of nano-sized enriched milk using in-vivo assay. *Food Chem.* **2017**, *214*, 606–613. [CrossRef] [PubMed]
82. Meza, B.E.; Zorrilla, S.E.; Olivares, M.L. Rheological methods to analyse the thermal aggregation of calcium enriched milks. *Int. Dairy J.* **2019**, *97*, 25–30. [CrossRef]
83. Mouratidou, T.; Vicente-Rodriguez, G.; Gracia-Marco, L.; Huybrechts, I.; Sioen, I.; Widhalm, K.; Valtueña, J.; González-Gross, M.; Moreno, L.A. Associations of Dietary Calcium, Vitamin D, Milk Intakes, and 25-Hydroxyvitamin D With Bone Mass in Spanish Adolescents: The HELENA Study. *J. Clin. Densitom.* **2013**, *16*, 110–117. [CrossRef] [PubMed]
84. Guiné, R.P.F.; Florença, S.G.; Correia, P.M.R. Portuguese Traditional Cheeses: Production and Characterization. In *Cheeses around the World: Types, Production, Properties and Cultural and Nutritional Relevance*; Nova Science Publishers: New York, NY, USA, 2019; pp. 115–161.
85. Ferreira, V.; Pires, I.S.C.; Miranda, L.S.; Ribeiro, M.C. Brazilian Cheeses: Diversity, Culture and Tradition. In *Cheeses around the World: Types, Production, Properties and Cultural and Nutritional Relevance*; Nova Science Publishers: New York, NY, USA, 2019; pp. 17–46.
86. Oluk, A.C.; Güven, M.; Hayaloglu, A.A. Proteolysis texture and microstructure of low-fat Tulum cheese affected by exopolysaccharide-producing cultures during ripening. *Int. J. Food Sci. Technol.* **2014**, *49*, 435–443. [CrossRef]
87. Wang, J.; Wu, T.; Fang, X.; Yang, Z. Manufacture of low-fat Cheddar cheese by exopolysaccharide-producing Lactobacillus plantarum JLK0142 and its functional properties. *J. Dairy Sci.* **2019**, *102*, 3825–3838. [CrossRef]
88. Ulbricht, T.L.; Southgate, D.A. Coronary heart disease: Seven dietary factors. *Lancet* **1991**, *338*, 985–992. [CrossRef]

89. Rasmussen, B.M.; Vessby, B.; Uusitupa, M.; Berglund, L.; Pedersen, E.; Riccardi, G.; Rivellese, A.A.; Tapsell, L.; Hermansen, K. KANWU Study Group Effects of dietary saturated, monounsaturated, and n-3 fatty acids on blood pressure in healthy subjects. *Am. J. Clin. Nutr.* **2006**, *83*, 221–226. [CrossRef]
90. Delicato, C.; Schouteten, J.J.; Dewettinck, K.; Gellynck, X.; Tzompa-Sosa, D.A. Consumers' perception of bakery products with insect fat as partial butter replacement. *Food Qual. Prefer.* **2020**, *79*, 103755. [CrossRef]
91. Bourrie, B.C.T.; Willing, B.P.; Cotter, P.D. The Microbiota and Health Promoting Characteristics of the Fermented Beverage Kefir. *Front. Microbiol.* **2016**, *7*, 674. [CrossRef]
92. Chen, M.; Ye, X.; Shen, D.; Ma, C. Modulatory Effects of Gut Microbiota on Constipation: The Commercial Beverage Yakult Shapes Stool Consistency. *J. Neurogastroenterol. Motil.* **2019**, *25*, 475–477. [CrossRef]
93. García-Burgos, M.; Moreno-Fernández, J.; Alférez, M.J.M.; Díaz-Castro, J.; López-Aliaga, I. New perspectives in fermented dairy products and their health relevance. *J. Funct. Foods* **2020**, *72*, 104059. [CrossRef]
94. Shah, N. Health Benefits of Yogurt and Fermented Milks. In *Manufacturing Yogurt and Fermented Milks, Second Edition*; John Willey & Sons: Hoboken, NJ, USA, 2007; pp. 327–351. ISBN 978-0-470-27781-2.
95. Redondo-Useros, N.; Gheorghe, A.; Díaz-Prieto, L.E.; Villavisencio, B.; Marcos, A.; Nova, E. Associations of Probiotic Fermented Milk (PFM) and Yogurt Consumption with Bifidobacterium and Lactobacillus Components of the Gut Microbiota in Healthy Adults. *Nutrients* **2019**, *11*, 651. [CrossRef]
96. De Moreno de Leblanc, A.; Perdigón, G. Yogurt feeding inhibits promotion and progression of experimental colorectal cancer. *Med. Sci. Monit.* **2004**, *10*, BR96–BR104.
97. Urbanska, A.M.; Bhathena, J.; Martoni, C.; Prakash, S. Estimation of the Potential Antitumor Activity of Microencapsulated Lactobacillus acidophilus Yogurt Formulation in the Attenuation of Tumorigenesis in Apc(Min/+) Mice. *Dig. Dis. Sci.* **2009**, *54*, 264–273. [CrossRef]
98. Guiné, R.P.F.; Rodrigues, A.P.; Ferreira, S.M.; Gonçalves, F.J. Development of Yogurts Enriched with Antioxidants from Wine. *J. Culin. Sci. Technol.* **2016**, *14*, 263–275. [CrossRef]
99. Stewart, H.; Dong, D.; Carlson, A. *Why Are Americans Consuming Less Fluid Milk? A Look at Generational Differences in Intake Frequency*; U.S. Department of Agriculture: Washington, DC, USA, 2013; pp. 1–2.
100. Capps, O.; Williams, G.W.; Salin, V. *Quantitative Evaluation of the Effectiveness of Marketing and Promotion Activities by the Milk Processor Education Program*; U.S. Department of Agriculture: Washington, DC, USA, 2016; pp. 1–109.
101. Wolf, C.A.; Malone, T.; McFadden, B.R. Beverage milk consumption patterns in the United States: Who is substituting from dairy to plant-based beverages? *J. Dairy Sci.* **2020**, *103*, 11209–11217. [CrossRef]
102. Santaliestra-Pasías, A.M.; González-Gil, E.M.; Pala, V.; Intemann, T.; Hebestreit, A.; Russo, P.; Van Aart, C.; Rise, P.; Veidebaum, T.; Molnar, D.; et al. Predictive associations between lifestyle behaviours and dairy consumption: The IDEFICS study. *Nutr. Metab. Cardiovasc. Dis.* **2020**, *30*, 514–522. [CrossRef]

Publisher's Note: MDPI stays neutral with regard to jurisdictional claims in published maps and institutional affiliations.

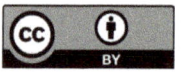

© 2020 by the authors. Licensee MDPI, Basel, Switzerland. This article is an open access article distributed under the terms and conditions of the Creative Commons Attribution (CC BY) license (http://creativecommons.org/licenses/by/4.0/).

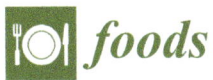

Article

Antimicrobial, Antioxidant, Sensory Properties, and Emotions Induced for the Consumers of Nutraceutical Beverages Developed from Technological Functionalised Food Industry By-Products

Egle Zokaityte [1,2], Vita Lele [1,2], Vytaute Starkute [1,2], Paulina Zavistanaviciute [1,2], Darius Cernauskas [2], Dovile Klupsaite [2], Modestas Ruzauskas [3,4], Juste Alisauskaite [1], Alma Baltrusaitytė [1], Mantvydas Dapsas [1], Karolina Siriakovaite [1], Simonas Trunce [1], Raquel P. F. Guiné [5], Pranas Viskelis [6], Vesta Steibliene [7] and Elena Bartkiene [1,2,*]

1. Department of Food Safety and Quality, Faculty of Veterinary, Lithuanian University of Health Sciences, Tilzes Str. 18, LT-47181 Kaunas, Lithuania; egle.zokaityte@lsmuni.lt (E.Z.); vita.lele@lsmuni.lt (V.L.); vytaute.starkute@lsmuni.lt (V.S.); paulina.zavistanaviciute@lsmuni.lt (P.Z.); juste.alisauskaite@stud.lsmu.lt (J.A.); alma.baltrusaityte@stud.lsmu.lt (A.B.); mantvydas.dapsas@stud.lsmu.lt (M.D.); karolina.siriakovaite@stud.lsmu.lt (K.S.); simonas.trunce@stud.lsmu.lt (S.T.)
2. Faculty of Animal Sciences, Institute of Animal Rearing Technologies, Lithuanian University of Health Sciences, Tilzes Str. 18, LT-47181 Kaunas, Lithuania; darius.cernauskas@lsmuni.lt (D.C.); dovile.klupsaite@lsmuni.lt (D.K.)
3. Department of Anatomy and Physiology, Faculty of Veterinary, Lithuanian University of Health Sciences, Tilzes Str. 18, LT-47181 Kaunas, Lithuania; modestas.ruzauskas@lsmuni.lt
4. Faculty of Veterinary, Institute of Microbiology and Virology, Lithuanian University of Health Sciences, Tilzes Str. 18, LT-47181 Kaunas, Lithuania
5. CERNAS Research Centre, Polytechnic Institute of Viseu, 3504-510 Viseu, Portugal; raquelguine@esav.ipv.pt
6. Lithuanian Research Centre for Agriculture and Forestry, Institute of Horticulture, Kauno Str. 30, LT-54333 Babtai, Lithuania; biochem@lsdi.lt
7. Psychiatry Clinic, Faculty of Medicine, Lithuanian University of Health Sciences, A. Mickeviciaus Str. 9, LT44307 Kaunas, Lithuania; vesta.steibliene@lsmuni.lt
* Correspondence: elena.bartkiene@lsmuni.lt; Tel.: +370-601-35837

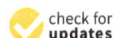

Received: 19 October 2020; Accepted: 4 November 2020; Published: 6 November 2020

Abstract: This study aims to develop nutraceutical beverages containing food processing by-products in their formulation, and determine the opinion of consumers. This is done by testing whether they know that the main ingredients of the product are by-products, performing an overall acceptability test of the developed beverages, and evaluating the emotions induced by the newly developed beverages for consumers. The main ingredients used for the preparation of added-value beverages were fermented milk permeate (containing galactooligosaccharides), extruded and fermented wheat bran (WB) (containing ≥6.0 $\log_{10}$ CFU g^{-1} viable antimicrobial properties showing lactic acid bacteria (LAB) strains), and different fruit/berry by-products (FBB) (as a source of compounds showing antioxidant properties). The definition of the quantities of bioactive ingredients was based on the overall acceptability of the prepared beverages, as well as on emotions induced in consumers by the tested beverages. Functional properties of the developed beverages were proofed by the evaluation of their antimicrobial and antioxidant properties, as well as viable LAB count during storage. Desirable changes in extruded and fermented WB were obtained: Fermentation reduced sugar concentration and pH in samples with predominant lactic acid isomer L(+). In addition, the viable LAB count in the substrate was higher than 6.0 $\log_{10}$ CFU g^{-1}, and no enterobacteria remained. By comparing the overall acceptability of the beverages enriched with WB, the highest overall acceptability was shown for the samples prepared with 10 g of the extruded and fermented WB (7.9 points). FBB showed desirable antimicrobial activity: Shepherd inhibited—2, sea buckthorn—3, blueberries—5, and raspberries—7 pathogens from the 10 tested. Comparing different beverage groups prepared with different types of FBB, in most cases (except sea buckthorn), by increasing FBB content the beverages overall acceptability was increased, and the highest score (on average, 9.5 points) was obtained for the samples prepared with 5.0 and 7.5 g of blueberries FBB. Moreover, a very strong positive correlation ($r = 0.8525$) was found between overall acceptability and emotion "happy" induced in consumers by the prepared beverages enriched with extruded and fermented WB and FBB. By comparing the samples prepared with the addition of WB with samples prepared with WB and FBB, it was observed that most FBB increased total phenolic compounds (TPC) content (on average, by 9.0%), except in the case of samples prepared with sea buckthorn. A very high positive correlation ($r = 0.9919$) was established between TPC and antioxidant activity. Finally, it can be stated that the newly developed nutraceutical beverages were acceptable for consumers, induced positive emotions, and possessed desirable antimicrobial and antioxidant properties, while being prepared in a sustainable and environmentally friendly manner.

Keywords: beverages; milk permeate; wheat bran; fruit/berry by-products; antimicrobial properties; antioxidant properties; overall acceptability; emotions induced for consumers

1. Introduction

According to future prognosis, the global population will increase to 8 billion by 2030 and more than nine billion by 2050, and such population growth will lead to the need for high-quality foods to be assured [1]. However, nowadays, a significant part of the world's population is suffering from malnutrition [1]. To ensure enough balanced food is available, the food industry must move to become a sustainable industry, in which by-products are very effectively recovered as high-value ingredients and (or) products. However, the food system is highly complex and is driven by many economic, cultural and environmental factors [1]. It should be mentioned that until now, many high-value food industry by-products are used as a low-value feedstock for livestock feeding. At the same time, many people are suffering from biologically active compounds (antioxidants, dietary fibre, etc.) deficiency [1]. As is the case with many food processing industries, by-product recovery can reduce the quantity of wastes that require treatment; however, new technologies and new product formulations should be developed. From another point of view, knowing that the main ingredients of the product are by-products, will the consumer choose it? For this reason, in our study, in addition to the overall acceptability standard test, evaluation of the emotions induced by the newly developed beverages for consumers were measured. Emotion is usually defined as a rapid reaction to a stimulus, which could be a food or drink [2]. The application of emotions evaluation has grown in the last years because it can be used for a prognosis about the emotions induced for consumers by the different food, as well as a choice of food. The emotions induced by food for consumers can be linked to health-related problems [3], and also, can be adapted for commercial product development, to ensure their popularity in the market.

The highest quantity of food-processing by-products is generated by fruit and vegetable, dairy, meat, poultry, olive oil, fermentation, and seafood industries [4]. For this reason, for the development of added-value beverages in this study, milk permeates, wheat bran, and fruit/berries by-products were chosen.

Milk permeate (MP) is a dairy industry by-product obtained during the milk protein concentrate production. The MP, containing a high concentration of lactose, can be used as a stock for galactooligosaccharides (GOS) production [5]. Our previous studies showed that MP fermentation with selected lactic acid bacteria (LAB) strains could lead to additional value formation, by lactose converting to GOS [5]. GOS are desirable compounds in food because consumption of prebiotics is a useful strategy in order to prevent many diseases, and GOS, as a nutraceutical compound, can lead to protective biological functions, e.g., antitumour [6].

Another food industry sectors that generate high quantities of by-products is the wheat processing industry [7–11]. Wheat is the most valuable crop in the world; however, wheat generates very large amounts of by-products (approximate 15% of wheat is not used efficiently), but could be potentially used for the production of value-added products. However, the addition of WB to food formulations usually induces adverse effects on sensory properties of the final product [12]. Extrusion is proposed to increase the acceptability of WB by changing its properties. Extrusion is a combination of thermal and mechanical treatments where the substrate is subjected to high temperature and shear forces for a short time. This process is used to texturise food materials and can have a positive influence on a functional value of WB, e.g., by decreasing antinutritional factors [13–16]. Moreover, as a high-temperature process, extrusion can lead to reduced microbial contamination, and during the Maillard reaction, the aroma changes to be more acceptable for consumers. Therefore, this process could be used for WB pre-treatment to improve it as a food ingredient, improve sensory properties, as well as to reduce microbial contamination. In addition, fermentation with selected LAB strains can lead to extruded WB having additional value, for example, by providing antimicrobial properties. For this reason, we hypothesise that extruded and fermented WB can be a useful ingredient for additional value beverages development.

Another industry that generates large amounts of by-products is fruit/berries industry. In this study, *Sambucus nigra* L., *Rubus idaeus* L., *Hippophae rhamnoides* L., and *Vaccinium myrtillus* L. by-products were used for the development of additional value beverages. *Sambucus nigra* L., known as elderberry, is a very popular species of the *Adoxaceae* family [17]. Elderberry is a very popular ingredient in many foods and beverage formulations: wine, juice, tea, liqueur, muffins, pancakes, jams and jellies, waffles, batter, etc. [18]. Elderberries are popular in folk and professional medicine, because of high quantities of bioactive compounds possessing desirable characteristics for health improvement [19–23]. Several papers have been published about their antioxidant activities [21,24–26].

Red raspberries (*Rubus idaeus* L.) are very popular worldwide and consumed as fresh or processed into a variety of products: confitures, juice, jams, etc. [27]. Due to their phenolic compounds and vitamin C, red raspberries possesses antitumoural, antibacterial, and antioxidant activities [28–34].

Sea buckthorn (*Hippophae rhamnoides* L.) is an ecologically and economically important plant [35]. Sea buckthorn berries contain a high amount of various hydrophilic and lipophilic compounds, carotenoids, polyphenols, organic, amino and fatty acids, minerals, etc. [36–40]. Sea buckthorn berries are used for high added-value juice and oil production [41]; therefore, the remaining pulp can be used for added-value products development. Blueberry (*Vaccinium myrtillus* L.) species are distributed all over the world [42]. These fruits are usually consumed in the fresh form, however, due to their short shelf life, they are used for jams, juices, wines, or liqueurs production [43]. These berries are conventionally used in medicine [44], because of their high content of phenolics and carotenoids, as well as vitamins. The European blueberry is an economically valuable wild berry, well-known for its richness of antioxidants (anthocyanins) [42,43]. Blueberries are used for various food and beverage preparation, including juice and wine, and these processes generate valuable by-products, which can be used for further added-value product development.

The aim of this study was to develop additional value beverages in a sustainable manner by using a formulation of food processing by-products. The main ingredients for additional value beverage preparation were fermented milk permeate (containing GOS), extruded and fermented wheat bran (WB) (containing ≥6.0 $\log_{10}$ CFU g^{-1} viable antimicrobial properties showing LAB), and different fruit/berry by-products (as a source of antioxidant properties showing compounds). The main selection of the quantities of bioactive ingredients was based on the prepared beverages 'overall acceptability, as well as on emotions induced by the tested beverages for consumers. Functional properties of the developed beverages were proofed by the evaluation of their antimicrobial and antioxidant properties, as well as viable LAB count in the developed drinks during the storage.

2. Materials and Methods

The whole experiment scheme is shown in Figure 1.

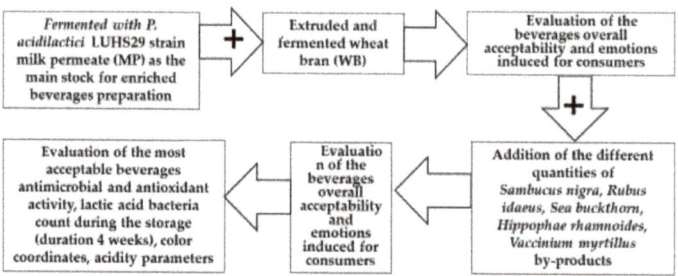

Figure 1. The experimental scheme.

2.1. Characteristics of Fermented Milk Permeate used for Beverages Preparation

Milk permeate (MP) was obtained from the Agricultural cooperative "Pienas LT", Biruliskes, Lithuania. Our previous studies showed that the highest concentration of galactooligosaccharides (GOS) and the most effective antimicrobial properties of MP could be obtained when *P. acidilactici* LUHS29 strain was used for MP fermentation [5]. Characteristics of the fermented MP, used in this study for enriched beverages preparation are shown in Table 1 (acidity parameters, LAB count, GOS concentration, overall acceptability and emotions induced for consumers) and Table 2 (antimicrobial properties).

2.2. Wheat Bran, Used for Beverages Enrichment, by Using it for Pre-Treatment Extrusion and Fermentation Processes

Wheat bran was obtained from the SME "Ustukiu malunas" (Pasvalys, Lithuania). Wheat bran samples (WB) were extruded at 130 °C, speed of the screw—25 rpm and fermented with *L. uvarum* LUHS245 strain. The LUHS245 strain, before the experiment, was stored at −80 °C in a Microbank system (Pro-Lab Diagnostics, Birkenhead, Wirral, UK) and grown in de Man, Rogosa and Sharpe (MRS) broth (CM 0359, Oxoid, Basingstoke, Hampshire, UK) at 30 °C for 48 h prior to use.

The following parameters for WB were established: pH, total titratable acidity (TTA), L(+) and D(-) lactic acid bacteria concentration, LAB, mould/yeast (M/Y), total bacteria (TBC), and total enterobacteria (TEC) counts; sugars concentration (fructose, glucose, sucrose, maltose); amino acids and biogenic amines concentration. Non-extruded and non-fermented WB samples were used as control.

Wheat Bran Analysis Methods

The pH was measured using a pH electrode (PP-15; Sartorius, Goettingen, Germany). The total titratable acidity (TTA) was evaluated for a 10 g sample of sample mixed with 90 mL of water, and the results were expressed in mL of 0.1 mol L^{-1} NaOH solution required to achieve a pH value of 8.2. For L(+) and D(−) lactic acid isomers concentration evaluation, a specific Megazyme assay Kit (Megazyme Int., Bray, Ireland) was used. The determination of LAB, total bacteria (TBC), enterobacteria (TEC), and mould/yeast (M/Y) counts in samples was performed according to Bartkiene et al. [45].

Table 1. Parameters after 48 h of milk permeate fermented with LUHS29 strain.

Milk Permeate Samples	pH	TTA, No.	LAB Count, $\log_{10}$ CFU mL^{-1}	Lactose, g 100 g^{-1}	GOS mg 100 mL^{-1}	
					G2	G3
MP$_{NF}$	5.88 ± 0.80 [b]	3.00 ± 0.14 [a]	nd	10.48 ± 0.28 [b]	nd	nd
MP$_{LUHS29}$	3.91 ± 0.23 [a]	9.50 ± 0.19 [b]	8.19 ± 0.23	5.05 ± 0.19 [a]	21.70 ± 0.33	5.10 ± 0.11

	Overall Acceptability	Emotions Induced by the Beverages (from 0 to 1)							
		Neutral	Happy	Sad	Angry	Surprised	Scared	Disgusted	Contempt	Valence
MP$_{NF}$	5.20 ± 0.18	0.370 ± 0.020 [b]	0.130 ± 0.003	0.180 ± 0.004 [b]	0.060 ± 0.001 [a]	0.03 ± 0.001 [b]	0.0010 ± 0.00002	0.00100 ± 0.00002	0.0900 ± 0.0020 [b]	0.080 ± 0.002 [a]
MP$_{LUHS29}$	5.30 ± 0.13	0.230 ± 0.004 [a]	0.14 ± 0.003	0.160 ± 0.003 [a]	0.130 ± 0.003 [b]	0.010 ± 0.0002 [a]	0.00100 ± 0.00002	0.00100 ± 0.00002	0.0300 ± 0.0006 [a]	0.130 ± 0.003 [b]

LAB, lactic acid bacteria; CFU, colony-forming units; TTA, total titratable acidity; MP, milk permeate; MP$_{LUHS29}$, fermented with LUHS29 (P. acidilactici); MP$_{NF}$, unfermented; GOS, galactooligosaccharides; nd, not determined; G2, galactobiose; G3, galactotriose. Data are represented as means ($n = 3$) ± SD. $^{a-b}$ Means with different letters in column are significantly different ($p \leq 0.05$).

Table 2. The diameter of inhibition zones (mm) of the prepared beverages against pathogenic and opportunistic strains of milk permeate fermented with LUHS29 strain.

Samples	Diameter of Inhibition Zones (DIZ) (mm)														
	Pathogenic and Opportunistic Bacteria Strains														
	1	2	3	4	5	6	7	8	9	10	11	12	13	14	15
MP$_{LUHS29}$	nd	nd	nd	nd	nd	nd	nd	nd	nd	12.7 ± 0.4	nd	nd	nd	nd	15.0 ± 0.1
MP$_{NF}$	nd	nd	nd	nd	nd	nd	nd	nd	nd	nd	nd	nd	nd	nd	nd

MP, milk permeate; MP$_{LUHS29}$, fermented with LUHS29 (P. acidilactici); MP$_{NF}$, unfermented; nd, not determined; 1, Klebsiella pneumonia; 2, Salmonella enterica; 3, Pseudomonas aeruginosa; 4, Acinetobacter baumannii; 5, Proteus mirabilis, 6, MRSA M87fox; 7, Enterococcus faecalis; 8, Enterococcus faecium; 9, Bacillus cereus; 10, Streptococcus mutans; 11, Enterobacter cloacae; 12, Citrobacter freundii; 13, Streptococcus epidermis, 14, Staphylococcus haemolyticus; 15, Pasteurella multocida. Data are represented as means ($n = 3$) ± SD.

To determine the sugar concentration, 2–3 g of sample was diluted with ~70 ml of distilled/deionised water, heated to 60 °C in a water bath for 15 min, clarified with 2.5 ml Carrez I (85 mM $K_4[Fe(CN)_6]$ × $3H_2O$) and 2.5 ml Carrez II (250 mM $ZnSO_4$ × $7H_2O$) solutions, and made up to 100 ml with distilled/deionised water. After 15 min, the samples were filtered through a filter paper and a 0.22 μm nylon syringe filter before analysis. A standard solution of a sugar's mixture was prepared by dissolving 0.2 g each of fructose (Hamburg, Germany), glucose (Sigma-Aldrich, Hamburg Germany), sucrose (Sigma-Aldrich, Hamburg Germany) and maltose (Sigma-Aldrich, Hamburg, Germany) in 100 mL of distilled/deionised water. A 2 mg mL^{-1} standard solution of sugars mixture was prepared following dilution with distilled/deionised water. Chromatographic conditions were as follows: The eluent was a mixture of 75 parts by volume of acetonitrile and 25 parts by volume water, the flow rate was 1.2 mL/min, 20 μL was injected. The YMC-Pack Polyamine II 250 × 4.6 mm, 5 μm (YMC Co., Ltd., Tokyo, Japan) column was used. The column temperature was set at 28 °C. Detection was performed using an Evaporative Light Scattering Detector ELSDLTII (Shimadzu Corp., Kyoto, Japan).

Free amino acids (FAA) were extracted using 0.1 M HCl. The extracts were analysed by gas chromatography with flame ionisation detection after an ion-exchange solid-phase extraction and chloroformate derivatisation using EZ:faast technology (Phenomenex) as described by Bartkiene et al. [46].

The extraction and determination of biogenic amines (BA) in wheat samples followed the procedures developed by Ben-Gigirey et al. [47] with some modifications, as described by Bartkiene et al. [48].

2.3. Fruits/Berries By-Products used for Milk Permeate Beverages Preparation

Four different fruit/berry by-products types (Shepherd/*Sambucus nigra*, Raspberries/*Rubus idaeus*, Sea buckthorns/*Hippophae rhamnoides*, Blueberries/*Vaccinium myrtillus*) were obtained from the Institute of Horticulture, Lithuanian Research Centre for Agriculture and Forestry (Babtai, Kaunas distr., Lithuania) in 2020. These by-products were vacuum dried in a vacuum dryer XF020 (France-Etuves, Chelles, France) at 45 ± 2.0 °C and a pressure of 6 × 10^{-3} mPa. The antimicrobial and antifungal properties for the selected fruit/berry by-products were evaluated.

Antimicrobial Properties of the Fruit/Berry By-Products Evaluation

The antimicrobial activity of fruit/berry by-products was evaluated against a variety of pathogenic and opportunistic bacterial strains (*Salmonella enterica Infantis* LT 101, *Staphylococcus aureus* LT 102, *E. coli* (hemolytic) LT 103, *Bacillus pseudomycoides* LT 104, *Aeromonas veronii* LT 105, *Cronobacter sakazakii* LT 106, *Hafnia alvei* LT 107, *Enterococcus durans* LT 108, *Kluyvera cryocrescens* LT 109, *Acinetobacter johnsonii* LT 110). The pathogenic and opportunistic bacterial strains used were obtained from the Lithuanian University of Health Sciences' (Kaunas, Lithuania) collection. The antimicrobial activity of the fruit/berry by-products was assessed by measuring the diameter of inhibition zones (DIZ, mm) in agarwell diffusion assays. Accordingly, a 0.5 McFarland unit density suspension of each pathogenic bacteria strain was inoculated onto the surface of cooled Mueller–Hinton agar (Oxoid, Basingstoke, UK) using sterile cotton swabs. Wells of 6 mm in diameter were punched in the agar and filled with the tested by-product. Before the experiment, the fruit/berry by-products were diluted with a sterile physiological solution (1 g of the by-product diluted with 2 mL of the physiological solution). The average DIZ was calculated from triplicate experiments.

2.4. Selection of the Optimal Quantities of Technologically Functionalised Wheat Bran for Milk Permeate Beverages Enrichment

The different quantities (2.5, 5.0, 7.5, and 10 g) of WB were added to the fermented MP samples (50 mL), and the most acceptable samples for the further enrichment with fruit/berry by-products were selected. In addition, emotions induced for consumers by the prepared beverages enriched with extruded and fermented WB were evaluated. Description of the overall acceptability and emotions induced for consumers by the prepared beverages are described below in Section 2.3.

Overall Acceptability and Emotions Induced for Consumers by the Prepared Beverage Enriched with Wheat Bran Beverages Evaluation

The overall acceptability of the beverages was established by 50 judges, according to International Standards Organisation method 8586-1 [49], using a 10-point scale ranging from 0 ("extremely dislike") to 10 ("extremely like"). Similarly, the prepared beverages were tested by applying FaceReader 6.0 software (Noldus Information Technology, Wageningen, The Netherlands), scaling nine emotion patterns (neutral, happy, sad, angry, surprised, scared, disgusted, contempt, and valence) according to Bartkiene et al. [50]. In the obvious measurement experiment, subjects were asked to rate the beverage samples during and after consumption with an intentional facial expression, which was recorded and then characterised by FaceReader 6.0. The participants were asked to taste the whole presented sample at once, take 15 s to reflect on the taste impressions, then give a signal with a hand and visualise the taste experience of the sample with a facial expression best representing their liking of the sample. The whole procedure was filmed using high-resolution Microsoft LifeCam Studio webcam mounted on a laptop facing the participants, and Media Recorder (Noldus Information Technology, Wageningen, The Netherlands) software. Special care was taken to ensure good illumination of participant's faces. The recordings, using a resolution of 1280 × 720 at 30 frames per second, were saved as AVI files and analysed frame by frame with FaceReader 6 software, scaling the nine basic emotion patterns (neutral, happy, sad, angry, surprised, scared, disgusted, contempt and valence) to 1 (maximum intensity of the fitted model). In addition, the FaceReader also analysed the valence, which indicates whether the person's emotional status is positive or negative. 'Happy' is the only positive emotion, while 'Sad', 'Angry', 'Scared', and 'Disgusted' are considered to be negative emotions. 'Surprised' can be either positive or negative. The valence is calculated as the intensity of 'Happy' minus the intensity of the negative emotion with the highest intensity. Valence scores ranged from -1 to 1. For each sample, the section of intentional facial expression (from the exact point at which the subject had finished raising their hand to give the signal until the subject started lowering their hand again) was extracted and used for statistical analysis.

2.5. Selection of the Optimal Quantities of Fruits/Berries By-Products for Milk Permeate Beverages Enrichment

The different quantities (2.5, 5.0, 7.5, 10 g) of fruit/berry by-products (Shepherd/*Sambucus nigra*, Raspberries/*Rubus idaeus*, Sea buckthorns/*Hippophae rhamnoides*, Blueberries/*Vaccinium myrtillus*) were tested. In addition to the optimal quantity of WB, the optimal quantity of the tested fruit/berry by-products was selected. First of all, the optimal quality was selected by the evaluation of overall acceptability and emotions induced for consumers by the prepared enriched with WB and fruit/berry by-products beverages (methods described in Section 2.3.

After an optimal (according to overall acceptability and induced emotions) fruit/berry by-products content selection, the most acceptable samples were analysed further, by evaluating prepared enriched beverages antimicrobial properties, LAB count during the storage, colour coordinates, and acidity parameters. Description of the above-mentioned methods is given in.

Antimicrobial Activity of the Prepared Beverages Enriched with Wheat Bran and Fruits/Berries By-Products

Antimicrobial activity of the prepared beverages enriched with extruded and fermented wheat bran and fruit/berry against a variety of pathogenic and opportunistic bacterial strains (*Salmonella enterica Infantis* LT 101, *Staphylococcus aureus* LT 102, *E. coli* (hemolytic) LT 103, *Bacillus pseudomycoides* LT 104, *Aeromonas veronii* LT 105, *Cronobacter sakazakii* LT 106, *Hafnia alvei* LT 107, *Enterococcus durans* LT 108, *Kluyvera cryocrescens* LT 109, *Acinetobacter johnsonii* LT 110) was evaluated. The used pathogenic and opportunistic bacterial strains were attained from the Lithuanian University of Health Sciences (Kaunas, Lithuania) collection. Antimicrobial activity was assessed by measuring the diameters of inhibition zones (DIZ, mm) in agar well diffusion assays. For this purpose, 0.5 McFarland unit density suspension of each pathogenic bacteria strain was inoculated onto the surface of cooled Mueller–Hinton agar (Oxoid, UK) using sterile cotton swabs. Wells of 6 mm in diameter were punched in the agar and filled with 50 µL of the prepared beverages samples. The average DIZ was calculated from triplicate experiments.

Acidity parameters (pH and TTA) of the prepared beverages enriched with extruded and fermented wheat bran and fruit/berries were evaluated immediately after preparing the beverages. The pH value of beverages was measured and recorded using a pH electrode (PP—15, Sartorius, Goettingen, Germany). The total titratable acidity (TTA) was determined of a 10 mL sample homogenised with 90 mL distilled water and expressed as the amount (mL) of 0.1 mol L^{-1} NaOH to obtain a pH value of 8.2.

The colour coordinates (L*, a*, b*) were assessed using a CIELAB system (Chromameter CR-400, Konica Minolta, Tokyo, Japan).

For the evaluation of LAB count, 10 mL of the beverage were homogenised with 90 mL of saline (9 g L^{-1} NaCl solution). Serial dilutions of 10^{-4} to 10^{-8} with saline were used for sample preparation. Sterile MRS agar (CM0361, Oxoid) of 5 mm thickness was used for bacterial growth on Petri dishes. The dishes were separately seeded with the sample suspension using surface sowing and were incubated under anaerobic conditions at 30 °C for 72 h. All results were expressed in $\log_{10}$ CFU mL^{-1} (colony forming units per mL of the sample) as the mean of three determinations. To determine the viability of LAB during four weeks of storage at +4 °C.

2.6. Statistical Analysis

The results were expressed as the mean ± standard deviation (SD). All analyses were performed at least in triplicate. Results were analysed using statistical package SPSS for Windows V15.0 (SPSS Inc., Chicago, IL, USA, 2007). The significance of differences between the samples was evaluated using Tukey range tests at a 5% level. A linear Pearson's correlation was used to quantify the strength of the relationship between the variables. The correlation coefficients were calculated using the statistical package SPSS. The results were recognised as statistically significant at $p \leq 0.05$.

3. Results

3.1. Parameters of the Extruded Wheat Bran

Acidity (pH, total titratable acidity (TTA), and lactic acid isomers concentration) and microbiological parameters (lactic acid bacteria (LAB), mould/yeast (M/Y), total bacteria (TBC), and total enterobacteria (TEC) count) of the extruded and fermented WB are shown in Table 3. In comparing fermented and non-fermented WB samples, after 24 h of fermentation, the samples' pH was reduced by 28.9%, and TTA increased by 94.3%, in comparison with non-fermented extruded samples. L(+)/D(−) ratio in fermented WB samples was 1.35, with predominant L(+) lactic acid. Lactic acid bacteria (LAB) count in fermented samples was, on average, 8.79 $\log_{10}$ CFU g^{-1}, however, significant reduction of M/Y count in fermented samples was not observed, compared with non-fermented ones. Enterobacteria did not remain in the fermented samples, however, extrusion was not a significant factor for TEC. Moreover, fermentation reduced sugar concentration in WB samples, and fructose, sucrose, and maltose did not remain after fermentation.

Technological microorganisms, such as LAB, produce a variety of organic acids in the substrate and lower the pH to levels that are inhibitory to many pathogenic and opportunistic microorganisms [51]. The increases of TTA and the reduction of pH improves food safety parameters as well. The levels of pH and TTA in the substrate are influenced by many factors, including processing methods and product properties.

Table 3. Acidity (pH, total titratable acidity (TTA), and lactic acid isomers concentration) and microbiological parameters (lactic acid bacteria (LAB), mould/yeast (M/Y), total bacteria (TBC), and total enterobacteria (TEC) count) of the extruded and fermented wheat bran.

Wheat by-Product Samples	pH	TTA, No.	Lactic Acid Content, g 100 g^{-1}		LAB	M/Y	TBC	TEC
			L(+)	D(−)	\multicolumn{4}{c}{log$_{10}$ CFU g^{-1}}			
	\multicolumn{2}{c}{Duration of Fermentation, 24 h}						
W$_{nonF}$	6.04 ± 0.01 c	0.10 ± 0.02 a	-	-	5.20 ± 0.12 a	4.26 ± 0.11	9.04 ± 0.14 b	5.69 ± 0.23 b
W$_{ex130}$/screwspeed25	5.91 ± 0.02 b	0.20 ± 0.03 b	-	-	5.34 ± 0.09 a	4.38 ± 0.19	8.46 ± 0.10 a	4.32 ± 0.14 a
W$_{ex130}$/screwspeed25Lu	4.20 ± 0.01 a	3.50 ± 0.10 c	0.275 ± 0.013	0.203 ± 0.007	8.79 ± 0.12 b	4.32 ± 0.07	8.84 ± 0.13 b	nd

	Fructose	Glucose	Sucrose	Maltose
	\multicolumn{4}{c}{g 100 g^{-1}}			
W$_{ex130}$/screwspeed25	0.11 ± 0.02	nd	0.81 ± 0.07	0.11 ± 0.01
W$_{ex130}$/screwspeed25Lu	nd	nd	nd	nd

W, wheat bran; $_{nonF}$, non-fermented; Lu, fermented with *Lactobacillus uvarum*; $_{ex130/screwspeed25}$—extruded at 130 °C, screw speed 25 rpm; TTA, total titratable acidity; LAB, lactic acid bacteria; M/Y, mould and yeast; TBC, total bacteria count; TEC, total enterobacteria count; CFU, colony-forming units; nd, not determined, not analysed. The data expressed as mean values (n = 3) ± SD; SD, standard deviation. $^{a-c}$ The mean values within a column with different letters are significantly different ($p \leq 0.05$).

The major metabolite of LAB is D(−) and/or L(+) lactic acid [52]. However, the studies revealed the microbiota metabolism of D(−) and L(+) lactic acid in fermented products are scarce. Data on the ratio of lactic acid isomers was published for sauerkraut and cheese [53,54]. Different LAB showed different production ratios of D and L lactic acid [52,55]. The accumulation of D(−) lactic acid may cause D-lactic acidosis in mammals [56,57]. For this reason, researchers aimed to reduce the accumulation of D(−) isomers in fermented foods during the fermentation.

The contamination of foods during the various processes of the production chain is always the point of concern; this is especially important for the outer layer of cereals, which are contaminated from the field. Moreover, the occurrence of some fungal species can be a signal of mycotoxin contamination [58–60]. Different methods, including thermal and non-thermal, are used to decrease the bacterial, as well as fungal contamination of the cereal-based products [58,61]. The most environmentally-friendly and efficient methods for cereal decontamination are fermentation processes. In addition, fermentation leads to some positive nutritional and sensory characteristics of the products [61]. Moreover, during the extrusion process, which includes a combination of high temperature and high pressure, toxin, as well as non-desirable microorganisms reduction in food can be observed [62].

It was published that WB contamination (TBC) before fermentation was 5 $\log_{10}$ CFU g^{-1}. For this reason, to ensure the stability of the fermentation process with *L. rhamnosus* 1473 strain, sterilisation step was included [63].

Finally, desirable changes in the fermented substrate were obtained: Fermentation reduced the sugar concentration and pH in the samples with predominant lactic acid isomer L(+), and also, the viable LAB count in the substrate was higher than 6.0 $\log_{10}$ CFU g^{-1} and enterobacteria did not remain.

The amino acids and biogenic amines (Bas) concentration in nontreated and extruded, as well as extruded and fermented cereal by-products, are shown in Table 4. Most of the analysed amino acids concentration after extrusion, as well as extrusion and fermentation in WB samples, remain similar as before treatment, however, some changes were established in glutamine, cysteine, tryptophan, phenylalanine and isoleucine content. Glutamine concentration in extruded and extruded/fermented WB samples was, on average, by 17.1% lower, compared with nontreated WB. An opposite tendency with cysteine concentration was found, and in comparison, nontreated and fermented/extruded WB samples, were on average, 15.0% higher in concentration in treated samples. However, tryptophan, phenylalanine, and isoleucine concentrations were reduced after extrusion and fermentation, on average, by 19.4, 21.4 and 20.0%, respectively. In opposite, lysine concentration in extruded and fermented samples was significantly higher (on average, by 23.5%).

Despite the fact that WB fermentation is a very popular process in the food and feed industry, however published studies are very scarce [64–66], and it is worthy of note that about an extrusion and fermentation combination for WB treatment was never reported before [63].

Overall, WB is the main by-product of the wheat milling industry, containing more than 15% protein [67]. It was published that the proteins can be derived from WB [68]. Despite the fact that endosperm biological value is higher in comparison with bran, however, WB proteins have a more favourable amino acid composition compared to endosperm proteins [69]. However, these proteins are located within cell wall polysaccharides, and for this reason, its digestion is pure [70]. Compared to endosperm, WB proteins contain a higher amount of lysine, arginine, and glycine [71]. The most dominant amino acids in WB are glutamic and aspartic acids, leucine, alanine, proline, arginine, and glycine [70]. However, such a high content of protein in WB can lead to biogenic amines (BA) formation, especially, during the fermentation processes [72].

In comparing Bas concentration in WB, phenylethylamine, tyramine, and spermidine were not found in the tested WB samples. However, putrescine and spermine concentration in WB was increased after extrusion and extrusion/fermentation processes (in extruded samples by 33.6%, in extruded and fermented WB by 36.1% higher, in comparison with nontreated WB). Cadaverine and histamine were found just in the nontreated WB (on average, 41.33 and 63.64 mg kg^{-1}, respectively). In opposite to putrescine, spermidine concentration after both treatments in WB was reduced (in extruded samples by 70.9%, in extruded and fermented WB by 70.1% lower, in compare with nontreated WB).

Table 4. The amino acids (g 100 g^{-1}) and biogenic amines (mg kg^{-1}) concentration in extruded and nontreated cereal by-products non-fermented and fermented with *L. uvarum* strain.

		W$_{nonF}$	W$_{ex130/}$ screwspeed25	W$_{ex130/}$ screwspeed25 Lu
The amino acids, g 100g^{-1}	Asp	0.43 ± 0.03 [a]	0.44 ± 0.03 [a]	0.48 ± 0.04 [a]
	Glu	1.75 ± 0.09 [b]	1.43 ± 0.09 [a]	1.47 ± 0.08 [a]
	Asn	nd	nd	nd
	Ser	0.29 ± 0.03 [a]	0.26 ± 0.02 [a]	0.26 ± 0.02 [a]
	His	0.12 ± 0.01 [b]	0.10 ± 0.01 [a]	0.11 ± 0.01 [a]
	Gly	0.27 ± 0.02 [a]	0.24 ± 0.02 [a]	0.26 ± 0.02 [a]
	Thr	0.25 ± 0.02 [a]	0.25 ± 0.02 [a]	0.26 ± 0.02 [a]
	Arg	0.31 ± 0.03 [b]	0.27 ± 0.02 [a]	0.27 ± 0.02 [a]
	Ala	0.24 ± 0.02 [a]	0.21 ± 0.02 [a]	0.23 ± 0.02 [a]
	Tyr	0.18 ± 0.01 [a]	0.19 ± 0.01 [a]	0.17 ± 0.01 [a]
	Cys	0.34 ± 0.03 [a]	0.38 ± 0.03 [b]	0.40 ± 0.03 [b]
	Val	0.34 ± 0.03 [a]	0.32 ± 0.03 [a]	0.34 ± 0.03 [a]
	Met	0.12 ± 0.01 [a]	0.13 ± 0.01 [a]	0.13 ± 0.01 [a]
	Trp	0.36 ± 0.03 [c]	0.32 ± 0.03 [b]	0.29 ± 0.02 [a]
	Phe	0.28 ± 0.02 [b]	0.24 ± 0.02 [a]	0.22 ± 0.02 [a]
	Ile	0.40 ± 0.04 [b]	0.32 ± 0.03 [a]	0.32 ± 0.03 [a]
	Leu	0.14 ± 0.01 [b]	0.10 ± 0.01 [a]	0.11 ± 0.01 [a]
	Lys	0.26 ± 0.02 [a]	0.29 ± 0.02 [a]	0.34 ± 0.03 [b]
	Pro	0.50 ± 0.04 [c]	0.27 ± 0.02 [b]	0.24 ± 0.02 [a]
BAs concentration, mg kg^{-1}	PHE	nd	nd	nd
	PUT	102.3 ± 2.6 [a]	154.1 ± 5.4 [b]	160.1 ± 4.0 [c]
	CAD	41.3 ± 1.6	nd	nd
	HIS	63.6 ± 2.2	nd	nd
	TYR	nd	nd	nd
	SPRMD	nd	nd	nd
	SPRM	111.9 ± 3.9 [c]	32.50 ± 0.8 [a]	33.6 ± 1.2 [b]

W, wheat bran; $_{nonF}$, non-fermented; Lu, fermented with *Lactobacillus uvarum*; $_{ex130/screwspeed25}$, extruded at 130 °C, screw speed 25 rpm; nd, not determined; Asp, aspartic acid, Ala, alanine, Gly, glycine, Val, valine, Leu, leucine, Ile, isoleucine, Thr, threonine, Ser, serine, Pro, proline Asn, asparagine, Met, methionine, Glu, glutamine, Phe, phenylalanine, Lys, lysine, His, histidine, Arg, arginine, Tyr, tyrosine, Trp, tryptophan, Cys, cysteine; Bas, biogenic amines; PHE, phenylethylamine; PUT, putrescine; CAD, cadaverine; HIS, histamine; TYR, tyramine; SPRMD, spermidine; SPRM, spermine. Data are represented as means (n = 3) ± SD. [a–c], mean values within a row denoted with different letters are significantly different ($p \leq 0.05$). nd, not determined.

Bas are non-volatile nitrogenous bases with an aliphatic, aromatic structure formed by the decarboxylation of free amino acids [73–75]. Depending on chemical structures, Bas are aromatic amines (histamine, tyramine, β-phenylethylamine, tryptamine and serotonin), aliphatic diamines (putrescine and cadaverine), and aliphatic polyamines (agmatine, spermidine, and spermine). It has been published that BA antioxidant properties are stronger than those of some antioxidant vitamins [76]. BA concentrations varied widely within food types [74,77–79], and they can be influenced by stock origin, processing, storage technology etc. [74,77,80]. It should be pointed out that the consumption of foods high BA concentrations may be deleterious to human health; for this reason, it is very important to estimate concentrations of BA in foods [74,77,80]. Bas are stable compounds [74], however, it has been published that the milling process influences BA distribution in different cereal fractions [81]. It has been reported that whole-grain wheat contains greater amounts of polyamines in comparison with bread [82]. Confirmed results on the BA content in different fractions of cereal grains are limited, however, it is known that histamine, putrescine, cadaverine, tyramine, spermidine and spermine are responsible for toxicological effects of foods [81]. As low molecular weight compounds, after ingestion, they rapidly appear in the blood and various organs and are can inducing several digestive, circulatory and respiratory symptoms [74].

It has been published that BA concentration in durum wheat cultivars is considerable, but not so high as in fish, meat, cheese, fermented vegetables, soy products, and alcoholic beverages, etc. [73,74,79]. Finally, despite that the cereals have low BA content in comparison to the other foods, together with other high-BA foods, they can enhance allergic reactions [73,74]. To prevent the non-desirable effects of food, it is very important to control BA in a wide range of products [74].

3.2. Antimicrobial Properties of the Fruits/Berries by-Products

The antimicrobial properties of the fruit/berry by-products are shown in Table 5. Selected for this experiment, fruit/berry by-products (shepherd, raspberries, sea buckthorn, blueberries) did not show inhibition properties against *Salmonella enterica Infantis* and *Kluyvera cryocrescens*. Only raspberry by-products inhibited *E. coli (hemolytic)*, *Aeromonas veronii* and *Cronobacter sakazakii*, with the diameter of inhibition zones (DIZ) being on average 12.9 mm. All the tested fruit/berry by-products inhibited *Enterococcus durans*, and the highest DIZ of the sea buckthorn against this pathogen was found (15.4 mm). Raspberries, sea buckthorn, and blueberries by-products showed antimicrobial properties against *Bacillus pseudomycoides* and *Acinetobacter johnsonii*, and the highest DIZ against both pathogens by raspberries by-products was found (on average, 15.4 mm). *Staphylococcus aureus* was inhibited by shepherd and blueberries by-products (DIZ, 13.3 and 9.2 mm, respectively). *Hafnia alvei* was inhibited by raspberries and blueberries by-products (DIZ 10.5 and 10.7 mm, respectively).

Sambucus nigra L. is well known because of its natural compounds, which reduces oxidative stress-induced diseases. Shepherd contains various organic acids, flavanol glycosides and anthocyanins [83,84]. The anthocyanins present in shepherd showed protective effects against influenza A and B virus and Helicobacter pylori infections [85–87], and work has been published about shepherd's antifungal, antitumour [88–94] and antimicrobial properties [95]. The main compounds responsible for shepherd's antimicrobial properties are polyphenols; extracts of shepherd possess antibacterial activity against E. coli and Pseudomonas pudita, however inhibition of *Bacillus cereus* and *Staphylococcus aureus* was not established in the literature.

Raspberry juice possesses antimicrobial and antifungal activity against *Staphylococcus aureus*, *Escherichia coli*, *Proteus vulgaris*, *Pseudomonas aeruginosa*, *Bacillus subtilis*, and *Candida albicans*. Antimicrobial activity of raspberries is explained by the presents of ellagitannins, whose content and composition may vary depending on the variety and geographical location, however, it has been published that raspberry extracts inhibited both Gram-positive and Gram-negative bacteria [96]. Sea buckthorn berries are rich in carotenoids, tocopherols, fatty acids, antioxidants, flavonoids, ascorbic and organic acids [97]. The main identified components are ascorbic acid, carotenoids and various phenolics, including proanthocyanins, gallic acid, ursolic acid, caffeic acid, cumaric acid, ferulic acid, catechin and epicatechin derivatives, quercetin, kaempferol, and isorhamnetin glycoside derivatives [98–101], which can be associated with pathogenic inhibition properties.

Blueberry fruits have revealed antimicrobial properties against *Citrobacter freundii* and *Enterococcus faecalis* [102]. It was published that blueberry leaves inhibited *S. aureus*, and this result can be related to high phenolic compounds content, which attacks an important number of bacteria, with the antimicrobial capacity depending on the interactions between polyphenols and bacterial cell surface [103,104]. *R. equi* was the most sensitive strain towards blueberry extracts, whereas *E. faecalis* Gram-positive strain was the most resistant one [105].

Fruit/berry by-products showed desirable antimicrobial activity: Shepherd inhibited 2, sea buckthorn —3, blueberries—5, and raspberries—7 pathogens from the 10 tested. Finally, in this study, shepherd by-products, and the obtained results showed that the tested by-products were very promising antimicrobial ingredients for nutraceuticals, pharmaceuticals, and food formulations.

Table 5. Antimicrobial properties of the fruit/berry by-products.

| Samples | The Diameter of Inhibition Zones (DIZ) (mm) ||||||||||
| | Pathogenic and Opportunistic Bacterial Strains ||||||||||
	1	2	3	4	5	6	7	8	9	10
Shepherd	n.d	13.3 ± 0.4 [b]	n.d	n.d	n.d	n.d	n.d	12.9 ± 0.4 [a]	n.d	n.d
Raspberries	n.d	n.d	12.0 ± 0.4	15.5 ± 0.3 [b]	14.4 ± 0.3	12.2 ± 0.2	10.5 ± 0.4	13.6 ± 0.3 [b]	n.d	15.3 ± 0.1 [c]
Sea buckthorn	n.d	n.d	n.d	14.3 ± 0.4 [a]	n.d	n.d	n.d	15.4 ± 0.2 [c]	n.d	13.4 ± 0.2 [b]
Blueberries	n.d	9.2 ± 0.2 [a]	n.d	14.2 ± 0.1 [a]	n.d	n.d	10.7 ± 0.21	12.4 ± 0.3 [a]	n.d	12.3 ± 0.4 [a]

Experiment Design

Bacillus pseudomycoides LT 104   *Acinetobacter johnsonii* LT 110   *Cronobacter sakazakii* LT 106

1. Shepherd by-products;
2. Raspberries by-products;
3. Sea buckthorn by-products;
4. Blueberry by-products; K–control.

1—*Salmonella enterica* Infantis LT 101; 2—*Staphylococcus aureus* LT 102; 3, E. coli (hemolytic) LT 103; 4—*Bacillus pseudomycoides* LT 104; 5—*Aeromonas veronii* LT 105; 6—*Cronobacter sakazakii* LT 106; 7—*Hafnia alvei* LT 107; 8—*Enterococcus durans* LT 108; 9—*Kluyvera cryocrescens* LT 109; 10—*Acinetobacter johnsonii* LT 110. The data expressed as mean values (n = 3) ± SD; SD, standard deviation. [a–c] The mear values within a column with different letters are significantly different ($p \leq 0.05$); n.d, not determined.

3.3. Overall Acceptability and Emotions Induced for Consumers by the Prepared Enriched with Wheat Bran Beverages

The overall acceptability and emotions induced for consumers by the prepared beverages enriched with extruded and fermented wheat bran (WB) are shown in Table 6. Comparing the overall acceptability of the prepared beverages enriched with the different treated WB, the highest overall acceptability of the samples, prepared with 10 g of the extruded and fermented WB, is shown (7.9 points).

Table 6. Overall acceptability and emotions induced for consumers by the prepared beverages enriched with extruded and fermented wheat bran.

	Beverages Samples					
	MP_{NF}	MP_F	$MP_{LUHS29+2.5WB}$	$MP_{LUHS29+5WB}$	$MP_{LUHS29+7.5WB}$	$MP_{LUHS29+10WB}$
	Overall Acceptability					
	5.2 ± 0.2 [b]	5.3 ± 0.1 [b]	4.2 ± 0.1 [a]	6.4 ± 0.1 [d]	6.2 ± 0.2 [c]	7.9 ± 0.2 [e]
	Emotions Induced by the Beverages (from 0 to 1)					
Neutral	0.37 ± 0.02 [c]	0.230 ± 0.004 [a]	0.470 ± 0.013 [d]	0.31 ± 0.01 [b]	0.46 ± 0.01 [d]	0.49 ± 0.01 [e]
Happy	0.130 ± 0.003 [c]	0.140 ± 0.003 [d]	0.060 ± 0.002 [b]	0.060 ± 0.002 [b]	0.01000 ± 0.0002 [a]	0.150 ± 0.004 [e]
Sad	0.180 ± 0.004 [e]	0.160 ± 0.003 [d]	0.070 ± 0.002 [c]	0.040 ± 0.001 [a]	0.060 ± 0.001 [b]	0.090 ± 0.003 [c]
Angry	0.060 ± 0.001 [d]	0.130 ± 0.003 [f]	0.030 ± 0.001 [c]	0.040 ± 0.001 [b]	0.100 ± 0.002 [e]	0.020 ± 0.001 [a]
Surprised	0.03 ± 0.001 [d]	0.0100 ± 0.0002 [c]	0.0030 ± 0.0001 [b]	0.080 ± 0.003 [e]	0.00100 ± 0.00002 [a]	0.00100 ± 0.00003 [a]
Scared	0.00100 ± 0.00002 [a]	0.00100 ± 0.00002 [a]	0.020 ± 0.001 [c]	0.0100 ± 0.0003 [b]	0.00100 ± 0.00002 [a]	0.00100 ± 0.00003 [a]
Disgusted	0.00100 ± 0.00002 [a]	0.00100 ± 0.00002 [a]	0.0020 ± 0.0001 [b]	0.00100 ± 0.00003 [a]	0.00100 ± 0.00002 [a]	0.0080 ± 0.0002 [c]
Contempt	0.090 ± 0.002 [d]	0.0300 ± 0.0006 [b]	0.050 ± 0.001 [c]	0.0100 ± 0.0003 [a]	0.140 ± 0.003 [e]	0.050 ± 0.001 [c]
Valence	0.080 ± 0.002 [c]	0.130 ± 0.003 [f]	0.090 ± 0.002 [d]	0.070 ± 0.002 [b]	0.0300 ± 0.0007 [a]	0.110 ± 0.003 [e]

MP_{NF}, non-fermented milk permeate; MP_F, milk permeate fermented with LUHS29 (*P. acidilactici*); WB, wheat bran extruded at 130 °C, screw speed 25 rpm and fermented with LUHS245 (*L. uvarum*); 2.5, 5, 7.5, and 10, quantity of WB used, g 50 mL^{-1}. Data are represented as means (n = 3) ± SD. [a–f] Means with different letters in column are significantly different ($p \leq 0.05$).

Today, scientific interest focuses not just on food's nutritional and functional value, but also on food-induced emotional responses, because, emotions are closely related to consumers' food choices [106,107]. It has been published that the disliking of unknown and/or non-traditional foods is strongly related to negative emotions [108]. It is also known that positive emotions, such as joy, happiness, and satisfaction, have a significant positive correlation with food's sensory properties [109]. According to Dalenberg et al. [110], emotional responses better-characterised food choices in comparison with liking. However, in comparison with other affective feelings, emotions were characterised by high intensity, rapid change, and were short-lasting [111].

In this study, between overall acceptability and the emotion "disgusted" was induced for consumers by the prepared beverages enriched with extruded and fermented WB, but very weak positive correlations were found (r = 0.1467), as well as weak positive correlations between overall acceptability and emotions "neutral", "happy", "sad", and "angry" were found (r = 0.2430, r = 0.2105, r = 0.2705, and r = 0.2439, respectively). The strongest (positive moderate) correlation between the overall acceptability and emotion "scared" was found (r = 0.5295). According to the results obtained, for the further experiment, samples prepared with 10 g of the extruded and fermented WB was chosen, as they showed the highest overall acceptability.

3.4. Overall Acceptability and Emotions Induced for Consumers by the Prepared Beverages Enriched with Wheat Bran and Fruits/Berries By-Product Beverages

Overall acceptability and emotions induced for consumers by the prepared beverages enriched with extruded and fermented WB and fruit/berry by-products are shown in Table 7. In comparison, different beverage groups prepared with different types of berries, in most of the cases (except sea buckthorn), by increasing the berries' content, the beverages' overall acceptability was increased, and the highest overall acceptability of the samples, prepared with 5.0 and 7.5 g of blueberry by-products was found (on average, 9.5 points).

Table 7. Overall acceptability and emotions induced for consumers by the prepared beverages enriched with extruded and fermented wheat bran and fruit/berry by-products.

Beverage Samples	Overall Acceptability	Emotions Induced by the Beverages (from 0 to 1)						
		Neutral	Happy	Sad	Angry	Surprised	Scared	Disgusted	Contempt	Valence
MP+10WB	7.9 ± 0.21 [e]	0.49 ± 0.01 [i]	0.150 ± 0.004 [c]	0.090 ± 0.002 [b]	0.0200 ± 0.0005 [a]	0.00100 ± 0.00003 [a]	0.00100 ± 0.00003 [a]	0.0080 ± 0.0002 [d]	0.050 ± 0.001 [b]	0.090 ± 0.002 [b]
2.5.ShepMP$_{LUHS29}$+10WB	3.2 ± 0.11 [b]	0.44 ± 0.02 [h]	0.080 ± 0.003 [a]	0.170 ± 0.006 [c]	0.070 ± 0.002 [b]	0.0090 ± 0.0003 [d]	0.00100 ± 0.00003 [a]	0.0020 ± 0.0001 [b]	0.110 ± 0.004 [e]	0.130 ± 0.004 [c]
5.0.ShepMP$_{LUHS29}$+10WB	7.6 ± 0.15 [e]	0.21 ± 0.01 [b]	0.190 ± 0.005 [d]	0.260 ± 0.007 [d]	0.070 ± 0.002 [b]	0.033 ± 0.001 [f]	0.00100 ± 0.00003 [a]	0.0030 ± 0.0001 [c]	0.100 ± 0.003 [e]	0.090 ± 0.002 [b]
7.5.ShepMP$_{LUHS29}$+10WB	8.0 ± 0.14 [f]	0.19 ± 0.00 [a]	0.34 ± 0.01 [f]	0.100 ± 0.002 [b]	0.110 ± 0.003 [c]	0.0050 ± 0.0001 [c]	0.00100 ± 0.00002 [a]	0.00100 ± 0.00002 [a]	0.050 ± 0.001 [b]	0.190 ± 0.004 [b]
2.5. RaspMP$_{LUHS29}$+10WB	2.6 ± 0.1 [a]	0.180 ± 0.006 [a]	0.050 ± 0.002 [a]	0.37 ± 0.01 [f]	0.170 ± 0.005 [d]	0.0020 ± 0.0001 [b]	0.00100 ± 0.00003 [a]	0.039 ± 0.001 [c]	0.35 ± 0.01 [i]	0.180 ± 0.006 [d]
5.0. RaspMP$_{LUHS29}$+10WB	7.3 ± 0.1 [d]	0.40 ± 0.01 [g]	0.180 ± 0.005 [d]	0.24 ± 0.01 [d]	0.020 ± 0.001 [a]	0.0020 ± 0.0001 [b]	0.00100 ± 0.00003 [a]	0.00100 ± 0.00003 [a]	0.060 ± 0.002 [c]	0.090 ± 0.002 [b]
7.5 RaspMP$_{LUHS29}$+10WB	8.6 ± 0.2 [g]	0.32 ± 0.01 [e]	0.360 ± 0.003 [f]	0.39 ± 0.01 [f]	0.020 ± 0.0004 [a]	0.0090 ± 0.0002 [d]	0.00100 ± 0.00002 [a]	0.00100 ± 0.00002 [a]	0.25 ± 0.01 [g]	0.320 ± 0.01 [f]
2.5. SeaMP$_{LUHS29}$+10WB	5.6 ± 0.2 [c]	0.47 ± 0.01 [h]	0.13 ± 0.00 [b]	0.25 ± 0.01 [d]	0.13 ± 0.004 [c]	0.0080 ± 0.0002 [d]	0.001 ± 0.00003 [a]	0.001 ± 0.00003 [a]	0.22 ± 0.01 [f]	0.47 ± 0.01 [g]
5.0 SeaMP$_{LUHS29}$+10WB	8.7 ± 0.2 [h]	0.32 ± 0.01 [e]	0.35 ± 0.00 [f]	0.40 ± 0.01 [f]	0.070 ± 0.002 [b]	0.00100 ± 0.00003 [a]	0.00100 ± 0.00003 [a]	0.00100 ± 0.00003 [a]	0.28 ± 0.01 [h]	0.32 ± 0.01 [f]
7.5 SeaMP$_{LUHS29}$+10WB	7.7 ± 0.2 [e]	0.26 ± 0.01 [c]	0.25 ± 0.01 [e]	0.30 ± 0.01 [e]	0.060 ± 0.002 [b]	0.0020 ± 0.0001 [b]	0.00100 ± 0.00003 [a]	0.00080 ± 0.00002 [d]	0.050 ± 0.001 [b]	0.260 ± 0.007 [e]
2.5 BluMP$_{LUHS29}$+10WB	7.3 ± 0.2 [d]	0.38 ± 0.01 [f]	0.190 ± 0.003 [d]	0.170 ± 0.005 [c]	0.0100 ± 0.0003 [a]	0.0150 ± 0.0004 [e]	0.00100 ± 0.00003 [a]	0.00100 ± 0.00002 [a]	0.080 ± 0.002 [d]	0.060 ± 0.002 [a]
5.0 BluMP$_{LUHS29}$+10WB	9.3 ± 0.17 [i]	0.28 ± 0.01 [d]	0.360 ± 0.003 [f]	0.190 ± 0.004 [c]	0.0100 ± 0.00002 [a]	0.00100 ± 0.00002 [a]	0.00100 ± 0.00002 [a]	0.00200 ± 0.00004 [b]	0.030 ± 0.001 [a]	0.28 ± 0.01 [e]
7.5 BluMP$_{LUHS29}$+10WB	9.6 ± 0.26 [j]	0.27 ± 0.01 [c]	0.480 ± 0.005 [g]	0.070 ± 0.002 [a]	0.0100 ± 0.0003 [a]	0.0340 ± 0.001 [f]	0.00100 ± 0.00003 [a]	0.0030 ± 0.0001 [a]	0.110 ± 0.003 [f]	0.060±0.002 [a]

2.5, 5.0, 7.5, quantities of fruit/berry by-products used, g 50 mL^{-1}; MP$_{NF}$, non-fermented milk permeate; MP$_F$, milk permeate fermented with LUHS29 (*P. acidilactici*); Shep, Shepherd/*Sambucus nigra*, Rasp, Raspberries/*Rubus idaeus*; Sea, Sea buckthorn/*Hippophae rhamnoides*; Blu, blueberries/*Vaccinium myrtillus*; WB, wheat bran extruded at 130 °C, screw speed 25 rpm and fermented with LUHS245 (*L. uvarum*). 10 WB, quantity of WB used, g 50 mL^{-1}. Data are represented as means ($n = 3$) ± SD. [a–i] Means with different letters in column are significantly different ($p \leq 0.05$).

Evaluation of the induced emotions by brands, packaging, etc. is generally performed to obtain information about product sales, brand loyalty, and consumer satisfaction [112]. However, the study of emotions induced by unpackaged foods and beverages in response to their sensory properties is more recent and very important for the development of product innovations [113,114]. It is suggested that the sensory properties of a product may correlate with emotions, and for this reason, a greater understanding of the relationship between sensory characteristics and emotions has become very important [115,116].

In this study, between overall acceptability and the emotion "happy" induced for consumers by the prepared beverages enriched with extruded and fermented WB and berries, there was a very strong positive correlations were found ($r = 0.8525$), as well as a strong negative correlation between overall acceptability and emotion "angry" was found ($r = -0.6842$). Moderate negative correlations between the overall acceptability and emotions "disgusted" and "contempt" were found ($r = -0.4134$ and $r = -0.4134$, respectively). Between overall acceptability and emotions "neutral" and "sad" very weak positive correlations were found ($r = 0.1136$ and $r = 0.1973$, respectively). According to overall acceptability results, for the further experiments, samples prepared with 20 g 50 mL^{-1} of WB and with the addition of 5.0 g 50 mL^{-1} of sea buckthorn and 7.5 g 50 mL^{-1} of shepherd, raspberries and blueberries were selected.

In the last decade, evaluation of emotions has been widely applied by the beverage industry in the product development cycle, for product improvement and optimisation, and changes in the formulation [117,118]. However, the literature in this area of application is scarce, since most manufacturers use this information internally to achieve a technical advantage against other competitors in the market [117]. Thomson et al. [119] published that specific sensory characteristics are associated with emotional conceptualisations in unbranded samples of dark chocolate, including associations of "cocoa" with "powerful" and "energetic", "bitter" with "confident", "adventurous" and "masculine", and "creamy" and "sweet" with "fun", "comforting" and "easy-going". However, Thomson et al. did not compare hedonic and emotional responses; for this reason, it is not possible to determine sensory-emotion linkages. However, a correlation between acceptability and emotional associations in food and beverages was reported [114,120–124].

In this study, also, a very strong positive correlation was found between overall acceptability and the emotion "happy", however, it should be mentioned that the beverages without fruit/berry by-products showed lower correlations between overall acceptability and induced emotions. It could be that more intensive sensory properties induced by the addition of fruit/berry by-products, induced stronger emotions for consumers, which were fixed, and in this study, by fruit/berry by-products induced emotions were positive.

3.5. Antimicrobial Activity of the Prepared Beverages Enriched with Wheat Bran and Fruits/Berries By-Products

The DIZ of the prepared beverages against pathogenic and opportunistic strains are shown in Table 8. All of the prepared beverages showed inhibition properties against *Salmonella enterica Infantis* and *Staphylococcus aureus*, however, all of the prepared beverages did not inhibit *Kluyvera cryocrescens*. Beverages, prepared with extruded and fermented WB, but without berries/fruits by-products inhibited 2 out of 10 tested pathogenic and opportunistic strains, however, beverages prepared with shepherd and sea buckthorn inhibited 9 out of 10, as well as beverages prepared with raspberry and blueberry by-products, which inhibited 8 out of 10 tested pathogenic and opportunistic strains. The highest DIZ of beverages prepared with shepherd against *E. coli* (hemolytic) and *Enterococcus durans* were found (13.4 and 12.3 mm, respectively), the highest DIZ of beverages prepared with raspberry by-products against *Bacillus pseudomycoides*, *Enterococcus durans*, and *Acinetobacter johnsonii* (DIZ, on average, 13.8 mm), the highest DIZ of beverages prepared with sea buckthorn by-products against *Enterococcus durans* and *Acinetobacter johnsonii* (DIZ, on average, 13.9 mm), and the highest DIZ of beverages prepared with blueberry by-products against *E. coli* (hemolytic) and *Enterococcus durans* (DIZ, on average, 14.8 mm).

Table 8. The diameter of inhibition zones (mm) of the prepared beverages against pathogenic and opportunistic strains.

Samples	The Diameter of Inhibition Zones (DIZ) (mm)										
	Pathogenic and Opportunistic Bacterial Strains										
	1	2	3	4	5	6	7	8	9	10
MP$_{LUHS29}$+10WB	9.1 ± 0.2 ^{a}	nd	nd	nd	10.1 ± 0.4 ^{b}	nd	nd	nd	nd	nd
MP$_{LUHS29}$+10WB+Shep7.5	10.2 ± 0.3 ^{b}	10.3 ± 0.4 ^{a}	13.4 ± 0.7 ^{c}	10.3 ± 0.4 ^{a}	9.0 ± 0.3 ^{a}	9.3 ± 0.1 ^{a}	9.2 ± 0.2 ^{a}	12.3 ± 0.3 ^{a}	nd	10.3 ± 0.4 ^{a}
MP$_{LUHS29}$+10WB+Rasp7.5	13.0 ± 0.2 ^{d}	10.1 ± 0.5 ^{a}	9.3 ± 0.3 ^{a}	13.6 ± 0.4 ^{c}	12.3 ± 0.6 ^{c}	9.6 ± 0.1 ^{a}	nd	13.4 ± 0.2 ^{b}	nd	14.3 ± 0.6 ^{d}
MP$_{LUHS29}$+10WB+Sea5.0	10.3 ± 0.4 ^{b}	11.0 ± 0.6 ^{ab}	10.2 ± 0.4 ^{b}	10.3 ± 0.3 ^{a}	12.4 ± 0.3 ^{c}	10.4 ± 0.2 ^{ab}	nd	14.5 ± 0.4 ^{c}	nd	13.2 ± 0.3 ^{c}
MP$_{LUHS29}$+10WB+Blu7.5	12.4 ± 0.3 ^{c}	12.6 ± 0.2 ^{c}	14.0 ± 0.3 ^{c}	12.1 ± 0.6 ^{b}	12.2 ± 0.2 ^{c}	12.3 ± 0.1 ^{b}	10.3 ± 0.2 ^{b}	15.6 ± 0.5 ^{d}	nd	12.1 ± 0.4 ^{b}

Salmonella enterica Infantis LT 101   *Staphylococcus aureus* LT 102   *E. coli* (hemolytic) LT 103

Bacillus pseudomycoides LT 104   *Aeromonas veronii* LT 105   *Cronobacter sakazakii* LT 106   *Acinetobacter johnsonii* LT 110

1. MP$_{LUHS29}$+10WB
2. MP$_{LUHS29}$+10WB+Shep7.5
3. MP$_{LUHS29}$+10WB+Rasp7.5
4. MP$_{LUHS29}$+10WB+Sea5
5. MP$_{LUHS29}$+10WB+Blu7.5

1, Salmonella enterica Infantis LT 101; 2, Staphylococcus aureus LT 102; 3, E. coli (hemolytic) LT 103; 4, Bacillus pseudomycoides LT 104; 5, Aeromonas veronii LT 105; 6, Cronobacter sakazakii LT 106; 7, Hafnia alvei LT 107; 8, Enterococcus durans LT 108; 9, Kluyvera cryocrescens LT 109; 10, Acinetobacter johnsonii LT 110; nd, not determined; MP$_{NF}$, non-fermented milk permeate; MP$_F$, milk permeate fermented with LUHS29 (*P. acidilactici*); Shep, Shepherd/*Sambucus nigra*, Rasp, Raspberries/*Rubus idaeus*; Sea, Sea buckthorns/*Hippophae rhamnoides*; Blu, blueberries/*Vaccinium myrtillus*; WB, wheat bran extruded at 130 °C, screw speed 25 rpm and fermented with LUHS245 (*L. uvarum*); 10WB, quantity of WB used, g 50 mL^{-1}; 5.0, 7.5, quantity of berries used, g 50 mL^{-1}. Data are represented as means (n = 3) ± SD. $^{a-d}$ Means with different letters in column are significantly different ($p \leq 0.05$); nd, not determined.

Finally, in all the cases, berries/fruits by-products increase beverages' antimicrobial properties, in comparison with beverages prepared just with extruded and fermented WB, and these results can be related to berries/fruits' bioactive compounds and antimicrobial properties, which are described above (Section 3.2). Moreover, during fermentation, LAB excreted a broad spectrum of antimicrobial compounds (organic acids, low molecular weight peptides, hydrogen peroxide, etc.) that inhibits the growth of pathogenic and opportunistic strains [125]. The antimicrobial activity of LAB against a variety of pathogenic and opportunistic strains was determined in several studies [126–131]. In the developed beverages, both antimicrobial ingredients: Viable LAB and fruit/berry by-products showed a symbiotic effect on pathogens inhibition.

3.6. LAB Count during the Storage, Colour Coordinates, and Acidity Parameters

The viable LAB count in prepared beverages during the four weeks of storage at +4 °C temperature is shown in Table 9. The LAB count after 24 h in beverages was, on average, 8.17 $\log_{10}$ CFU mL^{-1}, and after one and two weeks of storage, significant changes in the LAB counts were not found. However, after three weeks of storage, LAB count was reduced in the fermented milk permeate (without WB and berries/fruits by-products addition) samples (on average, by 10.3%). After four weeks of storage, higher than 6.0 $\log_{10}$ CFU mL^{-1} remain in two beverage groups: Beverages prepared with extruded and fermented WB (on average, 7.20 $\log_{10}$ CFU mL^{-1}) and in beverages prepared with extruded and fermented WB and 7.5 g 50 mL^{-1} of shepherd (on average, 6.93 $\log_{10}$ CFU mL^{-1}). Finally, three weeks storage time for beverages can be recommended, because during this time the viable LAB count in beverages remained higher than 6.0 $\log_{10}$ CFU mL^{-1}. In addition, the beverages prepared with extruded and fermented WB, and beverages prepared with extruded and fermented WB and 7.5 g 50 mL^{-1} of shepherd had their functional properties retained for longer, and for the above-mentioned beverages, four weeks storage time can be recommended.

Table 9. Viable lactic acid bacteria (LAB) count in prepared beverages during the four weeks of storage storage at +4 °C temperature.

Beverages Samples	LAB Count, $\log_{10}$ CFU mL^{-1}				
	24 h	1st Week	2nd Week	3rd Week	4th Week
MP$_{NF}$	n.d	n.d	n.d	n.d	n.d
MP$_F$	7.99 ± 0.22 [a]	7.89 ± 0.16 [a]	7.79 ± 0.19 [b]	6.99 ± 0.24 [a]	5.80 ± 0.17 [a]
MP$_{LUHS29+10WB}$	8.20 ± 0.18 [c]	8.01 ± 0.20 [b]	8.00 ± 0.28 [b]	8.01 ± 0.20 [b]	7.20 ± 0.21 [b]
MP$_{LUHS29+10WB}$+Shep7.5	8.33 ± 0.21 [d]	8.03 ± 0.15 [b]	7.83 ± 0.27 [b]	7.80 ± 0.27 [b]	6.93 ± 0.20 [b]
MP$_{LUHS29+10WB}$+Rasp7.5	8.17 ± 0.26 [b]	7.98 ± 0.19 [b]	7.91 ± 0.20 [b]	7.69 ± 0.19 [b]	5.88 ± 0.14 [a]
MP$_{LUHS29+10WB}$+Sea5.0	8.10 ± 0.12 [b]	7.99 ± 0.16 [b]	7.90 ± 0.27 [b]	7.54 ± 0.25 [b]	5.67 ± 0.13 [a]
MP$_{LUHS29+10WB}$+Blu7.5	8.15 ± 0.21 [b]	7.87 ± 0.29 [a]	7.31 ± 0.28 [a]	6.99 ± 0.27 [a]	5.94 ± 0.16 [a]

LAB, lactic acid bacteria; MP$_{NF}$, non-fermented milk permeate; MP$_F$, milk permeate fermented with LUHS29 (*P. acidilactici*); Shep, Shepherd/*Sambucus nigra*, Rasp, Raspberries/*Rubus idaeus*; Sea, Sea buckthorns/*Hippophae rhamnoides*; Blu—blueberries/*Vaccinium myrtillus*; WB, wheat bran extruded at 130 °C, screw speed 25 rpm and fermented with LUHS245 (*L. uvarum*); 10WB, quantity of WB used, g 50 mL^{-1}; 5.0, 7.5, quantity of berries used, g 50 mL^{-1}. The data expressed as mean values (n = 3) ± SD; SD, standard deviation. [a–d] The mean values within a column with different letters are significantly different ($p \leq 0.05$); n.d, not determined.

Colour coordinates, acidity and antioxidant parameters of the prepared beverages are shown in Table 10.

Table 10. Colour coordinates, acidity and antioxidant parameters of the prepared beverages.

Beverages Samples	Colour Coordinates, NBS			pH	TTA, °N	TPC, mg 100 g^{-1} d.m.	Antioxidant Activity, %
	L*	a*	b*				
MP$_{NF}$	27.3 ± 1.7 [b]	2.01 ± 0.06 [b]	1.11 ± 0.03 [b]	5.88 ± 0.2 [f]	3.0 ± 0.1 [a]	68.2 ± 3.7 [a]	14.1 ± 1.3 [a]
MP$_F$	31.4 ± 2.9 [c]	1.83 ± 0.05 [a]	1.34 ± 0.04 [c]	3.91 ± 0.02 [a]	9.5 ± 0.2 [d]	104.8 ± 5.9 [b]	21.7 ± 1.6 [b]
MP$_{LUHS29+10WB}$	39.1 ± 2.3 [f]	1.77 ± 0.06 [a]	1.92 ± 0.06 [d]	4.30 ± 0.01 [d]	8.5 ± 0.2 [c]	124.4 ± 4.1 [c]	25.8 ± 1.8 [c]
MP$_{LUHS29+10WB+Shep7.5}$	19.7 ± 1.6 [a]	5.31 ± 0.17 [c]	0.84 ± 0.03 [a]	4.26 ± 0.03 [d]	8.8 ± 0.2 [c]	132.5 ± 6.2 [d]	29.3 ± 1.9 [d]
MP$_{LUHS29+10WB+Rasp7.5}$	27.2 ± 1.8 [b]	15.6 ± 0.8 [e]	5.97 ± 0.26 [e]	4.17 ± 0.02 [b]	9.0 ± 0.3 [c]	141.7 ± 7.1 [e]	29.3 ± 1.7 [d]
MP$_{LUHS29+10WB+Sea5.0}$	30.4 ± 2.9 [c]	5.29 ± 0.23 [c]	15.5 ± 1.4 [f]	4.62 ± 0.02 [e]	7.9 ± 0.3 [b]	125.9 ± 4.5 [c]	26.1 ± 2.0 [c]
MP$_{LUHS29+10WB+Blu7.5}$	20.4 ± 1.6 [a]	6.36 ± 0.17 [d]	0.82 ± 0.02 [a]	4.20 ± 0.01 [c]	8.9 ± 0.2 [c]	132.8 ± 4.6 [d]	27.5 ± 1.6 [d]

L*, lightness; a*, redness (a* greenness); b*, yellowness (b* blueness); TTA, total titratable acidity; TPC, total phenolic compounds. MP$_{NF}$, non-fermented milk permeate; MP$_F$, milk permeate fermented with LUHS29 (*P. acidilactici*); Shep, Shepherd/*Sambucus nigra*, Rasp, Raspberries/*Rubus idaeus*; Sea, Sea buckthorn/*Hippophae rhamnoides*; Blu, blueberries/*Vaccinium myrtillus*; WB, wheat bran extruded at 130 °C, screw speed 25 rpm and fermented with LUHS245 (*L. uvarum*); 10 WB, quantity of WB used, g 50 mL^{-1}; 5.0, 7.5, quantity of berries used, g 50 mL^{-1}. The data expressed as mean values ($n = 3$) ± SD; SD, standard deviation. $^{a-f}$ The mean values within a column with different letters are significantly different ($p \leq 0.05$).

The highest lightness (L*) coordinates of the beverages prepared with extruded and fermented WB were established (39.1 NBS), the lowest L* (by 49.6% lower) of the beverages, prepared with WB and shepherd addition were found. The addition of raspberries increases redness (a*) of beverages, and in comparison with beverages groups with and without berries, beverages with raspberries had a* coordinates that were by 88.0 and 63.5% higher, respectively. The highest yellowness (b*) of the beverages prepared with the sea buckthorn was found (15.5 NBS), and in comparison with other beverages, this group showed, on average, 7.7 times higher b* coordinates. Colour characteristics are one from the main sensory properties, which have a strong relationship with consumers' acceptance and purchasing decisions regarding a product [132]. In addition, colour is a product quality indicator and influences the perception of taste, safety, as well as nutritional value [133].

Moderate positive correlations between overall acceptability and L*, between emotion "sad" and a*, and between the emotion "disgusted" and L* were found (Table 11). As well as moderate negative correlations between emotion "angry" and a*, it was also established between the emotion "surprised" and a* and b* colour coordinates. In addition, there were strong positive correlations between the emotion "neutral" and L*, between the emotion "happy" and a*, between the emotion "contempt" and a*, and between "valence" and a* and b* coordinates. The strong negative correlation between emotion "happy" and L* was established, as well as a very strong positive correlation between the emotion "sad" and b* and between emotion "contempt" and b*.

Table 11. Correlation coefficients between colour coordinates and overall acceptability and emotions induced for consumers by the tested beverages.

Colour Coordinates	Overall Acceptability	Neutral	Happy	Sad	Angry	Surprised	Scared	Disgusted	Contempt	Valence
Correlation Coefficients (R) between Colour Coordinates and Overall Acceptability and Emotions Induced for Consumers by the Tested Beverages.										
L*	−0.2472	0.7466	−0.6405	0.1461	−0.0861	−0.4778	0.2659	0.5806	−0.0196	0.0491
a*	0.5451	−0.1683	0.6144	0.5909	−0.4113	−0.0543	0.0369	−0.3109	0.6709	0.6530
b*	0.3512	0.0988	0.2708	0.8350	−0.0416	−0.4592	0.0483	−0.2360	0.8582	0.7929

L*, lightness; a*, redness (a* greenness); b*, yellowness (b* blueness).

In a comparison of the pH of the beverages prepared with functional additives, the lowest pH of the samples prepared with raspberries and blueberries was found to be 4.17 and 4.20, respectively, but it should be mentioned, that all the samples prepared with additives showed a higher pH than that fermented milk permeate (pH 3.91) without WB and/or fruits/berries. A very strong negative correlation was found between pH and TTA of the samples ($r = -0.94524$). In comparison, with total phenolic compound (TPC) content in samples, the highest TPC content in beverages prepared with the addition of raspberries was established (141.7 mg 100 g^{-1} d.m.). The lowest TPC content in non-fermented milk permeate was found (68.2 mg 100 g^{-1} d.m.), however, fermentation increased TPC in milk permeate samples, on average, by 34.9%, compared with samples prepared with extruded and fermented WB with fermented milk permeate without additives, where WB addition increased TPC content, on average, by 15.8%. When comparing the samples group prepared with the addition of extruded and fermented WB with samples prepared with WB and fruit/berry by-products, most fruits/berry by-products increased TPC content in the beverages (on average, by 9.0%), except samples prepared with sea buckthorn, in which TPC remained similar as before the addition of fruit/berry by-products. A very high positive correlation was established Between TPC and antioxidant activity of the samples ($r = 0.9919$).

The development of plant-derived nutraceutical beverages with antioxidant properties has been the intensively studied in recent years [134]. In this study, the main antioxidant properties in the developed beverages' ingredients were fruit/berry by-products, however, it should be mentioned that the LAB also excreted antioxidant property possessing compounds.

The modulation of the intestinal redox environment using viable bacteria possessing antioxidant properties has also been noted [135].

The health benefits of products containing desirable bioactive compounds have been previously published. Antioxidant characteristics of plants can be related to several anti-oxidative mechanisms of the chemical composition of plant tissues, as well as by micro- and macrocompounds interactions, including synergistic or opposite mechanisms of action [136].

The main compounds, which lead to shepherd antioxidant activity, are anthocyanins and flavanols [137]. Shepherd phenolics are depended on plant genetic differences, environmental conditions, degree of maturity, etc., and these factors are very important for industry because chemical composition is related to antioxidant capacity [138]. Raspberries are a good source of bioactive phytochemicals, especially phenolics, in which the general structure contains an aromatic ring with one or more hydroxyl groups, and these compounds are highly associated with antioxidant capacity [139]. The antioxidant capacity of phenolics is based on the ability of the phenolic ring to stabilise and delocalise unpaired electrons [140].

TPC in raspberries varied between 142 and 758 mg gallic acid equivalents (GAE) 100 g^{-1} fw [29]. The concentration of TPC in plants can be induced by many factors, including species, cultivar, ripening stage, soil, and climate [141,142], producing differences in the TPC found among the different studied species [96]. Moreover, in vitro antioxidant activity of the fruit/berries can be related to the high content of ascorbic acid [143–145]. It was reported that Sea buckthorns are rich in phenolics and flavonoids with potential antioxidant and antiproliferative activities and can be recommended in antioxidant and anticancer dietary supplement synthesis and utilisation in the food industry. Furthermore, it was published about blueberry antioxidant activity [102]. The effect of blueberry juice phytochemicals occurs through redox- and non-redox-regulated mechanisms and protects from oxidative damage factors related to bone remodelling and bone formation [146].

4. Conclusions

This study confirms that added-value products can be prepared from food industry by-products combinations. However, it should be mentioned that ingredients quantities and their pre-treatment must be carefully selected. In this study, in most cases (except sea buckthorn), by increasing FBB content the beverages overall acceptability was increased, and the highest was obtained for the samples prepared with 5.0 and 7.5 g of blueberries FBB. A very strong positive correlation ($r = 0.8525$) between overall acceptability, evaluated by points, and emotion "happy", induced for consumers by the prepared beverages, was found. Moreover, FBB is a good source to increase total phenolic compounds (TPC) content (in this study, on average, by 9.0%) in beverages. Finally, it can be stated that newly developed nutraceutical beverages are acceptable for consumers, induced positive emotions, as well as possessing desirable antimicrobial and antioxidant properties, and are prepared in an environmentally friendly and sustainable manner.

Author Contributions: Conceptualization and methodology: E.Z., E.B., R.P.F.G., M.R. and P.V.; investigation: E.Z., D.C., D.K., V.L., V.S. (Vytaute Starkute), P.Z., J.A., A.B., M.D., K.S. and S.T.; writing—original draft preparation: E.Z., D.C., V.L., V.S. (Vesta Steibliene) and P.Z.; writing—review and editing: E.B., R.P.F.G. and M.R.; visualization: E.Z., V.S. (Vesta Steibliene), P.Z., V.L. and P.V.; supervision: E.B. All authors have read and agreed to the published version of the manuscript.

Funding: This research received no external funding.

Acknowledgments: The authors gratefully acknowledge the EUREKA Network Project E!13309 "SUSFEETECH" (No. 01.2.2-MITA-K-702-05-0001) and COST Action 18101 SOURDOMICS—Sourdough biotechnology network towards novel, healthier and sustainable food and bioprocesses (https://sourdomics.com/; https://www.cost.eu/actions/CA18101/).

Conflicts of Interest: The authors declare no conflict of interest.

References

1. Sustainable Food Environment European Commission. Available online: https://ec.europa.eu/environment/archives/eussd/food.htm (accessed on 13 June 2020).
2. Meiselman, H.L. Emotions of Eating and Drinking. In *Handbook of Eating and Drinking: Interdisciplinary Perspectives*; Meiselman, H.L., Ed.; Springer International Publishing: Cham, Switzerland, 2020; pp. 349–370. ISBN 978-3-030-14504-0.
3. Bartkiene, E.; Steibliene, V.; Adomaitiene, V.; Lele, V.; Cernauskas, D.; Zadeike, D.; Klupsaite, D.; Juodeikiene, G. Corrigendum: The Perspectives Associated with the Computer-Based Diagnostic Method of Depressive Disorder. *Front. Psychiatry* **2019**, *10*, 10. [CrossRef] [PubMed]
4. Food Processing Industry-An Overview Science Direct Topics. Available online: https://www.sciencedirect.com/topics/earth-and-planetary-sciences/food-processing-industry (accessed on 2 July 2020).
5. Zokaityte, E.; Cernauskas, D.; Klupsaite, D.; Lele, V.; Starkute, V.; Zavistanaviciute, P.; Ruzauskas, M.; Gruzauskas, R.; Juodeikiene, G.; Rocha, J.; et al. Bioconversion of Milk Permeate with Selected Lactic Acid Bacteria Strains and Apple By-Products into Beverages with Antimicrobial Properties and Enriched with Galactooligosaccharides. *Microorganisms* **2020**, *8*, 1182. [CrossRef] [PubMed]
6. Fernández, J.; Moreno, F.J.; Olano, A.; Clemente, A.; Villar, C.J.; Lombó, F. A Galacto-Oligosaccharides Preparation Derived from Lactulose Protects Against Colorectal Cancer Development in an Animal Model. *Front. Microbiol.* **2018**, *9*, 2004. [CrossRef] [PubMed]
7. Germec, M.; Tarhan, K.; Yatmaz, E.; Tetik, N.; Karhan, M.; Demirci, A.; Turhan, I. Ultrasound-assisted dilute acid hydrolysis of tea processing waste for production of fermentable sugar. *Biotechnol. Prog.* **2016**, *32*, 393–403. [CrossRef] [PubMed]
8. Knauf, M.; Moniruzzaman, M. Lignocellulosic biomass processing: A perspective. *Int. Sugar J.* **2004**, *106*, 147–150.
9. Menon, V.; Rao, M. Trends in bioconversion of lignocellulose: Biofuels, platform chemicals & biorefinery concept. *Prog. Energy Combust. Sci.* **2012**, *38*, 522–550. [CrossRef]
10. Sharma, P.; Gujral, H.S.; Singh, B. Antioxidant activity of barley as affected by extrusion cooking. *Food Chem.* **2012**, *131*, 1406–1413. [CrossRef]
11. Germec, M.; Ozcan, A.; Turhan, I. Bioconversion of wheat bran into high value-added products and modelling of fermentations. *Ind. Crop. Prod.* **2019**, *139*, 111565. [CrossRef]
12. Guillon, F.; Champ, M. Structural and physical properties of dietary fibres, and consequences of processing on human physiology. *Food Res. Int.* **2000**, *33*, 233–245. [CrossRef]
13. Yang, Q.; Huang, X.; Zhao, S.; Sun, W.; Yan, Z.; Wang, P.; Li, S.; Huang, W.; Zhang, S.; Liu, L.; et al. Structure and Function of the Fecal Microbiota in Diarrheic Neonatal Piglets. *Front. Microbiol.* **2017**, *8*, 502. [CrossRef]
14. Gualberto, D.G.; Bergman, C.J.; Kazemzadeh, M.; Weber, C.W. Effect of extrusion processing on the soluble and insoluble fiber, and phytic acid contents of cereal brans. *Plant Foods Hum. Nutr.* **1997**, *51*, 187–198. [CrossRef]
15. Ralet, M.-C.; Thibault, J.-F.; Della Valle, G. Influence of extrusion-cooking on the physico-chemical properties of wheat bran. *J. Cereal Sci.* **1990**, *11*, 249–259. [CrossRef]
16. Kaur, J.; Debnath, J. Autophagy at the crossroads of catabolism and anabolism. *Nat. Rev. Mol. Cell Biol.* **2015**, *16*, 461–472. [CrossRef] [PubMed]
17. Applequist, W. A Brief Review of Recent Controversies in the Taxonomy and Nomenclature of Sambucus Nigra Sensu Lato. *Acta Hortic.* **2015**, *1061*, 25–33. [CrossRef]
18. Charlebois, D.; Byers, P.L.; Finn, C.E.; Thomas, A.L. *Elderberry: Botany, Horticulture, Potential*; Horticultural Reviews; Wiley: Hoboken, NJ, USA, 2010; Volume 37, pp. 213–280.
19. Manganelli, R.E.U.; Zaccaro, L.; Tomei, P. Antiviral activity in vitro of *Urtica dioica* L., *Parietaria diffusa* M. et K. and *Sambucus nigra* L. *J. Ethnopharmacol.* **2005**, *98*, 323–327. [CrossRef] [PubMed]
20. Lee, J.; Finn, C.E. Anthocyanins and other polyphenolics in American elderberry (*Sambucus canadensis*) and European elderberry (*S. nigra*) cultivars. *J. Sci. Food Agric.* **2007**, *87*, 2665–2675. [CrossRef]
21. Fazio, A.; Plastina, P.; Meijerink, J.; Witkamp, R.F.; Gabriele, B. Comparative analyses of seeds of wild fruits of Rubus and Sambucus species from Southern Italy: Fatty acid composition of the oil, total phenolic content, antioxidant and anti-inflammatory properties of the methanolic extracts. *Food Chem.* **2013**, *140*, 817–824. [CrossRef] [PubMed]

22. Sidor, A.; Gramza-Michałowska, A. Advanced research on the antioxidant and health benefit of elderberry (Sambucus nigra) in food—A review. *J. Funct. Foods* **2015**, *18*, 941–958. [CrossRef]
23. Viapiana, A.; Wesołowski, M. The Phenolic Contents and Antioxidant Activities of Infusions of *Sambucus nigra* L. *Plant Foods Hum. Nutr.* **2017**, *72*, 82–87. [CrossRef]
24. Dawidowicz, A.L.; Wianowska, D.; Baraniak, B. The antioxidant properties of alcoholic extracts from Sambucus nigra L. (antioxidant properties of extracts). *LWT* **2006**, *39*, 308–315. [CrossRef]
25. Paredes-López, O.; Cervantes-Ceja, M.L.; Vigna-Pérez, M.; Hernández-Pérez, T. Berries: Improving Human Health and Healthy Aging, and Promoting Quality Life—A Review. *Plant Foods Hum. Nutr.* **2010**, *65*, 299–308. [CrossRef]
26. Konieczynski, P.; Arceusz, A.; Wesolowski, M. Essential Elements and Their Relations to Phenolic Compounds in Infusions of Medicinal Plants Acquired from Different European Regions. *Biol. Trace Element Res.* **2015**, *170*, 466–475. [CrossRef] [PubMed]
27. Teng, J.; Jakeman, A.; Vaze, J.; Croke, B.; Dutta, D.; Kim, S. Flood inundation modelling: A review of methods, recent advances and uncertainty analysis. *Environ. Model. Softw.* **2017**, *90*, 201–216. [CrossRef]
28. Bowen-Forbes, C.S.; Zhang, Y.; Nair, M.G. Anthocyanin content, antioxidant, anti-inflammatory and anticancer properties of blackberry and raspberry fruits. *J. Food Compos. Anal.* **2010**, *23*, 554–560. [CrossRef]
29. De Souza, V.R.; Pereira, P.A.P.; Da Silva, T.L.T.; Lima, L.C.D.O.; Pio, R.; Queiroz, F. Determination of the bioactive compounds, antioxidant activity and chemical composition of Brazilian blackberry, red raspberry, strawberry, blueberry and sweet cherry fruits. *Food Chem.* **2014**, *156*, 362–368. [CrossRef]
30. Sariburun, E.; Şahin, S.; Demir, C.; Türkben, C.; Uylaşer, V. Phenolic Content and Antioxidant Activity of Raspberry and Blackberry Cultivars. *J. Food Sci.* **2010**, *75*, C328–C335. [CrossRef]
31. Bobinaitė, R.; Pataro, G.; Lamanauskas, N.; Šatkauskas, S.; Viškelis, P.; Ferrari, G. Application of pulsed electric field in the production of juice and extraction of bioactive compounds from blueberry fruits and their by-products. *J. Food Sci. Technol.* **2015**, *52*, 5898–5905. [CrossRef]
32. Diaconeasa, Z.; Florica, R.; Rugină, D.; Lucian, C.; Carmen, S. HPLC/PDA–ESI/MS Identification of Phenolic Acids, Flavonol Glycosides and Antioxidant Potential in Blueberry, Blackberry, Raspberries and Cranberries. *J. Food Nutr. Res.* **2014**, *2*, 781–785. [CrossRef]
33. Kula, M.; Majdan, M.; Głód, D.; Krauze-Baranowska, M. Phenolic composition of fruits from different cultivars of red and black raspberries grown in Poland. *J. Food Compos. Anal.* **2016**, *52*, 74–82. [CrossRef]
34. Mullen, W.; McGinn, J.; Lean, M.E.J.; MacLean, M.R.; Gardner, P.; Duthie, G.G.; Yokota, T.; Crozier, A. Ellagitannins, Flavonoids, and Other Phenolics in Red Raspberries and Their Contribution to Antioxidant Capacity and Vasorelaxation Properties. *J. Agric. Food Chem.* **2002**, *50*, 5191–5196. [CrossRef]
35. Sytařová, I.; Orsavová, J.; Snopek, L.; Mlček, J.; Byczyński, Ł.; Mišurcová, L. Impact of phenolic compounds and vitamins C and E on antioxidant activity of sea buckthorn (*Hippophaë rhamnoides* L.) berries and leaves of diverse ripening times. *Food Chem.* **2020**, *310*, 125784. [CrossRef] [PubMed]
36. Araya-Farias, M.; Makhlouf, J.; Ratti, C. Drying of Seabuckthorn (*Hippophae rhamnoides* L.) Berry: Impact of Dehydration Methods on Kinetics and Quality. *Dry. Technol.* **2011**, *29*, 351–359. [CrossRef]
37. Arif, S.; Ahmed, S.; Shah, A.; Hassan, L.; Awan, S.I.; Hamid, A.; Batool, F. Determination of optimum harvesting time for vitamin C, oil and mineral elements in berries sea buckthorn (*Hippophae rhamnoides*). *Pak. J. Bot.* **2010**, *42*, 3561–3568.
38. Fatima, T.; Kesari, V.; Watt, I.; Wishart, D.S.; Todd, J.F.; Schroeder, W.R.; Paliyath, G.; Krishna, P. Metabolite profiling and expression analysis of flavonoid, vitamin C and tocopherol biosynthesis genes in the antioxidant-rich sea buckthorn (*Hippophae rhamnoides* L.). *Phytochemistry* **2015**, *118*, 181–191. [CrossRef]
39. Stobdan, T.; Korekar, G.; Srivastava, R.B. Nutritional Attributes and Health Application of Seabuckthorn (*Hippophae rhamnoides* L.) A Review. *Curr. Nutr. Food Sci.* **2013**, *9*, 151–165. [CrossRef]
40. Tiitinen, K.; Yang, B.; Haraldsson, G.G.; Jonsdottir, S.; Kallio, H.P. Fast Analysis of Sugars, Fruit Acids, and Vitamin C in Sea Buckthorn (*Hippophaë rhamnoides* L.) Varieties. *J. Agric. Food Chem.* **2006**, *54*, 2508–2513. [CrossRef]
41. Beveridge, T.; Li, T.S.C.; Oomah, B.D.; Smith, A. Sea Buckthorn Products: Manufacture and Composition. *J. Agric. Food Chem.* **1999**, *47*, 3480–3488. [CrossRef] [PubMed]
42. Liu, S.; Marsol-Vall, A.; Laaksonen, O.; Kortesniemi, M.; Yang, B. Characterization and Quantification of Nonanthocyanin Phenolic Compounds in White and Blue Bilberry (*Vaccinium myrtillus*) Juices and Wines Using UHPLC-DAD–ESI-QTOF-MS and UHPLC-DAD. *J. Agric. Food Chem.* **2020**, *68*, 7734–7744. [CrossRef]

43. Pires, T.C.S.P.; Caleja, C.; Buelga, C.S.; Barros, L.; Ferreira, I.C. *Vaccinium myrtillus* L. Fruits as a Novel Source of Phenolic Compounds with Health Benefits and Industrial Applications-A Review. *Curr. Pharm. Des.* **2020**, *26*, 1917–1928. [CrossRef]
44. Elias, M.; Madureira, J.; Santos, P.; Carolino, M.; Margaça, F.; Verde, S.C. Preservation treatment of fresh raspberries by e-beam irradiation. *Innov. Food Sci. Emerg. Technol.* **2020**, *66*, 102487. [CrossRef]
45. Bartkiene, E. Possible Uses of Lactic acid Bacteria for Food and Feed Production. *Agric. Res. Technol. Open Access J.* **2017**, *4*, 4. [CrossRef]
46. Bartkiene, E.; Bartkevics, V.; Starkute, V.; Krungleviciute, V.; Cizeikiene, D.; Zadeike, D.; Juodeikiene, G.; Maknickiene, Z. Chemical composition and nutritional value of seeds of *Lupinus luteus* L., *L. angustifolius* L. and new hybrid lines of *L. angustifolius* L. *Zemdirb. Agric.* **2016**, *103*, 107–116. [CrossRef]
47. Ben-Gigirey, B.; De Sousa, J.M.V.B.; Villa, T.G.; Barros-Velazquez, J. Histamine and Cadaverine Production by Bacteria Isolated from Fresh and Frozen Albacore (*Thunnus alalunga*). *J. Food Prot.* **1999**, *62*, 933–939. [CrossRef] [PubMed]
48. Bartkiene, E.; Bartkevičs, V.; Rusko, J.; Starkute, V.; Bendoraitiene, E.; Zadeike, D.; Juodeikiene, G. The effect of Pediococcus acidilactici and Lactobacillus sakei on biogenic amines formation and free amino acid profile in different lupin during fermentation. *LWT* **2016**, *74*, 40–47. [CrossRef]
49. 14:00–17:00 ISO 8586-1:1993. Available online: https://www.iso.org/cms/render/live/en/sites/isoorg/contents/data/standard/01/58/15875.html (accessed on 18 September 2020).
50. Bartkiene, E.; Zokaityte, E.; Lele, V.; Sakiene, V.; Zavistanaviciute, P.; Klupsaite, D.; Bendoraitiene, J.; Navikaite-Snipaitiene, V.; Ruzauskas, M. Technology and characterisation of whole hemp seed beverages prepared from ultrasonicated and fermented whole seed paste. *Int. J. Food Sci. Technol.* **2019**, *55*, 406–419. [CrossRef]
51. Sanni, A. The need for process optimization of African fermented foods and beverages. *Int. J. Food Microbiol.* **1993**, *18*, 85–95. [CrossRef]
52. Garvie, I.E. Bacterial lactate dehydrogenases. *Microbiol. Rev.* **1980**, *44*, 106–139. [CrossRef]
53. Jin, Y.; Compaan, A.; Bhattacharjee, T.; Huang, Y. Granular gel support-enabled extrusion of three-dimensional alginate and cellular structures. *Biofabrication* **2016**, *8*, 025016. [CrossRef]
54. Mozuriene, E.; Bartkiene, E.; Juodeikiene, G.; Žadeikė, D.; Basinskiene, L.; Maruška, A.; Stankevičius, M.; Ragažinskienė, O.; Damašius, J.; Cizeikiene, D. The effect of savoury plants, fermented with lactic acid bacteria, on the microbiological contamination, quality, and acceptability of unripened curd cheese. *LWT* **2016**, *69*, 161–168. [CrossRef]
55. Manome, A.; Okada, S.; Uchimura, T.; Komagata, K. The ratio of L-form to D-form of lactic acid as a criteria for the identification of lactic acid bacteria. *J. Gen. Appl. Microbiol.* **1998**, *44*, 371–374. [CrossRef] [PubMed]
56. Kowlgi, N.G.; Chhabra, L. D-Lactic Acidosis: An Underrecognized Complication of Short Bowel Syndrome. *Gastroenterol. Res. Pr.* **2015**, *2015*, 1–8. [CrossRef]
57. Monroe, G.R.; Van Eerde, A.M.; Tessadori, F.; Duran, K.J.; Savelberg, S.M.C.; Van Alfen, J.C.; Terhal, P.A.; Van Der Crabben, S.N.; Lichtenbelt, K.D.; Fuchs, S.A.; et al. Identification of human D lactate dehydrogenase deficiency. *Nat. Commun.* **2019**, *10*, 1477. [CrossRef]
58. Khaneghah, A.M.; Moosavi, M.H.; Oliveira, C.A.; Vanin, F.; Sant'Ana, A.S. Electron beam irradiation to reduce the mycotoxin and microbial contaminations of cereal-based products: An overview. *Food Chem. Toxicol.* **2020**, *143*, 111557. [CrossRef]
59. Heshmati, A.; Zohrevand, T.; Khaneghah, A.M.; Nejad, A.S.M.; Sant'Ana, A.S. Co-occurrence of aflatoxins and ochratoxin A in dried fruits in Iran: Dietary exposure risk assessment. *Food Chem. Toxicol.* **2017**, *106*, 202–208. [CrossRef]
60. Khaneghah, A.M.; Fakhri, Y.; Sant'Ana, A.S. Impact of unit operations during processing of cereal-based products on the levels of deoxynivalenol, total aflatoxin, ochratoxin A, and zearalenone: A systematic review and meta-analysis. *Food Chem.* **2018**, *268*, 611–624. [CrossRef]
61. Zhu, C.; Bortesi, L.; Baysal, C.; Twyman, R.; Fischer, R.; Capell, T.; Schillberg, S.; Christou, P. Characteristics of Genome Editing Mutations in Cereal Crops. *Trends Plant Sci.* **2017**, *22*, 38–52. [CrossRef] [PubMed]
62. Peng, X.; Zhang, S.; Li, L.; Zhao, X.; Ma, Y.; Shi, D. Long-term high-solids anaerobic digestion of food waste: Effects of ammonia on process performance and microbial community. *Bioresour. Technol.* **2018**, *262*, 148–158. [CrossRef]

63. Spaggiari, M.; Ricci, A.; Calani, L.; Bresciani, L.; Neviani, E.; Dall'Asta, C.; Lazzi, C.; Galaverna, G. Solid state lactic acid fermentation: A strategy to improve wheat bran functionality. *LWT* **2020**, *118*, 108668. [CrossRef]
64. Arte, E.; Rizzello, C.G.; Verni, M.; Nordlund, E.; Katina, K.; Coda, R. Impact of Enzymatic and Microbial Bioprocessing on Protein Modification and Nutritional Properties of Wheat Bran. *J. Agric. Food Chem.* **2015**, *63*, 8685–8693. [CrossRef]
65. Messia, M.; Reale, A.; Maiuro, L.; Candigliota, T.; Sorrentino, E.; Marconi, E. Effects of pre-fermented wheat bran on dough and bread characteristics. *J. Cereal Sci.* **2016**, *69*, 138–144. [CrossRef]
66. Prückler, M.; Lorenz, C.; Endo, A.; Kraler, M.; Dürrschmid, K.; Hendriks, K.; Silva, F.; Auterith, E.; Kneifel, W.; Michlmayr, H. Comparison of homo and heterofermentative lactic acid bacteria for implementation of fermented wheat bran in bread. *Food Microbiol.* **2015**, *49*, 211–219. [CrossRef]
67. Laddomada, B.; Caretto, S.; Mita, G. Wheat Bran Phenolic Acids: Bioavailability and Stability in Whole Wheat-Based Foods. *Molecules* **2015**, *20*, 15666–15685. [CrossRef]
68. De Brier, N.; Gomand, S.V.; Donner, E.; Paterson, D.; Delcour, J.A.; Lombi, E.; Smolders, E. Distribution of Minerals in Wheat Grains (*Triticum aestivum* L.) and in Roller Milling Fractions Affected by Pearling. *J. Agric. Food Chem.* **2015**, *63*, 1276–1285. [CrossRef] [PubMed]
69. Di Lena, G.; Vivanti, V.; Quaglia, G.B. Amino acid composition of wheat milling by-products after bioconversion by edible fungi mycelia. *Food/Nahrung* **1997**, *41*, 285–288. [CrossRef]
70. Balandrán-Quintana, R.R.; Mercado-Ruiz, J.N.; Mendoza-Wilson, A.M. Wheat Bran Proteins: A Review of Their Uses and Potential. *Food Rev. Int.* **2015**, *31*, 279–293. [CrossRef]
71. Zhu, K.; Huang, S.; Peng, W.; Qian, H.; Zhou, H.-M. Effect of ultrafine grinding on hydration and antioxidant properties of wheat bran dietary fiber. *Food Res. Int.* **2010**, *43*, 943–948. [CrossRef]
72. Alzuwaid, N.T.; Sissons, M.; Laddomada, B.; Fellows, C.M. Nutritional and functional properties of durum wheat bran protein concentrate. *Cereal Chem. J.* **2019**, *97*, 304–315. [CrossRef]
73. Feddern, V.; Mazzuco, H.; Fonseca, F.N.; De Lima, G.J.M.M. A review on biogenic amines in food and feed: Toxicological aspects, impact on health and control measures. *Anim. Prod. Sci.* **2019**, *59*, 608. [CrossRef]
74. Ruiz-Capillas, C.; Herrero, A.M. Impact of Biogenic Amines on Food Quality and Safety. *Foods* **2019**, *8*, 62. [CrossRef]
75. Wink, M. Modes of Action of Herbal Medicines and Plant Secondary Metabolites. *Medicines* **2015**, *2*, 251–286. [CrossRef] [PubMed]
76. Ali, M.A.; Poortvliet, E.; Strömberg, R.; Yngve, A. Polyamines in foods: Development of a food database. *Food Nutr. Res.* **2011**, *55*, 5572. [CrossRef]
77. Buyukuslu, N.; Hizli, H.; Esin, K.; Garipagaoglu, M. A Cross-Sectional Study: Nutritional Polyamines in Frequently Consumed Foods of the Turkish Population. *Foods* **2014**, *3*, 541–557. [CrossRef]
78. Gg, H.; Gd, H.; Az, W. Effect of Refined Milling on the Nutritional Value and Antioxidant Capacity of Wheat Types Common in Ethiopia and a Recovery Attempt with Bran Supplementation in Bread. *J. Food Process. Technol.* **2015**, *6*, 6. [CrossRef]
79. Ladero, V.; Calles-Enriquez, M.; Fernandez, M.; Alvarez, M.A. Toxicological Effects of Dietary Biogenic Amines. *Curr. Nutr. Food Sci.* **2010**, *6*, 145–156. [CrossRef]
80. Ozogul, F.; Ozogul, Y. Biogenic amine content and biogenic amine quality indices of sardines (*Sardina pilchardus*) stored in modified atmosphere packaging and vacuum packaging. *Food Chem.* **2006**, *99*, 574–578. [CrossRef]
81. Karayigit, B.; Colak, N.; Ozogul, F.; Gundogdu, A.; Inceer, H.; Bilgiçli, N.; Ayaz, F.A. The biogenic amine and mineral contents of different milling fractions of bread and durum wheat (*Triticum* L.) cultivars. *Food Biosci.* **2020**, *37*, 100676. [CrossRef]
82. Okamoto, S.; Hijikata-Okunomiya, A.; Wanaka, K.; Okada, Y.; Okamoto, U. Enzyme-Controlling Medicines: Introduction. *Semin. Thromb. Hemost.* **1997**, *23*, 493–501. [CrossRef] [PubMed]
83. Nakajima, J.-I.; Tanaka, I.; Seo, S.; Yamazaki, M.; Saito, K. LC/PDA/ESI-MS Profiling and Radical Scavenging Activity of Anthocyanins in Various Berries. *J. Biomed. Biotechnol.* **2004**, *2004*, 241–247. [CrossRef] [PubMed]
84. Wu, X.; Gu, L.; Prior, R.L.; McKay, S. Characterization of Anthocyanins and Proanthocyanidins in Some Cultivars of Ribes, Aronia, and Sambucu sand Their Antioxidant Capacity. *J. Agric. Food Chem.* **2004**, *52*, 7846–7856. [CrossRef]
85. Jing, P.; Bomser, J.A.; Schwartz, S.J.; He, J.; Magnuson, B.A.; Giusti, M.M. Structure−Function Relationships of Anthocyanins from Various Anthocyanin-Rich Extracts on the Inhibition of Colon Cancer Cell Growth. *J. Agric. Food Chem.* **2008**, *56*, 9391–9398. [CrossRef]

86. Zafra-Stone, S.; Yasmin, T.; Bagchi, M.; Chatterjee, A.; Vinson, J.A.; Bagchi, D. Berry anthocyanins as novel antioxidants in human health and disease prevention. *Mol. Nutr. Food Res.* **2007**, *51*, 675–683. [CrossRef] [PubMed]
87. Zakay-Rones, Z.; Thom, E.; Wollan, T.; Wadstein, J. Randomized Study of the Efficacy and Safety of Oral Elderberry Extract in the Treatment of Influenza A and B Virus Infections. *J. Int. Med. Res.* **2004**, *32*, 132–140. [CrossRef] [PubMed]
88. Bhattacharya, S.; Christensen, K.B.; Olsen, L.C.B.; Christensen, L.P.; Grevsen, K.; Færgeman, N.J.; Kristiansen, K.; Young, J.F.; Oksbjerg, N. Bioactive Components from Flowers of Sambucus nigral. Increase Glucose Uptake in Primary Porcine Myotube Cultures and Reduce Fat Accumulation in Caenorhabditis elegans. *J. Agric. Food Chem.* **2013**, *61*, 11033–11040. [CrossRef] [PubMed]
89. Beaux, D.; Fleurentin, J.; Mortier, F. Effect of extracts of Orthosiphon stamineus benth, Hieracium pilosella l., Sambucus nigra l. and Arctostaphylos uva-ursi l. spreng. in rats. *Phytother. Res.* **1998**, *12*, 498–501. [CrossRef]
90. Chen, L.; Hu, J.Y.; Wang, S.Q. The role of antioxidants in photoprotection: A critical review. *J. Am. Acad. Dermatol.* **2012**, *67*, 1013–1024. [CrossRef]
91. Chrubasik, C.; Maier, T.; Dawid, C.; Torda, T.; Schieber, A.; Hofmann, T.; Chrubasik, S. An observational study and quantification of the actives in a supplement with Sambucus nigra and Asparagus officinalis used for weight reduction. *Phytother. Res.* **2008**, *22*, 913–918. [CrossRef]
92. Folmer, F.; Basavaraju, U.; Jaspars, M.; Hold, G.; El-Omar, E.; Dicato, M.; Han, B.W. Anticancer effects of bioactive berry compounds. *Phytochem. Rev.* **2013**, *13*, 295–322. [CrossRef]
93. Gray, A.M.; Abdel-Wahab, Y.H.A.; Flatt, P.R. The Traditional Plant Treatment, Sambucus nigra (elder), Exhibits Insulin-Like and Insulin-Releasing Actions In Vitro. *J. Nutr.* **2000**, *130*, 15–20. [CrossRef]
94. Picon, P.D.; Picon, R.V.; Costa, A.F.; Sander, G.B.; Amaral, K.M.; Aboy, A.L.; Henriques, A.T. Randomized clinical trial of a phytotherapic compound containing Pimpinella anisum, Foeniculum vulgare, *Sambucus nigra*, and *Cassia augustifolia* for chronic constipation. *BMC Complement. Altern. Med.* **2010**, *10*, 17. [CrossRef]
95. Omulokoli, E.; Khan, B.; Chhabra, S. Antiplasmodial activity of four Kenyan medicinal plants. *J. Ethnopharmacol.* **1997**, *56*, 133–137. [CrossRef]
96. Schulz, M.; Chim, J.F. Nutritional and bioactive value of Rubus berries. *Food Biosci.* **2019**, *31*, 100438. [CrossRef]
97. Tiitinen, K.M.; Hakala, A.M.A.; Kallio, H.P. Quality Components of Sea Buckthorn (*Hippophaë rhamnoides*) Varieties. *J. Agric. Food Chem.* **2005**, *53*, 1692–1699. [CrossRef] [PubMed]
98. Arimboor, R.; Kumar, K.S.; Arumughan, C. Simultaneous estimation of phenolic acids in sea buckthorn (Hippophaë rhamnoides) using RP-HPLC with DAD. *J. Pharm. Biomed. Anal.* **2008**, *47*, 31–38. [CrossRef] [PubMed]
99. Bal, L.M.; Meda, V.; Naik, S.; Satya, S. Sea buckthorn berries: A potential source of valuable nutrients for nutraceuticals and cosmoceuticals. *Food Res. Int.* **2011**, *44*, 1718–1727. [CrossRef]
100. Teleszko, M.; Wojdyło, A.; Rudzińska, M.; Oszmiański, J.; Golis, T. Analysis of Lipophilic and Hydrophilic Bioactive Compounds Content in Sea Buckthorn (*Hippophaë rhamnoides* L.) Berries. *J. Agric. Food Chem.* **2015**, *63*, 4120–4129. [CrossRef]
101. Guo, R.; Guo, X.; Li, T.; Fu, X.; Liu, R.H. Comparative assessment of phytochemical profiles, antioxidant and antiproliferative activities of Sea buckthorn (*Hippophaë rhamnoides* L.) berries. *Food Chem.* **2017**, *221*, 997–1003. [CrossRef]
102. Burdulis, D.; Šarkinas, A.; Jasutienė, I.; Stackevicené, E.; Nikolajevas, L.; Janulis, V. Comparative study of anthocyanin composition, antimicrobial and antioxidant activity in bilberry (*Vaccinium myrtillus* L.) and blueberry (*Vaccinium corymbosum* L.) fruits. *Acta Pol. Pharm. Drug Res.* **2009**, *66*, 399–408.
103. Bouarab-Chibane, L.; Forquet, V.; Lantéri, P.; Clément, Y.; Léonard-Akkari, L.; Oulahal, N.; Degraeve, P.; Bordes, C. Antibacterial Properties of Polyphenols: Characterization and QSAR (Quantitative Structure–Activity Relationship) Models. *Front. Microbiol.* **2019**, *10*, 829. [CrossRef]
104. Coppo, E.; Marchese, A. Antibacterial activity of polyphenols. *Curr. Pharm. Biotechnol.* **2014**, *15*, 380–390. [CrossRef]
105. Ștefănescu, B.-E.; Călinoiu, L.-F.; Ranga, F.; Fetea, F.; Mocan, A.; Vodnar, D.C.; Crișan, G. Chemical Composition and Biological Activities of the Nord-West Romanian Wild Bilberry (*Vaccinium myrtillus* L.) and Lingonberry (*Vaccinium vitis-idaea* L.) Leaves. *Antioxidants* **2020**, *9*, 495. [CrossRef]

106. Piqueras-Fiszman, B.; Jaeger, S.R. The impact of the means of context evocation on consumers' emotion associations towards eating occasions. *Food Qual. Prefer.* **2014**, *37*, 61–70. [CrossRef]
107. Piqueras-Fiszman, B.; Jaeger, S.R. Emotion responses under evoked consumption contexts: A focus on the consumers' frequency of product consumption and the stability of responses. *Food Qual. Prefer.* **2014**, *35*, 24–31. [CrossRef]
108. Shim, H.-K.; Lee, C.L.; Valentin, D.; Hong, J.-H. How a combination of two contradicting concepts is represented: The representation of premium instant noodles and premium yogurts by different age groups. *Food Res. Int.* **2019**, *125*, 108506. [CrossRef]
109. Cardello, A.V.; Meiselman, H.L.; Schutz, H.G.; Craig, C.; Given, Z.; Lesher, L.L.; Eicher, S. Measuring emotional responses to foods and food names using questionnaires. *Food Qual. Prefer.* **2012**, *24*, 243–250. [CrossRef]
110. Dalenberg, J.R.; Gutjar, S.; Ter Horst, G.J.; De Graaf, K.; Renken, R.J.; Jager, G. Evoked Emotions Predict Food Choice. *PLoS ONE* **2014**, *9*, e115388. [CrossRef]
111. Spinelli, S.; Monteleone, E. Emotional Responses to Products. In *Technology and Nutrition, Methods in Consumer Research*; Woodhead Publishing: Sawston/Cambridge, UK, 2018; pp. 261–296. ISBN 978-0-08-102089-0.
112. Smith, D.C.; Aaker, D.A. Managing Brand Equity: Capitalizing on the Value of a Brand Name. *J. Mark.* **1992**, *56*, 125–128. [CrossRef]
113. Meiselman, H.L. A review of the current state of emotion research in product development. *Food Res. Int.* **2015**, *76*, 192–199. [CrossRef]
114. Spinelli, S.; Masi, C.G.; Zoboli, G.P.; Prescott, J.M.; Monteleone, E. Emotional responses to branded and unbranded foods. *Food Qual. Prefer.* **2015**, *42*, 1–11. [CrossRef]
115. Moskowitz, H.R. Sensory Drivers of Liking and Sensory Preference Segmentation. In Proceedings of the ACS Symposium Series, American Chemical Society (ACS). *Chem. Taste* **2002**, *825*, 214–226. [CrossRef]
116. Guinard, J.-X. Internal and External Preference Mapping: Understanding Market Segmentation and Identifying Drivers of Liking. In Proceedings of the ACS Symposium Series, American Chemical Society (ACS). *Chem. Taste* **2002**, *825*, 227–242. [CrossRef]
117. King, S.C. Emotions Elicited by Foods. In *Emotion Measurement*; Woodhead Publishing: Sawston/Cambridge, UK, 2016; pp. 455–472. ISBN 9780081005088.
118. Van Zyl, H. *Emotion in Beverages. Emotion Measurement*; Woodhead Publishing: Sawston/Cambridge, UK, 2016; pp. 473–499. ISBN 978-0-08-1005088.
119. Thomson, D.M.; Crocker, C.; Marketo, C.G. Linking sensory characteristics to emotions: An example using dark chocolate. *Food Qual. Prefer.* **2010**, *21*, 1117–1125. [CrossRef]
120. Spinelli, S.; Masi, C.; Dinnella, C.; Zoboli, G.P.; Monteleone, E. How does it make you feel? A new approach to measuring emotions in food product experience. *Food Qual. Prefer.* **2014**, *37*, 109–122. [CrossRef]
121. Gutjar, S.; Dalenberg, J.R.; De Graaf, C.; De Wijk, R.A.; Palascha, A.; Renken, R.J.; Jager, G. What reported food-evoked emotions may add: A model to predict consumer food choice. *Food Qual. Prefer.* **2015**, *45*, 140–148. [CrossRef]
122. Mora, M.; Urdaneta, E.; Chaya, C. Emotional response to wine: Sensory properties, age and gender as drivers of consumers' preferences. *Food Qual. Prefer.* **2018**, *66*, 19–28. [CrossRef]
123. Jaeger, S.R.; Xia, Y.; Le Blond, M.; Beresford, M.K.; Hedderley, D.I.; Cardello, A.V. Supplementing hedonic and sensory consumer research on beer with cognitive and emotional measures, and additional insights via consumer segmentation. *Food Qual. Prefer.* **2019**, *73*, 117–134. [CrossRef]
124. Mora, M.; Giussani, B.; Pagliarini, E.; Chaya, C. Improvement of an emotional lexicon for the evaluation of beers. *Food Qual. Prefer.* **2019**, *71*, 158–162. [CrossRef]
125. Gálvez, A.; López, R.L.; Pulido, R.P.; Burgos, M.J.G. *Listeria Monocytogenes in the Food Processing Environment*; SpringerBriefs in Food, Health, and Nutrition; Springer: Cham, Switzerland, 2014; pp. 3–14. [CrossRef]
126. Cizeikiene, D.; Juodeikiene, G.; Paskevicius, A.; Bartkiene, E. Antimicrobial activity of lactic acid bacteria against pathogenic and spoilage microorganism isolated from food and their control in wheat bread. *Food Control.* **2013**, *31*, 539–545. [CrossRef]

127. Bartkiene, E.; Lele, V.; Sakiene, V.; Zavistanaviciute, P.; Ruzauskas, M.; Bernatoniene, J.; Jakstas, V.; Viskelis, P.; Zadeike, D.; Juodeikiene, G. Improvement of the antimicrobial activity of lactic acid bacteria in combination with berries/fruits and dairy industry by-products. *J. Sci. Food Agric.* **2019**, *99*, 3992–4002. [CrossRef]
128. Bartkiene, E.; Krungleviciute, V.; Antanaitis, R.; Kantautaite, J.; Ruzauskas, M.; Vaskeviciute, L.; Siugzdiniene, R.; Kucinskiene, J.; Juodeikiene, G.; Kucinskas, A.; et al. Antimicrobial activity of lactic acid bacteria multiplied in an alternative substrate and their influence on physiological parameters of new-born calves. *Veterinární Med.* **2016**, *61*, 653–662. [CrossRef]
129. Barbosa, A.A.T.; Mantovani, H.C.; Jain, S. Bacteriocins from lactic acid bacteria and their potential in the preservation of fruit products. *Crit. Rev. Biotechnol.* **2017**, *37*, 852–864. [CrossRef]
130. Elsanhoty, R.; Ghonamy, A.; El-Adly, N.; Ramadan, M.F. Impact of Lactic Acid Bacteria and Bifidobacterium on the Survival of Bacillus subtilus During Fermentation of Wheat Sourdough. *J. Food Process. Preserv.* **2016**, *41*, e13086. [CrossRef]
131. Rumjuankiat, K.; Keawsompong, S.; Nitisinprasert, S. Bacterial contaminants from frozen puff pastry production process and their growth inhibition by antimicrobial substances from lactic acid bacteria. *Food Sci. Nutr.* **2016**, *5*, 454–465. [CrossRef] [PubMed]
132. Hernandez, B.; Sáenz, C.; Alberdi, C.; Diñeiro, J.M. CIELAB color coordinates versus relative proportions of myoglobin redox forms in the description of fresh meat appearance. *J. Food Sci. Technol.* **2016**, *53*, 4159–4167. [CrossRef]
133. Palacios-Morillo, A.; Jurado, J.M.; Alcázar, A.; Pablos, F. Differentiation of Spanish paprika from Protected Designation of Origin based on color measurements and pattern recognition. *Food Control.* **2016**, *62*, 243–249. [CrossRef]
134. Ştefănescu, B.-E.; Călinoiu, L.F.; Ranga, F.; Fetea, F.; Mocan, A.; Vodnar, D.C.; Crisan, G. The Chemical and Biological Profiles of Leaves from Commercial Blueberry Varieties. *Plants* **2020**, *9*, 1193. [CrossRef]
135. Amaretti, A.; Di Nunzio, M.; Pompei, A.; Raimondi, S.; Rossi, M.; Bordoni, A. Antioxidant properties of potentially probiotic bacteria: In vitro and in vivo activities. *Appl. Microbiol. Biotechnol.* **2012**, *97*, 809–817. [CrossRef]
136. Goud, N.S.; Prasad, G. Antioxidant, Antimicrobial Activity and Total Phenol and Flavonoids Analysis of Sambucus Nigra (Elderberry). *Int. J. Curr. Pharm. Res.* **2020**, *12*, 35–37. [CrossRef]
137. Rice-Evans, C.; Miller, N.; Paganga, G. Antioxidant properties of phenolic compounds. *Trends Plant Sci.* **1997**, *2*, 152–159. [CrossRef]
138. Zadernowski, R.; Naczk, M.; Nesterowicz, J. Phenolic Acid Profiles in Some Small Berries. *J. Agric. Food Chem.* **2005**, *53*, 2118–2124. [CrossRef]
139. Yang, J.W.; Choi, I.S. Comparison of the phenolic composition and antioxidant activity of Korean black raspberry, Bokbunja, (*Rubus coreanus* Miquel) with those of six other berries. *CyTA J. Food* **2016**, *15*, 1–8. [CrossRef]
140. Hidalgo, G.-I.; Almajano, M.P. Red Fruits: Extraction of Antioxidants, Phenolic Content, and Radical Scavenging Determination: A Review. *Antioxidants* **2017**, *6*, 7. [CrossRef]
141. Lee, J.; Dossett, M.; Finn, C.E. Rubus fruit phenolic research: The good, the bad, and the confusing. *Food Chem.* **2012**, *130*, 785–796. [CrossRef]
142. Lazar, T.; Taiz, L.; Zeiger, E. Plant physiology. *Ann. Bot.* **2003**, *91*, 750–751. [CrossRef]
143. Gao, X.; Ohlander, M.; Jeppsson, N.; Björk, L.; Trajkovski, V. Changes in Antioxidant Effects and Their Relationship to Phytonutrients in Fruits of Sea Buckthorn (*Hippophae rhamnoides* L.) during Maturation. *J. Agric. Food Chem.* **2000**, *48*, 1485–1490. [CrossRef]
144. Kim, J.-S.; Kwon, Y.-S.; Sa, Y.-J.; Kim, M.-J. Isolation and Identification of Sea Buckthorn (*Hippophae rhamnoides*) Phenolics with Antioxidant Activity and α-Glucosidase Inhibitory Effect. *J. Agric. Food Chem.* **2011**, *59*, 138–144. [CrossRef]

145. Rösch, D.; Bergmann, M.; Knorr, A.D.; Kroh, L.W. Structure–Antioxidant Efficiency Relationships of Phenolic Compounds and Their Contribution to the Antioxidant Activity of Sea Buckthorn Juice. *J. Agric. Food Chem.* **2003**, *51*, 4233–4239. [CrossRef]
146. Domazetovic, V.; Marcucci, G.; Falsetti, I.; Bilia, A.R.; Vincenzini, M.T.; Brandi, M.L.; Iantomasi, T. Blueberry Juice Antioxidants Protect Osteogenic Activity against Oxidative Stress and Improve Long-Term Activation of the Mineralization Process in Human Osteoblast-Like SaOS-2 Cells: Involvement of SIRT1. *Antioxidants* **2020**, *9*, 125. [CrossRef]

Publisher's Note: MDPI stays neutral with regard to jurisdictional claims in published maps and institutional affiliations.

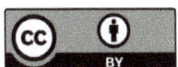 © 2020 by the authors. Licensee MDPI, Basel, Switzerland. This article is an open access article distributed under the terms and conditions of the Creative Commons Attribution (CC BY) license (http://creativecommons.org/licenses/by/4.0/).

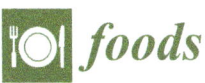

Article

Perceived Risk of Fish Consumption in a Low Fish Consumption Country

Ágoston Temesi [1,*], **Dawn Birch** [2], **Brigitta Plasek** [1], **Burak Atilla Eren** [1] **and Zoltán Lakner** [1]

1. Department of Food Chain Management, Institute of Agribusiness, Szent István University, 1118 Budapest, Hungary; plasek.brigitta@etk.szie.hu (B.P.); eren.burak.atilla@hallgato.uni-szie.hu (B.A.E.); lakner.zoltan@etk.szie.hu (Z.L.)
2. USC Business School, University of the Sunshine Coast, Sippy Downs, Queensland 4556, Australia; dbirch@usc.edu.au
* Correspondence: temesi.agoston@etk.szie.hu; Tel.: +36-1-305-7178

Received: 18 August 2020; Accepted: 10 September 2020; Published: 12 September 2020

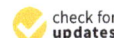

Abstract: Among the numerous health benefits of fish consumption, perhaps the most recognized is the role of omega-3 fatty acids in the prevention of cardiovascular disease. Cardiovascular disease is prevalent in Hungary, which has the lowest fish consumption in Europe. Increasing fish consumption is the aim of most European countries and given the high incidence of cardiovascular disease in Hungary, it is of particular importance. A significant reduction of the VAT for fish in 1 January 2018 aimed to increase fish consumption in Hungary. However, despite reduced VAT, the price of fish in Hungary rose from 2017 to 2018. The aim of our research is to explore perceived risks that serve to exacerbate Hungarian consumers' low fish consumption, and to measure their effects to identify potential strategies to most effectively increase fish consumption. We applied partial least squares structural equation modeling (PLS-SEM) to analyze responses provided by 1042 survey participants (collected with face-to-face interviews, using quota sampling in 2014) to explore variables of fish consumption associated with perceived risk including psychological, physical, social, and functional risks. Our model is the first one that applies detailed perceived risk categories to measure those effects on low fish consumption. The results indicate that psychological risk associated with negative past experiences have both a direct, and through functional risk, an indirect significant negative effect on fish consumption. Conversely, neither social nor physical risk impede Hungarian fish consumption. We conclude that the seafood industry could benefit from targeted interventions that seek to reduce functional risk-perception of the person responsible for preparing fish in the household.

Keywords: perceived risk; functional risk; psychological risk; social risk; physical risk; negative past experiences; structural equation modeling; consumer behavior

---

1. Introduction

Whilst in 2004, Olsen noted a surprisingly low volume of research on fish consumption from the perspective of marketing and consumer behavior [1], a more recent review by Carlucci et al. (2015) identified 49 relevant studies [2]. In more recent times, consumer research on barriers to fish consumption have been conducted across the globe [3] and in specific continents including Europe [4,5], Africa [6], Asia [7], Australia [8], South-America [9,10]. In their review, Carlucci et al. (2015) identified the main barriers of fish consumption to be associated with unpleasant sensory qualities of fish, low convenience, consumer lack of confidence in selecting and preparing fish, concerns about potential health risks, low availability of fish and high prices [2].

Understanding barriers to fish consumption is especially important in countries where consumption is markedly low, and in some cases, decreasing. Of concern, Eumofa (2019) data reveals long-range stagnation of fish consumption in some Central-European countries. For example, Hungary has the lowest annual per capita fish consumption in Europe (5.6 kg) with only 5% of expenditure on animal proteins in 2018 being for fish and seafood. Likewise, only 9% of expenditure on animal proteins in the Czech Republic in 2018 was spent on fish and seafood [11].

Fish consumption is important due to numerous positive health benefits for example, reduced incidence of disease such as breast cancer (e.g., [12]), sarcopenia [13], and mental illnesses such as depression [14], as well as, neurological diseases (e.g., [15]). In particular, researchers emphasize the preventive role of omega-3 fatty acids and role of fish consumption in reducing cardiovascular disease [16–19]. We argue there may be a direct correlation between health problems in Hungary and very low fish consumption, with Hungary reporting the worst data for cardiovascular disease within the European Union [20,21].

Seeking to increase fish consumption, the Hungarian government reduced the VAT for fish by 22% in 1 January 2018. In Hungary, carp is one of the most popular species of fish [22,23]. Changes in the price of a slice of carp, in monthly intervals in 2017 and 2018 (the year before and after the reduced VAT) are illustrated in Figure 1.

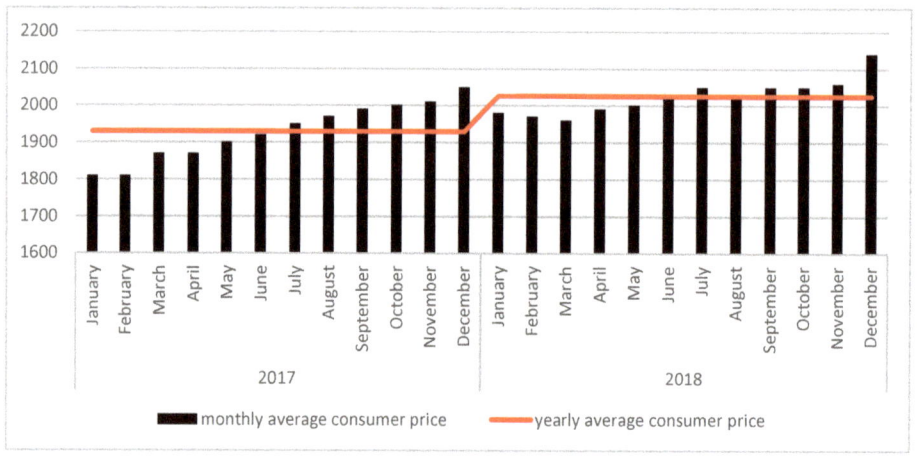

Figure 1. Monthly and yearly national average consumer price of a carp slice or fillet HUF/kg Source: [24].

The data reveals that the reduction of VAT in January 2018 successfully lowered the rising price of a carp slice; however by July 2018, only 7 months later, the price reached the previous 2017 price level. Hence, the reduction of VAT only temporarily reduced and then constrained the price, potentially explained by opportunistic behavior on behalf of Hungarian fish mongers. Given the latest fish consumption data available from FAO, Eumofa, and EC are from 2017, it is not possible to state whether the reduced VAT led to any increase in fish consumption in Hungary. However, while price (representing financial risk for the consumer), has been identified as a major barrier to fish consumption, other risks including functional, social, physical and psychological risks associated with fish consumption also influence fish consumption [25,26], and these risks are the focus of this paper.

1.1. Conceptual Model

Numerous studies have investigated reasons for lower-than-optimal fish consumption across the globe [2]. Several studies have explored the effect of food neophobia on fish consumption, and concluded that a higher degree of food neophobia negatively influenced fish consumption both for children [27,28] and adults [28–32]. Jaeger et al. [32] showed in the case of 112 analyzed foods—among them different forms of fish—that food neophobia has a significant effect on both the frequency of the given food's intake and on the preferences related to it. Many papers have been premised on the theory of planned behavior [33], for example, in Indonesia [34], Peru [10], Croatia [35], Bangladesh [36], Vietnam [37,38] and Belgium [39]. Data analysis for fish consumption studies has frequently involved the use of structural equation modeling (SEM) [38,40–45]. SEM was used by Pieniak et al. [46] and Siddique [36] and Schaefer et al. [47] used regression based on the variables of "risk perception" and "perceived risk", however, these two variables only explained a fraction of the effect. In an Australian study, Birch and Lawley [25] applied perceived risk theory [48,49] to explore the role of various categories of perceived risk on fish consumption, but they did not attempt modeling. Categories of perceived risk were first identified by Jacoby and Kaplan [50], distinguishing functional (or performance risk), physical, social, financial and psychological risks. In a consumer context, Murphy and Enis (p. 31 [51]) define risk as the "monetary and nonmonetary price of the product" with financial risk being monetary and social, psychological, physical, functional being nonmonetary.

In line with a study of perceived barriers to fish consumption in Australia conducted by Birch and Lawley [25], we investigate non-monetary risks associated with fish consumption in Hungary including physical, social, psychological (negative past experiences) and functional (occurring during cooking) risks.

1.1.1. Physical Risks

Fish consumption may involve various physical risks including choking on bones, allergic reactions, spoiled fish and contaminants such as heavy metals [25,47,52]. An increase in consumers' perception of the physical risk of consuming fish may be expected as freshwater contamination becomes better detected [53–56]. While communication of potential physical risk associated with fish consumption (e.g., mercury) is important [57], Anual et al. argue that consumers should be informed about contaminants in a way that equips them with the knowledge to more effectively manage the risk rather than resulting in decreased fish consumption [58]. Given potential perceived physical risks associated with fish consumption, we hypothesize:

Hypothesize 1 (H1). *Physical risks directly and negatively influence fish consumption.*

1.1.2. Social Risks

Fish consumption studies have investigated the role of social norms and social risks in mitigating fish consumption [5,25,39,59–61]. For example, in a Belgian study ($n = 429$) conducted by Verbeke and Vackier [39], one quarter of respondents not living alone indicated that they served a fish dish less frequently because of the resistance of the household members, and specifically concluded that the presence of a teenager in the household negatively influences fish consumption. Likewise, in an Australian study ($n = 899$), Birch and Lawley [25] found that nearly a third of the Australian respondents not living alone also served fish less frequently if other members of the household disliked fish. In Pinho et al.'s research [5], the barrier of the "taste preference of family and friends" proved to be a significant factor with households of three or more people. Zhou et al. [61] confirmed the findings of Myrland et al. [59], and Verbeke and Vackier [39] and concluded that the presence of a teenager in the household negatively influences fish consumption. Given the potential for dislike of fish by others to reduce fish consumption, we hypothesize:

Hypothesize 2 (H2). *Social risks directly and negatively influence fish consumption.*

1.1.3. Psychological Risks

Past experience influences intention to eat fish [42]. Fish consumption in childhood has been found to influence fish consumption in adulthood with studies indicating that regular childhood fish consumption leads to higher fish consumption as an adult (e.g., [41,62,63]). Conversely, too frequent fish consumption in childhood may result in aversion towards fish as a food in adulthood [62]. Negative past experiences associated with dislike of the sensory qualities of fish (bones, smell, appearance, taste, texture, etc.) have been found to lead to lower fish consumption [2,8,25,59]. In Hungary, a key source of unpleasant sensorial experiences may potentially be linked to consumption of primarily freshwater fish (that may have a muddy taste) [6], given Hungary is landlocked country. Given negative past experiences may influence fish consumption, we hypothesize:

Hypothesize 3 (H3). *Psychological risk associated with negative past experiences directly and negatively influences fish consumption.*

1.1.4. Functional Risks

Functional risk has been found to be a major barrier to fish consumption [25]. Numerous studies highlight the importance of knowledge in increasing fish consumption [1,4,43,64]. Hence, increasing consumer knowledge and confidence around selecting, cooking and serving fish (especially younger consumers) may lead to increased fish consumption [8,63]. Lack of knowledge and confidence may arise from low familiarity that has been found, for example, to be a key barrier to consumption of seafood such as shrimp and mussels [65]. Contini et al. emphasized the role of cooking skills on intention to consume fish [40], however, lack of knowledge of the person responsible for cooking in terms of fish preparation may not have the same significance in all countries, and rather may be more closely related to consumption frequency [66]. In our study, we specifically explore the functional risks that emerge during the preparation of fish dishes by the person responsible for cooking within the household. Given the potential for functional risk to influence fish consumption, we hypothesize:

Hypothesize 4 (H4). *Functional risk arising during the preparation of fish directly and negatively influences fish consumption.*

1.1.5. Interaction Effects

Badr. et al.'s study revealed that consumers regard the preparation of freshwater fish to be particularly difficult, requiring knowledge and skills [6]. The lack of these can easily result in improperly prepared fish meals. Poorly prepared fish arising from functional risk likely leads to a less than pleasing consumption experience, thus increasing the likelihood of psychological risk. According to the results of Laureati et al. [28] whether kids like a fish dish depends greatly on its cooking method. They connect all of this to neophobia and note that choosing the right recipe can significantly contribute to reducing it. Hence, we hypothesize:

Hypothesize 5 (H5). *Functional risk that arises during cooking directly and positively influence psychological risk due to negative past experiences.*

Poorly prepared fish may also lead to lower familiarity and acceptance of fish by other members of the household thus increasing social risk due to food acculturation effects. The effect of which is amplified further as the acceptance of unknown fish and fish meals will be more difficult due to higher perceived risk [67] and may result in the younger generation regarding the preparation of fish meals as even more difficult [39,45,68]. Hence, we hypothesize:

Hypothesize 6 (H6). *Functional risk that arise during preparation directly and positively influence (facilitate) the development of social risk.*

The aim of the present research is to apply the theory of perceived risk and contribute to the increasingly sophisticated modelling that seeks to explain complex fish consumption behavior. The context for the study is in a very low fish consumption country, namely Hungary, with the aim of identifying the role of perceived risk and inform strategies for reducing identified perceived risks in order to increase fish consumption. Figure 2 presents the conceptual model for the study indicating direct and indirect effects.

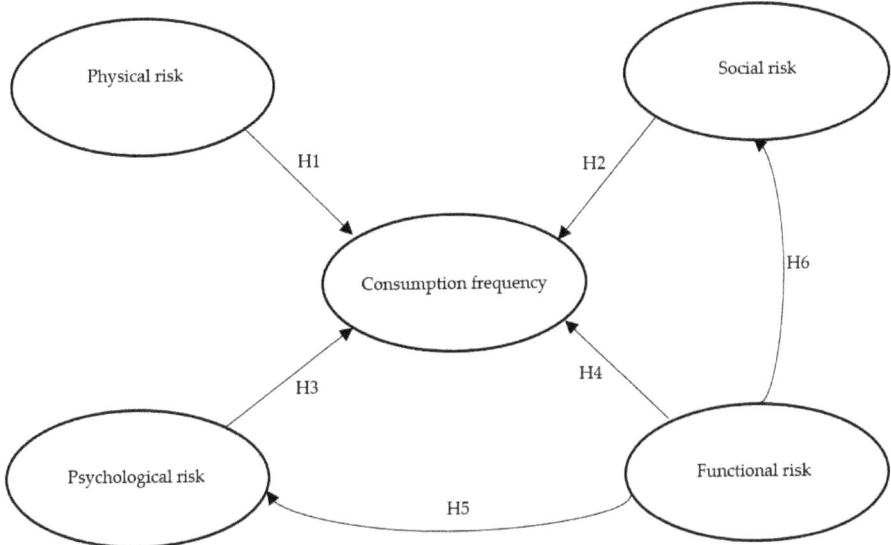

Figure 2. Conceptual framework.

2. Materials and Methods

A face to face state-wide paper-based survey of 1063 Hungarian consumers was conducted between 22nd September to 10th October 2014 in public places of 8 big cities of Hungary, namely in Budapest, Székesfehérvár, Pécs, Győr, Miskolc, Debrecen, Szolnok, and Szeged, using a standardized questionnaire. Due to the refusal to answer certain questions, we discarded the responses of 21 respondents, and thus analyzed the data from 1042 respondents. The respondents were motivated with a small non-food gift for participating in the survey. Before completing the survey, the respondents provided verbal consent to their answers being recorded. At the beginning of the survey we also informed them in writing that their answers will later be analyzed, but at the same time the responses would remain anonymous, and we did not collect any specific demographic data about the respondents. They had the option to refuse to answer any question or stop answering the survey at any point. The data is representative of the general population with respect to age and gender as a result of quota-sampling. A respondent profile is presented in Table 1.

Table 1. Demographic and income properties of respondents ($n = 1042$).

Variables		Composition of the Sample	Composition of the Population *
Gender	Male	46.8%	46.9%
	Female	53.0%	53.1%
	Missing	0.2%	
Age group	18–25	11.6%	11.5%
	26–35	17.8%	15.3%
	36–45	18.1%	19.5%
	46–55	16.4%	15.8%
	56 or older	35.9%	37.9%
	Missing	0.2%	

Table 1. Cont.

Education	Elementary	6.6%	
	Trade/vocational	16.3%	
	Secondary	32.1%	
	Tertiary	42.6%	
	Missing	2.3%	
Region	Northern Hungary	6.9%	11.6%
	Northern Great Plains	12.8%	14.9%
	Southern Great Plains	14.7%	12.8%
	Central Hungary	32.2%	30.7%
	Central Transdanubia	10.0%	10.8%
	Western Transdanubia	10.7%	10.0%
	Southern Transdanubia	8.5%	9.1%
	Missing	4.2%	
Perceived income status	Very tight	2.5%	
	Tight	11.7%	
	Average	58.4%	
	Good	20.6%	
	Very good	4.0%	
	Missing	2.7%	

* Source: [69].

In the two main parts of the questionnaire, we queried about the frequency of fish consumption and agreement with attitude statements.

Attitude statements for the survey were replicated or modified to the Hungarian consumption context based on the work of Birch and Lawley [25]. The degree of agreement was measured on a 5-point Likert-scale with ends labelled 1 = completely disagree and 5 = completely agree. The research focused on barriers of fish consumption and all the attitude statements are associated with perceived risk. The following attitude statements were included in the investigation (Table 2):

Table 2. Items and constructs.

Psychological risk
I like the taste of fish—reverse coded
I came to like fish already as a child–reverse coded
I have had good experiences in eating sea fish in the past – reverse coded
I have had good experiences in eating freshwater fish in the past–reverse coded
Physical risk
I am concerned that spoiled fish will be sold to me
I am concerned that fish may not have been handled in a hygienic way
I am concerned that fish contains a lot of contaminants from sea
I am concerned that fish contains a lot of contaminants from freshwaters
Functional risk
The person who cooks in our household does not know how to prepare freshwater fish
The person who cooks in our household does not know how to prepare saltwater fish
It is hard for the person who cooks in our household to bring him/herself to cook from fish that (s)he does not know
Social risk
Other adults in my household do not like fish
One or more children in my household do not like fish
Resistance by other members of my household makes it hard to serve fish as often as I want

Partial least square based structural equation modeling (PLS-SEM) was performed with the help of the SmartPLS software [70]. We built a reflective model, with frequency of consumption as a dependent variable measured with the question—How often did you consume a whole portion (10–15 dekagrams) of fish in the past year?

3. Results

3.1. Frequency of Fish Consumption

Typically, health guidelines recommend consumption of two servings of fish per week. For the grouping of frequency of consumption, we used the categorization of Birch and Lawley [25], regular fish consumers (2–3 times per week to at least once a week), light fish consumers (about once per fortnight), and very light fish consumers (once per month). Confirming the very low average fish consumption in Hungary, 12% ($n = 120$) of respondents report never consuming fish. Only 47% of respondents consume fish at least once per month. We categorized respondents who consume fish less than once per month but at least once a year ($n = 440$, 42%) as "extremely light" fish consumers. They may be the ones who typically, but not exclusively, consume the traditional Christmas fish dishes (fish soup, carp in breadcrumbs) in Hungary, so they are familiar with fish dishes, but consume them only on holidays. Very light fish consumers ($n = 263$) accounted for 25% of those surveyed and light fish consumers accounted for a further 10% ($n = 107$), while regular fish consumers ($n = 112$) only accounted for 11% of the respondents. Consumption frequency characteristics of the sample are introduced in Table 3.

Table 3. Consumption frequency of the sample ($n = 1042$).

Consumption Frequency		n	%
Regular	(2–3 times per week to at least once a week)	112	11%
Light	(About once per fortnight)	107	10%
Very light	(Once per month)	263	25%
Extremely light	(Less than once per month but at least once a year)	440	42%
Never	(Never)	120	12%

3.2. Measurement of Model

The attitude statements of the research tested were built into the model. The factor loadings of the items and the values belonging to the background variables of the model are shown in Table 4.

The values of the model confirm its reliability. Composite Reliability values fall between 0.767 and 0.823 and exceed the expected value of 0.7 in all cases [71]. The values of average variance extracted (AVE) vary between 0.505 and 0.565, and thus exceed the expected score of 0.5 [72]. Finally, Cronbach's alpha scores exceed 0.7 [73]. Although some factor loadings do not exceed 0.7, retaining them is in accordance with the recommendation of Hair et al. [74], who argue that items with factor loadings between 0.4 and 0.7 should be examined to determine whether discarding them will result in worse indices for the model. Moreover, in all cases, the values substantially exceed the value (<0.5) that Bagozzi and Yi consider the threshold for rejection [75]. The Collinearity Statstics show, that the VIF values for all items are below the threshold of 3 [72].

Considering the fact that we built a reflective model, the indices of the structural model were calculated with Consistent PLS Algorithm. Our results indicate that the model is a good fit (SRMR = 0.061, NFI = 0.856), and is consistent with the recommendation of Hu and Bentler [76], in that the SRMR score should remain below 0.8. Tables 5 and 6 show the results of the discriminant validity. Table 5 displays the Fornell-Larcker test of discriminant validity, while Table 6 shows the Heterotrait-Monotrait Ratio (HTMT).

Table 4. Construct reliability and validity.

Construct and Indicators	Factor Loading
Psychological risk (CR = 0.823, AVE = 0.539, CA = 0.823)	
I like the taste of fish—reverse coded	0.776
I came to like fish already as a child—reverse coded	0.634
I have had good experiences in eating sea fish in the past—reverse coded	0.733
I have had good experiences in eating freshwater fish in the past—reverse coded	0.783
Physical risk (CR = 0.803, AVE = 0.505, CA = 0.801)	
I am concerned that spoiled fish will be sold to me	0.667
I am concerned that fish may not have been handled in a hygienic way	0.730
I am concerned that fish contains a lot of contaminants from sea	0.670
I am concerned that fish contains a lot of contaminants from freshwaters	0.772
Functional risk (CR = 0.767, AVE = 0.525, CA = 0.762)	
The person who cooks in our household does not know how to prepare freshwater fish	0.782
The person who cooks in our household does not know how to prepare saltwater fish	0.729
It is hard for the person who cooks in our household to bring him/herself to cook from fish that (s)he does not know	0.657
Social risk (CR = 0.789, AVE = 0.565, CA = 0.787)	
Other adults in my household do not like fish	0.582
One or more children in my household do not like fish	0.697
Resistance by other members of my household makes it hard to serve fish as often as I want	0.933

* CR = composite reliability, AVE = average variance extracted, CA = Cronbach's alpha.

Table 5. Fornell-Larcker test of discriminant validity.

	Functional Risk	Psychological Risk	Consumption Frequency	Physical Risk	Social Risk
Functional risk	**0.724**				
Psychological risk	0.327	**0.734**			
Consumption frequency	−0.179	−0.353	**1.000**		
Physical risk	0.284	0.127	−0.005	**0.711**	
Social risk	0.389	0.349	−0.157	0.214	**0.751**

Square roots of the average variance extracted (AVE) shown on diagonal (in bold).

Table 6. Heterotrait-monotrait (HTMT) criterion for discriminant validity.

	Functional Risk	Psychological Risk	Consumption Frequency	Physical Risk	Social Risk
Functional risk					
Psychological risk	0.330				
Consumption frequency	0.179	0.352			
Physical risk	0.287	0.128	0.026		
Social risk	0.390	0.345	0.152	0.215	

Table 5 shows that the specific values of the square roots of the average variance extracted in the constructs are in all cases higher than the correlation values in the same columns or rows [77], whereas the values in Table 6 are remarkably lower than the 0.85 threshold [78], which means that discriminant validity has been established.

3.3. Structural Model Assessment

Bootstrapping procedure has been used to test level of significance and t statistics. Our first hypothesis (H1), the direct and negative relationship between the perception of physical risk and consumption frequency was not confirmed by our model ($\beta = 0.064$, $p = 0.070$). Similarly, the hypothesized direct and negative relationship between the perception of social risk and consumption frequency (H2) could also not be verified ($\beta = -0.026$, $p = 0.465$). The direct and negative effects of unpleasant experiences as psychological risk on consumption frequency (H3) were verified ($\beta = -0.326$, $p < 0.001$), as was the perceived functional risk during cooking (H4) ($\beta = -0.081$, $p = 0.043$), although Cohen's f-square is very low. The hypothesized relationships between risks were also confirmed in our research. Our results show a direct and positive relationship between functional risk perceived during cooking and the psychological risk associated with negative past experiences (H5) ($\beta = 0.327$, $p < 0.001$), as well as between functional risk perceived during cooking and the perception of social risk (H6) ($\beta = 0.389$, $p < 0.001$). Table 7 and Figure 3 summarize our results.

Table 7. Results for structural equation modelling.

	Direct Effect	Indirect Effect	Total Effect	Cohen's f²	T Statistics	p Values	Supported?
Physical risk → Consumption frequency	β = 0.064		0.064	0.004	1.813	p = 0.070	no
Social risk → Consumption frequency	β = −0.026		−0.026	0.001	0.732	p = 0.465	no
Psychological risk → Consumption frequency	β = −0.326		−0.326	0.102	9.868	p < 0.001	yes
Functional risk → Consumption frequency	β = −0.081	β = −0.117	−0.197	0.006	2.026	p = 0.043	yes
Functional risk → Psychological risk	β = 0.327		0.327	0.120	8.129	p < 0.001	yes
Functional risk → Social risk	β = 0.389		0.389	0.179	10,014	p < 0.001	yes

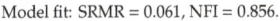

Model fit: SRMR = 0.061, NFI = 0.856.

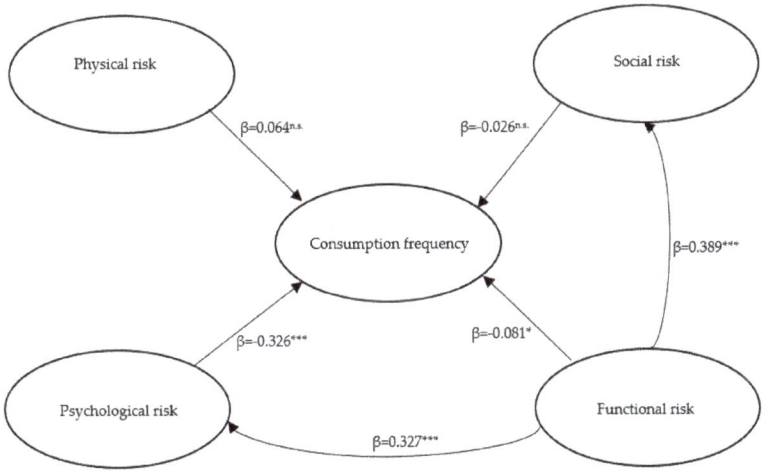

Figure 3. Results of structural equation modeling. β = standardized regression coefficient; * $p < 0.05$, *** $p < 0.001$, n.s. not significant.

The values of R^2, adjusted R^2 and Q^2 in Table 8 illustrate the explanatory power of the model.

Table 8. Coefficient determination (R^2), Adjusted R^2 and Q^2

Construct	R^2	Adjusted R^2	Q^2
Physical risk			
Social risk	0.152	0.151	0.064
Psychological risk	0.107	0.106	0.043
Functional risk			
Consumption frequency	0.133	0.130	0.102

The explanatory power of the model for consumption frequency is 13% (adjusted R^2 = 0.130), which is low but acceptable see [71,79]. Stone-Geisser's Q^2 values [74,80,81] are greater than 0, which means that each element of the endogenous constructs has predictive relevance. (Psychological risk = 0.043, Consumption frequency = 0.102, Social risk = 0.064).

4. Discussion

The aim of this research was to explore perceived risks that hinder fish consumption and their relative importance in Hungary, which has the lowest fish consumption in Europe. Our model is the first one that applies detailed perceived risk categories to measure those effects on low fish consumption. The structural equation model built to test the hypotheses did not support a direct and negative effect of either physical or social risk on fish consumption. Interestingly and contrary to expectations, perceived physical risk (perceived lack of hygiene, contamination, or spoiled fish) has a slight positive relationship with fish consumption. This may be explained by higher levels of involvement with fish and greater knowledge about fish among people who consume more fish. However, this awareness of potential physical risk is managed and does not hinder their fish consumption.

We observed a direct and negative relationship between functional risk arising during preparing fish and psychological risk associated with negative past experiences and frequency of consumption. Based on our model, we did not find a direct effect of functional risk on frequency of consumption, as Cohen's f^2 value is extremely low. However, indirectly, through negative past experiences, functional risk has a significant negative effect on frequency of consumption. This is consistent with the findings of Laureati et al. [28], who find cooking methods and choosing the right recipe to be of key importance regarding young people's acceptance of fish dishes.

Likewise, while functional risk increases perceptions of social risk, functional risk does not have an indirect effect on the frequency of fish consumption through social risk. Thus it appears that in effect, fish consumption in Hungary is not influenced by the fact whether others in the household like fish dishes.

Our results indicate that the fish industry could benefit from targeted interventions that reduce perceptions of functional risk. This would involve focusing on educating the person responsible for preparing fish within households to improve their skills in preparing fish dishes, or semi-prepared products, which can help boost their confidence and be more successful. This will likely lead to higher levels of household consumption of fish leading to greater familiarity and acceptance of fish for meals, thus mitigating social risk. Moreover, increased self-efficacy with fish preparation will likely lead to better (sensory) experiences and thus reduce perceived psychological risk associated with fish.

5. Limitations and Further Research

Our study is the first to use perceived risks as background variables for structural equation modeling to explain fish consumption frequency. The explanatory power of the model (R^2) is small, as we used the elements of perceived risk that only partially explain fish consumption and willingness to purchase fish. Our findings are consistent with Siddique [36] who found the effect of perceived risk on dry fish consumption to be 18%. In accordance with the aim of the research, further research will build broader models including other constructs explaining fish consuming behavior, such as habit, or food neophobia. Further researches will focus not only on risks but other barriers and also drivers of fish consumption will show better explanatory power when using new factors. This study focused on Hungary based on concern about being the lowest fish consumption country within Europe and high incidence of cardiovascular disease that would benefit from increased fish consumption. Future studies could test the model in other countries with similarly low fish consumption and health issues.

Author Contributions: Conceptualization, Á.T. and Z.L.; Methodology, Á.T. and B.P.; Formal Analysis, Á.T.; Investigation, Á.T.; Resources, Á.T.; Data Curation, Á.T. and B.P.; Writing—Original Draft Preparation, Á.T., Z.L. and B.A.E.; Writing—Review & Editing, D.B.; Supervision, D.B. and Z.L.; Funding Acquisition, Á.T. All authors have read and agreed to the published version of the manuscript.

Funding: The Project is supported by the European Union and co-financed by the European Social Fund (grant agreement no. EFOP-3.6.3-VEKOP-16-2017-00005) and supported by the Hungarian Government through the project of "Complex break points in the development of competitiveness of the aquaculture sector" (project number: VKSZ_12-1-2013-0078).

Acknowledgments: The authors would like to express their gratitude to Péter Palotás, an expert in fish processing, and to Gyula Kasza, for his help with conducting the survey, and to Victor Vijay, who provided instrumental help during the work on structural equation modeling.

Conflicts of Interest: The authors declare no conflict of interest.

References

1. Olsen, S.O. Antecedents of seafood consumption behavior: An overview. *J. Aquat. Food Prod. Technol.* **2004**, *13*, 79–91. [CrossRef]
2. Carlucci, D.; Nocella, G.; De Devitiis, B.; Viscecchia, R.; Bimbo, F.; Nardone, G. Consumer purchasing behaviour towards fish and seafood products. Patterns and insights from a sample of international studies. *Appetite* **2015**, *84*, 212–227. [CrossRef] [PubMed]
3. Supartini, A.; Oishi, T.; Yagi, N. Changes in fish consumption desire and its Factors: A Comparison between the United Kingdom and Singapore. *Foods* **2018**, *7*, 97. [CrossRef] [PubMed]
4. Skuland, S.E. Healthy eating and barriers related to social class. The case of vegetable and fish consumption in Norway. *Appetite* **2015**, *92*, 217–226. [CrossRef] [PubMed]
5. Pinho, M.G.M.; Mackenbach, J.D.; Charreire, H.; Oppert, J.M.; Bárdos, H.; Glonti, K.; Rutter, H.; Compernolle, S.; De Bourdeaudhuij, I.; Beulens, J.W.J.; et al. Exploring the relationship between perceived barriers to healthy eating and dietary behaviours in European adults. *Eur. Nutr.* **2018**, *57*, 1761–1770. [CrossRef]
6. Badr, L.M.; Salwa, O.; Ahmed, Y. Perceived barriers to consumption of freshwater fish in Morocco. *Br. Food J.* **2015**, *117*, 274–285. [CrossRef]
7. Hosseini, S.M.; Adeli, A.; Vahedi, M. Evaluating factors and barriers affecting on per capita fish consumption in Sari. *J. Fish.* **2016**, *69*, 341–350.
8. Christenson, J.K.; O'Kane, G.M.; Farmery, A.K.; McManus, A. The barriers and drivers of seafood consumption in Australia: A narrative literature review. *Int. J. Consum. Stud.* **2017**, *41*, 299–311. [CrossRef]
9. Maciel, E.S.; Sonati, J.G.; Lima, L.K.F.; Savay-da-Silva, L.K.; Galvão, J.A.; Oetterer, M. Similarities and distinctions of fish consumption in Brazil and Portugal measured through electronic survey. *Int. Food Res. J.* **2016**, *23*, 395–402.
10. Higuchi, A.; Davalos, J.; Hernani-Merino, M. Theory of planned behavior applied to fish consumption in modern Metropolitan Lima. *Food Sci. Technol.* **2017**, *37*, 202–208. [CrossRef]
11. EUMOFA. The EU Fish Market, 2019 Edition. Available online: https://www.eumofa.eu/documents/20178/314856/EN_The+EU+fish+market_2019.pdf/ (accessed on 6 April 2020).
12. Zheng, J.S.; Hu, X.J.; Zhao, Y.M.; Yang, J.; Li, D. Intake of fish and marine n-3 polyunsaturated fatty acids and risk of breast cancer: Meta-analysis of data from 21 independent prospective cohort studies. *BMJ* **2013**, *346*, f3706. [CrossRef] [PubMed]
13. Rondanelli, M.; Rigon, C.; Perna, S.; Gasparri, C.; Iannello, G.; Akber, R.; Naso, M.; Freije, A.M. Novel Insights on Intake of Fish and Prevention of Sarcopenia: All Reasons for an Adequate Consumption. *Nutrients* **2020**, *12*, 307. [CrossRef] [PubMed]

14. Supartini, A.; Oishi, T.; Yagi, N. Sex differences in the relationship between sleep behavior, fish consumption, and depressive symptoms in the general population of South Korea. *Int. J. Environ. Res. Public Health* **2017**, *14*, 789. [CrossRef] [PubMed]
15. Raji, C.A.; Erickson, K.I.; Lopez, O.L.; Kuller, L.H.; Gach, H.M.; Thompson, P.M.; Riverol, M.; Becker, J.T. Regular fish consumption and age-related brain gray matter loss. *Am. J. Prev. Med.* **2014**, *47*, 444–451. [CrossRef] [PubMed]
16. Mozaffarian, D.; Bryson, C.L.; Lemaitre, R.N.; Burke, G.L.; Siscovick, D.S. Fish intake and risk of incident heart failure. *J. Am. Coll. Cardiol.* **2005**, *45*, 2015–2021. [CrossRef] [PubMed]
17. Raatz, S.K.; Silverstein, J.T.; Jahns, L.; Picklo, M.J. Issues of fish consumption for cardiovascular disease risk reduction. *Nutrients*, **2013**, *5*, 1081–1097. [CrossRef] [PubMed]
18. Owen, A.J.; Abramson, M.J.; Ikin, J.F.; McCaffrey, T.A.; Pomeroy, S.; Borg, B.M.; Gao, C.; Brown, D.; Ofori-Asenso, R. Recommended Intake of Key Food Groups and Cardiovascular Risk Factors in Australian Older, Rural-Dwelling Adults. *Nutrients* **2020**, *12*, 860. [CrossRef]
19. Ghasemi Fard, S.; Wang, F.; Sinclair, A.J.; Elliott, G.; Turchini, G.M. How does high DHA fish oil affect health? A systematic review of evidence. *Crit. Rev. Food Sci. Nutr.* **2019**, *59*, 1684–1727. [CrossRef]
20. EUROSTAT. Cardiovascular Diseases Statistics (November 2019). Available online: https://ec.europa.eu/eurostat/statistics-explained/index.php/Cardiovascular_diseases_statistics#Deaths_from_cardiovascular_diseases (accessed on 6 April 2020).
21. EHN. European Cardiovascular Disease Statistics. 2017. Available online: www.ehnheart.org/cvd-statistics/cvd-statistics-2017.html (accessed on 6 April 2020).
22. FAO Yearbook. *Fishery and Aquaculture Statistics 2017*; Food and Agriculture Organization of the United Nations: Rome, Italy, 2019. Available online: http://www.fao.org/3/ca5495t/CA5495T.pdf (accessed on 18 August 2020).
23. Palotás, P.; Jónás, G.; Lehel, J.; Friedrich, L. Preservative Effect of Novel Combined Treatment with Electrolyzed Active Water and Lysozyme Enzyme to Increase the Storage Life of Vacuum-Packaged Carp. *J. Food Qual.* **2020**, *2020*, 4861471. [CrossRef]
24. HCSO. Egyes Termékek és Szolgáltatások Havi, Országos Fogyasztói Átlagára (Average Countrywide Monthly Prices of Products and Services). Hungarian Central Statistical Office 2017–2018. Available online: https://www.ksh.hu/docs/hun/xstadat/xstadat_evkozi/e_qsf005e.html (accessed on 18 April 2020).
25. Birch, D.; Lawley, M. Buying seafood: Understanding barriers to purchase across consumption segments. *Food Qual. Prefer.* **2012**, *26*, 12–21. [CrossRef]
26. Snoj, B.; Korda, A.P.; Mumel, D. The relationships among perceived quality, perceived risk and perceived product value. *J. Prod. Brand Manag.* **2004**, *13*, 156–167. [CrossRef]
27. Helland, S.H.; Bere, E.; Bjørnarå, H.B.; Øverby, N.C. Food neophobia and its association with intake of fish and other selected foods in a Norwegian sample of toddlers: A cross-sectional study. *Appetite* **2017**, *114*, 110–117. [CrossRef] [PubMed]
28. Laureati, M.; Cattaneo, C.; Bergamaschi, V.; Proserpio, C.; Pagliarini, E. School children preferences for fish formulations: The impact of child and parental food neophobia. *J. Sens. Stud.* **2016**, *31*, 408–415. [CrossRef]
29. Smith, S.; Varble, S.; Secchi, S. Fish consumers: Environmental attitudes and purchasing behavior. *J. Food Prod. Mark.* **2017**, *23*, 267–282. [CrossRef]
30. Siegrist, M.; Hartmann, C.; Keller, C. Antecedents of food neophobia and its association with eating behavior and food choices. *Food Qual. Prefer.* **2013**, *30*, 293–298. [CrossRef]
31. Varble, S.; Secchi, S. Human consumption as an invasive species management strategy. A preliminary assessment of the marketing potential of invasive Asian carp in the US. *Appetite* **2013**, *65*, 58–67. [CrossRef]
32. Jaeger, S.R.; Rasmussen, M.A.; Prescott, J. Relationships between food neophobia and food intake and preferences: Findings from a sample of New Zealand adults. *Appetite* **2017**, *116*, 410–422. [CrossRef]
33. Ajzen, I. The theory of planned behavior. *Organ. Behav. Hum. Decis. Process.* **1991**, *50*, 179–211. [CrossRef]
34. Fiandari, Y.R.; Surachman, S.; Rohman, F.; Hussein, A.S. Perceived value dimension in repetitive fish consumption in Indonesia by using an extended theory of planned behavior. *Br. Food J.* **2019**, *121*, 1220–1235. [CrossRef]
35. Tomić, M.; Matulić, D.; Jelić, M. What determines fresh fish consumption in Croatia? *Appetite* **2016**, *106*, 13–22. [CrossRef]

36. Siddique, M.A.M. Explaining the role of perceived risk, knowledge, price, and cost in dry fish consumption within the theory of planned behavior. *J. Glob. Mark.* **2012**, *25*, 181–201. [CrossRef]
37. Thong, N.T.; Olsen, S.O. Attitude toward and consumption of fish in Vietnam. *J. Food Prod. Mark.* **2102**, *18*, 79–95. [CrossRef]
38. Tuu, H.H.; Olsen, S.O.; Thao, D.T.; Anh, N.T.K. The role of norms in explaining attitudes, intention and consumption of a common food (fish) in Vietnam. *Appetite* **2008**, *51*, 546–551. [CrossRef] [PubMed]
39. Verbeke, W.; Vackier, I. Individual determinants of fish consumption: Application of the theory of planned behaviour. *Appetite* **2005**, *44*, 67–82. [CrossRef]
40. Contini, C.; Boncinelli, F.; Gerini, F.; Scozzafava, G.; Casini, L. Investigating the role of personal and context-related factors in convenience foods consumption. *Appetite* **2018**, *126*, 26–35. [CrossRef] [PubMed]
41. Thorsdottir, F.; Sveinsdottir, K.; Jonsson, F.H.; Einarsdottir, G.; Thorsdottir, I.; Martinsdottir, E. A model of fish consumption among young consumers. *J. Consum. Mark.* **2012**, *29*, 4–12. [CrossRef]
42. Mitterer-Daltoé, M.L.; Carrillo, E.; Queiroz, M.I.; Fiszman, S.; Varela, P. Structural equation modelling and word association as tools for a better understanding of low fish consumption. *Food Res. Int.* **2013**, *52*, 56–63. [CrossRef]
43. Rortveit, A.W.; Olsen, S.O. Combining the role of convenience and consideration set size in explaining fish consumption in Norway. *Appetite* **2009**, *52*, 313–317. [CrossRef]
44. Olsen, S.O.; Scholderer, J.; Brunsø, K.; Verbeke, W. Exploring the relationship between convenience and fish consumption: A cross-cultural study. *Appetite* **2007**, *49*, 84–91. [CrossRef]
45. Olsen, S.O. Understanding the relationship between age and seafood consumption: The mediating role of attitude, health involvement and convenience. *Food Qual. Prefer.* **2003**, *14*, 199–209. [CrossRef]
46. Pieniak, Z.; Verbeke, W.; Scholderer, J.; Brunsø, K.; Olsen, S.O. Impact of consumers' health beliefs, health involvement and risk perception on fish consumption. *Br. Food J.* **2008**, *110*, 898–915. [CrossRef]
47. Schaefer, A.M.; Zoffer, M.; Yrastorza, L.; Pearlman, D.M.; Bossart, G.D.; Stoessel, R.; Reif, J.S. Mercury Exposure, Fish Consumption, and Perceived Risk among Pregnant Women in Coastal Florida. *Int. J. Environ. Res. Public Health* **2019**, *16*, 4903. [CrossRef] [PubMed]
48. Bauer, R.A. Consumer behaviour as risk taking. In *Dynamic Marketing for a Changing World, Proceedings of the 43rd Conference of the American Marketing Association, Chicago, IL, USA, June 1960*; Hancock, R.S., Ed.; American Marketing Association: Chicago, IL, USA, 1960; pp. 389–398.
49. Mitchell, V.W. Consumer perceived risk: Conceptualisations and models. *Eur. J. Mark.* **1999**, *33*, 163–195. [CrossRef]
50. Jacoby, J.; Kaplan, L.B. The Components of Perceived Risk. In *SV—Proceedings of the Third Annual Conference of the Association for Consumer Research, Chicago, IL, USA, 3–5 November 1972*; Venkatesan, M., Ed.; Association for Consumer Research; pp. 382–393. Available online: https://www.acrwebsite.org/volumes/12016/volumes/sv02/SV-02 (accessed on 18 August 2020).
51. Murphy, P.E.; Enis, B.M. Classifying products strategically. *J. Mark.* **1986**, *50*, 24–42. [CrossRef]
52. Neale, E.P.; Nolan-Clark, D.; Probst, Y.C.; Batterham, M.J.; Tapsell, L.C. Comparing attitudes to fish consumption between clinical trial participants and non-trial individuals. *Nutr. Diet.* **2012**, *69*, 124–129. [CrossRef]
53. Babcsányi, I.; Tamás, M.; Szatmári, J.; Hambek-Oláh, B.; Farsang, A. Assessing the impacts of the main river and anthropogenic use on the degree of metal contamination of oxbow lake sediments (Tisza River Valley, Hungary). *J. Soils Sediments* **2020**, *20*, 1662–1675. [CrossRef]
54. Li, J.; Miao, X.; Hao, Y.; Xie, Z.; Zou, S.; Zhou, C. Health Risk Assessment of Metals (Cu, Pb, Zn, Cr, Cd, As, Hg, Se) in Angling Fish with Different Lengths Collected from Liuzhou, China. *Int. J. Environ. Res. Public Health* **2020**, *17*, 2192. [CrossRef]
55. Hacon, S.S.; Dórea, J.G.; Fonseca, M.D.F.; Oliveira, B.A.; Mourão, D.S.; Gonçalves, R.A.; Mariani, C.F.; Bastos, W.R. The influence of changes in lifestyle and mercury exposure in riverine populations of the Madeira River (Amazon Basin) near a hydroelectric project. *Int. J. Environ. Res. Public Health* **2014**, *11*, 2437–2455. [CrossRef]
56. Pico, Y.; Belenguer, V.; Corcellas, C.; Díaz-Cruz, M.S.; Eljarrat, E.; Farré, M.; Gago-Ferrero, P.; Huerta, B.; Navarro-Ortega, A.; Petrovic, M.; et al. Contaminants of emerging concern in freshwater fish from four Spanish Rivers. *Sci. Total Environ.* **2019**, *659*, 1186–1198. [CrossRef]

57. Krabbenhoft, C.A.; Manente, S.; Kashian, D.R. Evaluation of an Educational Campaign to Improve the Conscious Consumption of Recreationally Caught Fish. *Sustainability* **2019**, *11*, 700. [CrossRef]
58. Anual, Z.F.; Maher, W.; Krikowa, F.; Hakim, L.; Ahmad, N.I.; Foster, S. Mercury and risk assessment from consumption of crustaceans, cephalopods and fish from West Peninsular Malaysia. *Microchem. J.* **2018**, *140*, 214–221. [CrossRef]
59. Myrland, Ø.; Trondsen, T.; Johnston, R.S.; Lund, E. Determinants of seafood consumption in Norway: Lifestyle, revealed preferences, and barriers to consumption. *Food Qual. Prefer.* **2000**, *11*, 169–188. [CrossRef]
60. Olsen, S.O. Consumer involvement in seafood as family meals in Norway: An application of the expectancy-value approach. *Appetite* **2001**, *36*, 173–186. [CrossRef]
61. Zhou, L.; Jin, S.; Zhang, B.; Zeng, Q.; Wang, D. Determinants of fish consumption by household type in China. *Br. Food J.* **2015**, *117*, 1273–1288. [CrossRef]
62. Altintzoglou, T.; Hansen, K.B.; Valsdottir, T.; Odland, J.Ø.; Martinsdóttir, E.; Brunsø, K.; Luten, J. Translating barriers into potential improvements: The case of new healthy seafood product development. *J. Consum. Mark.* **2010**, *27*, 224–235. [CrossRef]
63. Birch, D.; Lawley, M. The role of habit, childhood consumption, familiarity, and attitudes across seafood consumption segments in Australia. *J. Food Prod. Mark.* **2014**, *20*, 98–113. [CrossRef]
64. Pieniak, Z.; Verbeke, W.; Scholderer, J. Health-related beliefs and consumer knowledge as determinants of fish consumption. *J. Hum. Nutr. Diet.* **2010**, *23*, 480–488. [CrossRef]
65. Thong, N.T.; Solgaard, H.S. Consumer's food motives and seafood consumption. *Food Qual. Prefer.* **2017**, *56*, 181–188. [CrossRef]
66. Brunsø, K.; Verbeke, W.; Olsen, S.O.; Jeppesen, L.F. Motives, barriers and quality evaluation in fish consumption situations. *Br. Food J.* **2009**, *111*, 699–716. [CrossRef]
67. Fischer, A.R.; Frewer, L.J. Consumer familiarity with foods and the perception of risks and benefits. *Food Qual. Prefer.* **2009**, *20*, 576–585. [CrossRef]
68. Sveinsdóttir, K.; Martinsdóttir, E.; Green-Petersen, D.; Hyldig, G.; Schelvis, R.; Delahunty, C. Sensory characteristics of different cod products related to consumer preferences and attitudes. *Food Qual. Prefer.* **2009**, *20*, 120–132. [CrossRef]
69. HCSO. Hungarian Microcensus Data 2016. 2020. Available online: https://www.ksh.hu/mikrocenzus2016/kotet_3_demografiai_adatok (accessed on 23 April 2020).
70. Ringle, C.M.; Wende, S.; Becker, J.M. SmartPLS 3. Boenningstedt: SmartPLS GmbH. Available online: http://www.smartpls.com (accessed on 18 August 2020).
71. Hair, J.F.; Ringle, C.M.; Sarstedt, M. PLS-SEM: Indeed a silver bullet. *J. Mark. Theory Pract.* **2011**, *19*, 139–152. [CrossRef]
72. Hair, J.F.; Risher, J.J.; Sarstedt, M.; Ringle, C.M. When to use and how to report the results of PLS-SEM. *Eur. Bus. Rev.* **2019**, *31*, 2–24. [CrossRef]
73. Cortina, J.M. What is coefficient alpha? An examination of theory and applications. *J. Appl. Psychol.* **1993**, *78*, 98. [CrossRef]
74. Hair, J.F., Jr.; Hult, G.T.M.; Ringle, C.; Sarstedt, M. *A Primer on Partial Least Squares Structural Equation Modeling (PLS-SEM)*; Sage Publications: New York, NY, USA, 2016.
75. Bagozzi, R.P.; Yi, Y. On the evaluation of structural equation models. *J. Acad. Mark. Sci.* **1988**, *16*, 74–94. [CrossRef]
76. Hu, L.T.; Bentler, P.M. Cutoff criteria for fit indexes in covariance structure analysis: Conventional criteria versus new alternatives. *Struct. Equ. Model. A Multidiscip. J.* **1999**, *6*, 1–55. [CrossRef]
77. Fornell, C.; Larcker, D.F. Evaluating structural equation models with unobservable variables and measurement error. *J. Mark. Res.* **1981**, *18*, 39–50. [CrossRef]
78. Henseler, J.; Ringle, C.M.; Sarstedt, M. A new criterion for assessing discriminant validity in variance-based structural equation modeling. *J. Acad. Mark. Sci.* **2015**, *43*, 115–135. [CrossRef]
79. Diaz-Ruiz, R.; Costa-Font, M.; Gil, J.M. Moving ahead from food-related behaviours: An alternative approach to understand household food waste generation. *J. Clean. Prod.* **2018**, *172*, 1140–1151. [CrossRef]
80. Stone, M. Cross-validatory choice and assessment of statistical predictions. *J. R. Stat. Soc. Ser. B Methodol.* **1974**, *36*, 111–133. [CrossRef]
81. Geisser, S. A predictive approach to the random effect model. *Biometrika* **1974**, *61*, 101–107. [CrossRef]

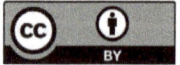

© 2020 by the authors. Licensee MDPI, Basel, Switzerland. This article is an open access article distributed under the terms and conditions of the Creative Commons Attribution (CC BY) license (http://creativecommons.org/licenses/by/4.0/).

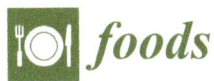

Article

Perceptions about Healthy Eating and Emotional Factors Conditioning Eating Behaviour: A Study Involving Portugal, Brazil and Argentina

Ana Paula Cardoso [1,*], Vanessa Ferreira [2], Marcela Leal [3], Manuela Ferreira [4], Sofia Campos [1] and Raquel P. F. Guiné [5]

1. CI&DEI Research Centre, School of Education, Polytechnic Institute of Viseu, 3504-510 Viseu, Portugal; sofiamargaridacampos@gmail.com
2. Department of Nutrition, School of Nursing, UFMG University, Belo Horizonte, BR 30130-100, Brazil; vanessa.nutr@gmail.com
3. Faculty of Health Sciences, School of Nutrition, Maimonides University, Buenos Aires, AR C1405, Argentina; leal.nutricion@gmail.com
4. UICISA:E Research Centre, School of Health, Polytechnic Institute of Viseu, 3504-510 Viseu, Portugal; mmcferreira@gmail.com
5. CERNAS Research Centre, School of Agriculture, Polytechnic Institute of Viseu, 3504-510 Viseu, Portugal; raquelguine@esav.ipv.pt
* Correspondence: a.p.cardoso@esev.ipv.pt

Received: 3 August 2020; Accepted: 2 September 2020; Published: 4 September 2020

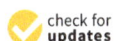

Abstract: This study analysed the perceptions about healthy eating as well as some emotional factors conditioning eating behaviour in a sample of people from Portugal, Brazil and Argentina. This is a descriptive cross-sectional study involving a non-probabilistic sample of 2501 participant. Data was collected through a questionnaire applied to adult citizens residing in their respective countries. For data analysis chi-square tests were used, and associations were evaluated by Cramer's coefficients. Moreover, a tree classification analysis was conducted for variables related with perceptions about healthy eating and emotional conditioning of eating behaviour. The results revealed that participants' perceptions are generally in agreement with healthy eating. However, significant differences were found between countries ($p = 0.018$) and by levels of education ($p < 0.0005$), with a more accurate perception for Portugal and at the university level. The existence of statistically significant associations between all sociodemographic variables considered and the conditioning of eating behaviour by emotional motivations should be noted. Tree classification analysis showed that the most important discriminant sociodemographic variable for perceptions about healthy eating was education, followed by professional area and country, while the most relevant discriminants for emotional conditioning of eating behaviour were country and then living environment and sex. Thus, it is important to consider these variables in initiatives that aim to promote adherence to behaviours that contribute to the health and well-being of the population.

Keywords: perceptions; healthy eating; emotional motivations; individual differences

1. Introduction

Human behaviour regarding food is associated with a large number of interrelated factors [1], including those of a psychological and social nature. This constitutes an inseparable act of human survival and encompasses two functions, maintain the level of nutrients necessary for the body and provide the pleasure that is derived from the act of eating through the release of serotonin and dopamine [2]. Emotions are part of the evolution of the human species and, obviously, of the development of children, adolescents and adults, constituting a fundamental part of learning. Emotions are adaptive because they prepare, predispose and guide behaviours towards positive or negative experiences, besides behaviours of survival and reproduction [3].

Human beings need a varied diet so that it is balanced and healthy [4]. This is an object of study that has been the target of an increasing number of investigations, since unhealthy eating behaviour is an important risk factor for health and mortality [5]. In the literature, there is not a consensus on organic farming being an important part of a healthful diet. Nevertheless, organic farming's importance is increasing in the dietary patterns of some citizens in the countries studied and is considered important for the health of their population [6–8]. Some studies support the association between organic farming and health, like for example Costa et al. [9] report that organic farming is safer than conventional farming, because this last can cause DNA damage in people exposed to pesticides. Additionally, organic food contains higher levels of nutrients and bioactive substances that improve consumers' health and wellness [10–13]. Organic diets have the benefit of exposing consumers to considerably lower levels of chemicals, which can cause several human diseases like cancer, autism, and infertility [14–19]. Data form pesticide residues' monitoring clearly show that foods from organic farming have lower levels of pesticide residues when compared with foods grown in conventional farming systems [20,21].

Throughout the human developmental trajectory, all actions and thoughts are mediated by emotions. For example, eating can be motivated by positive (e.g., happiness) and negative (e.g., anger, depression) emotions, coupled with the desire to nourish [22]. Gibson [23] showed that negative emotions and depression have an influence on food. Although the typical response to stress is to eat less, some studies [24,25] have shown that eating more also appears in atypical depression.

A better understanding of the factors involved in food choices is essential to promote a healthy change in dietary behaviour [26]. Lazarevich et al. [27] conducted a study where emotional nutrition was identified as a mediating variable between depression and Body Mass Index (BMI) in young men and women. Intervention proposals in adequate nutritional education must therefore bear in mind the management of emotions and the detection of individuals vulnerable to depression and other emotional risks. While there are several papers that relate obesity and other eating disorders with emotional factors, we did not find any with the specificity of this investigation, conducted simultaneously on the different countries involved in this study.

The present study is part of the project entitled "Psychosocial motivations associated with food choices and practices" (EATMOT), which aims to analyse the different psychological and social motivations that determine people's eating patterns, whether in relation to their eating choices or habits. It is essential to understand these factors if we intend to intervene in this area, either in terms of health promotion or in terms of disease prevention or treatment. Some of the aspects to be explored in the scope of this project include factors related to perceptions and eating habits, in areas such as emotional aspects or cultural influences.

Although eating behaviour results from a lifelong learning process, this does not invalidate that the subjects' food preferences change over time and according to their experience and learning [4]. This reinforces the importance of understanding the influence of different types of variables, including sociodemographic ones, on eating behaviour. Hence, the main objective of this study in particular was to analyse the perceptions corresponding to healthy eating and emotional conditions linked to the eating behaviour of people from three countries (Portugal, Argentina and Brazil). It was also analysed to what extent aspects such as country of residence, age, sex, education level, living environment, marital status, or area of study or work can influence the participants' perceptions.

2. Materials and Methods

2.1. Data Collection

The questionnaire used in this study was first validated for the Portuguese population [28–30] and then applied in other countries, after translation and adaptation. The questionnaire was applied in Brazil in Portuguese and translated into Spanish, following a back-translation methodology for validation. For the translation process, all the issues related to the possible cultural influences in the interpretation of the questions were verified. Moreover, in the case of Brazil, although speaking the same language, some adaptations were made in order to better suit the Brazilian way of speaking the Portuguese language.

In order to measure respondents' perceptions about healthy eating and also about the emotional factors conditioning eating behaviour, their opinion on a set of statements was asked using a 5-point Likert scale, ranging from 1 = strongly disagree to 5 = strongly agree [31].

The questionnaire was applied, after informed consent, only to adults (18 years or older). All participants were volunteers, and their answers were collected and treated as anonymous. All ethical considerations were completely obeyed when designing the questionnaire and collecting the data, which was kept strictly confidential in such a way that none of the responses could ever be associated with the participant. The survey was approved by the Ethical Committee of Polytechnic Institute of Viseu, with reference no 04/2017.

2.2. Data Analysis

The data collected through the descriptive and cross-sectional study were analysed statistically, using the SPSS - Statistical Package for the Social Sciences from IBM - International Business Machines Inc. (version 24, Armonk, Nova York, EUA). Descriptive statistics was used for exploratory data analysis, and inferential statistics was also used, by means of the Chi-square test, to evaluate the association between some sociodemographic variables and the perceptions under study. Cramer's V coefficient was used to assess the strength of the associations between the tested variables [32]. This coefficient varies from 0 to 1 and can be interpreted as $V \approx 0.1$—weak association, $V \approx 0.3$—moderate association, $V \approx 0.5$ or over—strong association [33].

The responses obtained were transformed into new variables with two levels: value 1 (grouping the responses of agree and strongly agree) and value 0 (grouping the responses of strongly disagree and disagree). In the 1st case, that is, to measure respondents' perceptions of healthy eating, the scale defined was as follows: "correct perceptions" (1) and "incorrect perceptions" (0); in the 2nd case, that is, to measure the emotional conditioning factors of eating behaviour, the scale was used: "conditioned" (1) and "non-conditioned" (0) eating behaviour. Responses corresponding to "no opinion" (value 3 of the scale) were not considered for this particular purpose.

The variables measuring the perceptions of healthy eating and emotional conditioning factors were analysed by tree classification analysis in order to evaluate the relative importance of the different sociodemographic variables. For this, a Classification and Regression Trees (CRT) algorithm with cross-validation was used. The classification algorithm (CRT) bases the decision process on some specified criteria, in this case defined according to the high numbers of responses. The minimum change in improvement was 0.0004, and the minimum number of cases for parent nodes was 100 and for child nodes was 50. These parameters allow the decision-making process (and this is why the classification tree can also be termed as decision tree) which happens in any of the nodes. Therefore, a parent node is a node that originates branches to other nodes, while a terminal node is that which corresponds to a stopping point. The decision to stop is derived from one of these conditions: Either the next improvement is lower that the threshold defined (0.0004), or the number of cases in the next nodes is lower than 50 (defined as minimum for child nodes).

The level of significance considered in data analysis was 5% ($p < 0.05$).

3. Results

3.1. Sample Characterization

Table 1 summarizes the sociodemographic data of the sample, that included elements from Portugal (52.2%), Argentina (20.9%) and Brazil (26.6%). There were 2501 participants in the study, of which 69.8% were female and 30.2% male, grouped by the following age groups: 43.3% of young adults (18 ≤ years ≤ 30), 39.5% of adults (31 ≤ years ≤ 50), 14.5% of senior adults (51 ≤ years ≤ 65) and 2.6% of elderly (years ≥ 66).

Table 1. Sociodemographic characterization of the sample (N = 2501).

Variable	Groups	%	Variable	Groups	%
Age [1]	Young adults	43.4	Country	Argentina	20.9
	Adults	39.5		Brazil	26.6
	Senior adults	14.5		Portugal	52.5
	Elderly	2.6	Living environment	Rural	9.6
Sex	Women	69.8		Urban	84.4
	Men	30.2		Suburban	6.0
Education	Basic school	0.6	Area of study/work	Nutrition	10.7
	Secondary school	39.6		Food	5.1
	University degree	59.8		Agriculture	2.2
Marital status	Single	46.7		Sport	3.3
	Married	44.1		Psychology	2.6
	Divorced	6.5		Health	19.8
	Widowed	2.8		Others	56.4

[1] Young adults: 18 ≤ years ≤ 30, Adults: 31 ≤ years ≤ 50, Senior adults: 51 ≤ years ≤ 65, Elderly: years ≥ 66.

Most participants (59.8%) had higher education, 39.6% had completed secondary school level of education, and only 0.6% had the lowest level of education (basic school). Regarding marital status, 46.7% were single, 44.1% were married, 6.5% were divorced, and 2.8% were widowed. With regard to the environment in which they live, 84.4% lived in urban areas, 9.6% in rural areas and 6.0% in a suburban area.

The area of study or professional activity of the participants was also analysed, according to previously defined categories. It was found that 56.4% were not related to any of the listed areas and that the other respondents were distributed by the areas of health (19.8%), nutrition (10.7%), food (5.1%), sport (3.3%), psychology (2.6%) and agriculture (2.2%).

3.2. Perceptions About Healthy Diet

The participants revealed, in general, a perception concordant with healthy eating, as can be seen in Table 2. The high agreement of respondents in relation to some items, such as number 3 about the importance of fruits and vegetables (25.1% agree, 73.1% strongly agree), number 4 about balanced and varied diet (22.5% agree, 75.0% strongly agree), number 5 about not avoiding any foods (35.0% agree, 24.7% strongly agree) or number 9 about the value of foods from organic farming (37.4% agree, 32.6% strongly agree), is highlighted. For these items, agreement is indicative of correct perceptions about healthy diet. In the opposite way, the high disagreement with inverted items also stands out, i.e., disagreement with items that are indicative of wrong perceptions of healthy diet, such as numbers 2 (15.7% strongly disagree, 56.9% disagree) or 10 (13.3% strongly disagree, 50.7% disagree), respectively, about totally avoiding sugary or fat foods. Regarding items such as numbers 1, 6 and 8, the participants were very divided, with similar numbers for those who were for and those who were against aspects such as the diets based on counting calories, the price of healthy foods or the value of tradition to healthy dietary patterns.

Table 2. Perceptions about healthy eating (Scale from 1 = strongly disagree to 5 = strongly agree).

Perceptions about Healthy Eating	Percentage of Answers according to Scale Points				
	1 (%)	2 (%)	3 (%)	4 (%)	5 (%)
1. Healthy eating is based on counting calories	17.2	27.9	18.2	25.6	11.1
2. We should never consume sugary products	15.7	56.9	14.2	10.6	2.6
3. Fruits and vegetables are important for a healthy diet	0.6	0.2	1.1	25.1	73.1
4. A healthy diet must be balanced, varied and complete	0.6	0.2	1.8	22.5	75.0
5. We can eat everything as long as it is in small quantities	4.4	24.4	11.5	35.0	24.7
6. I believe that a healthy diet is expensive	16.8	28.4	21.9	24.1	8.8
7. In my opinion it is strange that some people have cravings for sweets	31.7	50.7	12.4	4.0	1.2
8. I believe that tradition is very important for healthy eating	10.8	25.0	25.1	30.3	8.9
9. I believe that food coming from organic farming is healthier	1.5	5.7	22.8	37.4	32.6
10. We should never consume high fat foods	13.3	50.7	17.9	13.5	4.6

Considering the influence of the seven sociodemographic variables analysed (age, sex, education, marital status, country, living environment and area of study/work) on the perceptions about healthy eating, it was observed that only in two cases there were significant differences between groups, i.e., there were statistically significant associations between perceptions and country of residence and between perceptions and education level (Table 3). The results of the Chi-square test revealed a statistically significant association between the perceptions of healthy eating and the country of residence ($p = 0.018$). For this association, the analysis of the adjusted residues indicated that the differences were in Portugal, with a more correct perception, and in Brazil, with a more incorrect perception, with values of the adjusted residues positive and greater than two. Nevertheless, despite being significant, this association is weak ($V = 0.057$).

Table 3. Perceptions about healthy eating according to country and level of education.

Variable	Perception		Chi-Square Test	Cramer's Coefficient
	Correct	Incorrect		
	(%)	(%)	p	V
Country				
Argentina	90.8	9.2	0.018	0.057
Brazil	89.7	10.3		
Portugal	93.2	6.8		
Education				
Basic school	93.3	6.7	<0.0005	0.092
Secondary school	88.7	11.3		
University degree	93.8	6.2		

In the case of the variables, perception versus level of education (Table 3), the association was also significant ($p < 0.0005$) and weak ($V = 0.092$). Participants with a university degree showed a more correct perception about healthy eating than those with secondary school, according to the adjusted residues. The results further show that the perceptions about healthy eating are high for participants with the lowest level of education, basic school. This is a little surprising, and it might be due to the fact that there was not a real representative number of people with the lowest level of education, and this might be biasing the results. Hence, to confirm a possible trend of increasing education being associated with better perceptions of healthy eating, further studies should be made with more people from lower levels of education. Nevertheless, this is very difficult because the world trend, as guidance form the United Nations, is to increase the levels of education in all countries, including those under development.

The variable measuring the perceptions about healthy eating was submitted to a tree classification analysis for assessment of the relative importance of the possible influential variables. Figure 1 presents the tree obtained, and which highlights the relative importance of the sociodemographic variables to define the perceptions of the participants about a healthy diet. The estimated risk for this tree was 0.082 (with standard error 0.005) for resubstitution, and equal values were also obtained for cross-validation. The obtained tree (Figure 1) has 11 nodes, from which 6 are terminal.

or studies in the field of psychology those who have eating behaviour more conditioned by emotional aspects (weak association: V = 0.154).

Table 5. Emotional conditionings of eating behaviour according to sociodemographic variables.

Variable	Eating Habits		Chi-Square Test	Cramer's Coefficient
	Conditioned	Not Conditioned		
	(%)	(%)	p	V
Country				
Argentina	33.2	66.8	<0.0005	0.166
Brazil	36.4	63.6		
Portugal	20.4	79.6		
Education				
Basic school	26.7	73.3	0.006	0.064
Secondary school	30.8	69.2		
University degree	25.0	75.0		
Age [1]				
Young adults	34.0	66.0	<0.0005	0.156
Adults	25.3	74.7		
Senior adults	15.2	84.8		
Elderly	12.5	87.5		
Sex				
Women	31.6	68.4	<0.0005	0.146
Men	17.4	82.6		
Marital status				
Single	34.1	65.9	<0.0005	0.160
Married	21.0	79.0		
Divorced	30.4	69.6		
Widowed	7.2	92.8		
Living environment				
Rural	37.7	62.3	<0.0005	0.116
Urban	25.1	74.9		
Suburban	41.6	58.4		
Area of study/work				
Nutrition	37.6	62.4	<0.0005	0.154
Food	37.8	62.2		
Agriculture	20.4	79.6		
Sport	26.8	73.2		
Psychology	46.2	53.8		
Health	32.2	67.8		
Others	22.1	77.9		

[1] Young adults: 18 ≤ years ≤ 30, Adults: 31 ≤ years ≤ 50, Senior adults: 51 ≤ years ≤ 65, Elderly: years ≥ 66.

Moreover, the variable measuring the emotional conditioning of eating behaviour was submitted to a tree classification analysis and the obtained results are shown in Figure 2. The estimated risk for this tree was 0.273 (with standard error 0.009) for resubstitution and 0.281 (with standard error 0.009) for cross-validation. The obtained tree has 18 nodes, being 9 of them terminal. The results showed that for the whole number of cases (node 0) 72.7% of participants have eating behaviours not conditioned by emotional factors. For this variable, the first discriminant was country, separating Portugal (79.6% not conditioned) from Brazil and Argentina. While for Portugal the next discriminant was living environment (Urban: 15.1% conditioned), for the other countries the next discriminant was sex (women more conditioned by emotional factors than men: 39.1% and 24.0%, respectively). For the women in Brazil and Argentina with professions or studies related to food, nutrition or agriculture, education was the following discriminant, separating those with a university degree as being less susceptible to condition their eating behaviours in function of emotional aspects (31.1% conditioned against 45.1% for those with less education). For participants from Portugal living in urban areas, the next discriminant was marital status, separating the single and divorced as being more conditioned (25.0) than the married or widowed (9.1%). For these groups of single and divorced people, the next discriminant was professional area, with participants linked with food, health, nutrition and psychology showing more conditioned eating habits (35.2%).

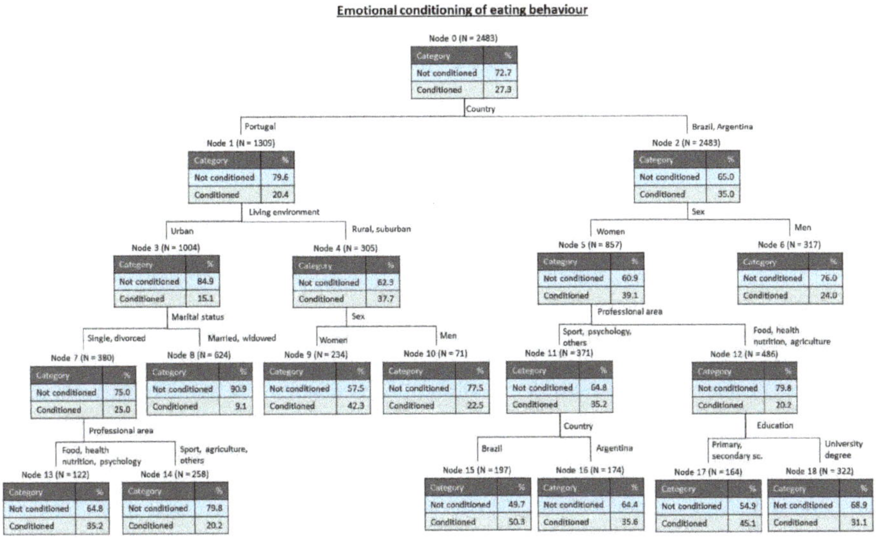

Figure 2. Tree classification for the emotional conditionings of eating behaviour.

4. Discussion

The results revealed that the participants' perceptions about healthy eating were, in general, correct. Significant differences were found by country and level of education, with adult citizens residing in Portugal and those with higher education showing a more correct perception of what healthy eating should be. These results are in line with those of the study by Ferrão et al. [30]. They are also consistent with the results of Lê et al. [34] who showed an association between a high educational level and adherence to a healthy diet. High agreement regarding the importance of fruits and vegetables in the diet as well as of a varied and balanced diet or disagreement as to the avoidance of sugary or fatty foods in the three countries was observed. This generalized opinion can be explained by the European influence shared by these countries, despite the cultural specificities of each one, and the well spread information about the health benefits of fruits and vegetables [35,36] while fats, particularly saturated fat, and sugars may contribute for important health morbidities like diabetes, heart diseases and obesity [37–39]. In relation to the differences between countries in particular, the more correct perception of what is the healthy diet in Portugal may be associated with the Mediterranean diet [40] that characterizes the gastronomic tradition of Portugal, in contrast to Brazil and Argentina. There is not one global definition of healthy diet; however, as discussed earlier, there are worldwide recommendations and recognition of some unhealthy foods, which leaves some space for country differences. The correct perception of healthy eating, associated with a greater nutritional knowledge, is recognized as an important factor in the promotion of adequate eating behaviours, as some scientific evidence suggests [41,42]. This emphasizes the relevance of training aimed at increasing food literacy, with a view to better stimulate suitable food choices in the general population. For this purpose, additional studies must be carried out in order to better understand how information should be provided in each of the participating countries. It is suggested that the results of this work be discussed among health professionals (including those linked with psychology) to analyse the best way of action according to the specificities of each country regarding health policies, health care systems, educational systems and their coordination towards a common objective. This must be done separately in each of the countries, given their social, cultural and political differences. These differences should be communicated to the proper organisms to include them in education campaigns, designed in the different countries according to their specificity. Regarding the emotional factors conditioning eating behaviour, the need for emotional management is transversal to the different cultures. Therefore, the organizers of health-promoting initiatives in each of these countries should organize dynamic and interactive sessions, in which participants have the opportunity to exchange their own experiences and recognize the association between emotions and eating behaviours, as well as the importance of an adequate emotional eating management, in order to develop emotional skills to achieve a healthier diet. More specifically, some authors [25,27,43] highlight the application of 3rd Generation Therapies to regulate emotions as a means of balancing dietary changes. The most referred techniques are cognitive-behavioural psychotherapies, mindfulness and acceptance and commitment, as they are those that have the greatest impact and that present the best results.

In this study, statistically significant associations were found between the emotional motivations for eating behaviour and all sociodemographic variables (country, living environment, age, sex, educational level, marital status and area of study/work). In the investigation by Chambers et al. [44], the results revealed that different emotional motivations are related to food, namely, eating to relieve stress, weight control, emotional comfort and eating sweets to relieve depressive states. The same authors state that food choices and their quantity and quality vary according to the individual's particular characteristics and according to a specific emotional status. However, Ashurst et al. [45] mention that, despite the importance of affective processes in eating behaviour, it is still difficult to predict how emotions affect the act of eating. They highlight the importance of individual differences and emphasize that previous research did not focus much on the overlapped variability of changes in eating behaviour induced by emotions, justified, on one hand, by the differences between the individuals and, on the other hand, by their emotions according to a particular moment or experience.

Our results showed that food can serve as emotional consolation, help deal with stress and fight loneliness or boredom. In an investigation carried out with university students, Bennett et al. [46] found that food is often used as a way to distract attention from negative emotions. According to Boggiano [47], eating behaviour that deals with negative emotions is called "emotional eating" and individuals with emotional eating behaviour eat for reasons other than physiological needs. These individuals generally continue to eat to achieve the balance of the homeostatic shift of energy in a positive direction, especially in case of emotional situations.

Bennett et al. [46] found that when participants reported negative emotions, they were more likely to consume meat/proteins and sweets. However, our results are not so conclusive on this, because only a small percentage of participants assumed that when they felt depressed their cravings for sweets increased.

Young adults, women, residents in Brazil or Argentina, those who live in rural areas, those who are single or divorced, those who have secondary education, or whose area of study or work is related with nutrition, psychology, food or health are the ones that evidence a higher degree of conditioning in their eating behaviour according to emotional aspects. These results are, to some extent, in line with those of the research by Bartkiene et al. [48], which indicated that age, education level and sex are associated with emotional motivations for eating. The works by Bennett et al. [46] and Guiné et al. [49] also reported gender differences in the emotional factors driving eating behaviour.

Significant differences were found in the perceptions about healthy eating for countries and education levels, with more correct perceptions for people from Portugal and with a university degree. A plausible explanation for these differences has to do with the gastronomic tradition of each country, with emphasis on the prevalence of the Mediterranean diet in Portugal, as discussed earlier, considered one of the healthiest [50]. Regarding the educational level, attending higher education drives the students to a constant search for new information and development of the critical thinking, and this allows greater awareness also about the benefits of healthy eating and the constant need to search for more correct information about food and its effects [51,52].

Other variables, like area of study/work, living environment or marital status, showed also differences in the way emotional aspects influence eating behaviour. It has been referred that different social statuses are linked to different behaviours on several aspects and also linked with food and eating habits. The cultural context proved to be a determining factor in the selection of the type of food consumed and quantities ingested, which is in line with the investigation by Castro et al. [53] who compared the eating behaviours of French, American and German university students and found that there were marked differences between these cultures in terms of quantity, composition, diurnal rhythm and pattern of food intake between the different cultures.

According to literature, a more personalized analysis is required in the design of proposals that aim to promote adherence to healthy eating behaviours [48]. Decision-makers and professionals responsible for organizing health-promoting initiatives should therefore seek to increase citizens' food literacy levels and address the diversity of individual variables, such as sex, age, education level, living environment and culture of origin, in the design of training proposals, in order to undertake more effective actions in adhering to behaviours that contribute to the health and well-being of the population.

5. Conclusions and Limitations

The results of this study indicated that, in general, the participants' perceptions about healthy eating are in line with the preconized principles of a healthy diet, particularly regarding the importance of consuming fruits and vegetables, of practicing a balanced, varied and complete diet, and of consuming foods from organic farming. Significant differences were found in the perceptions about healthy eating for countries and education levels, with more correct perceptions for people from Portugal and with a university degree.

Concerning the emotional factors and the way they influence eating patterns, a low level of influence was found, particularly in aspects related with the role of food as consolation or as a way to deal with stress. The emotional conditionings of eating behaviour were found to significantly vary according to all sociodemographic variables tested.

Tree classification analysis revealed that the most important discriminant for perceptions about healthy eating was education, followed by professional area and country, while the most relevant discriminants for emotional conditioning of eating behaviour were country followed by living environment and sex.

One of the limitations of this study derives from the fact that it covers a sample that, although vast, is not probabilistic, therefore does not give sufficient guarantees to be representative of the entire population. Additionally, derived from being a convenience sample, the representativeness of all groups was not even, as for example for sex or education levels. Therefore, these results must be understood as exploratory and further studies should be undertaken for proper generalization of the results. Another limitation has to do with the fact that the questionnaire was only validated for Portugal, despite having the collaboration of researchers from the other countries involved in the work of translation and adaptation to the cultural context.

Author Contributions: Conceptualization, R.P.F.G.; methodology, R.P.F.G., A.P.C.; software, R.P.F.G.; validation, R.P.F.G.; formal analysis, R.P.F.G.; investigation, A.P.C., R.P.F.G., V.F., M.L.; resources, R.P.F.G.; data curation, R.P.F.G.; writing—original draft preparation, A.P.C., R.P.F.G.; writing—review and editing, A.P.C., R.P.F.G., S.C., M.F., V.F., M.L.; visualization, R.P.F.G.; supervision, R.P.F.G.; project administration, R.P.F.G.; funding acquisition, R.P.F.G. All authors have read and agreed to the published version of the manuscript.

Funding: This research was funded by FCT—Foundation for Science and Technology, Portugal, and CI&DETS Research Centre (Polytechnic Institute of Viseu, Portugal) grant number PROJ/CI&DETS/CGD/0012. The APC was funded by FCT—Foundation for Science and Technology (Portugal), grants number UIDB/00681/2020 and UIDB/05507/2020.

Acknowledgments: Thanks' to FCT—Foundation for Science and Technology, Portugal, within the scope of the projects Refª UIDB/00681/2020 and UIDB/05507/2020. Furthermore, we would like to thank the Centre for Studies in Education and Innovation (CI&DEI), the Centre for Natural Resources and Society (CERNAS), and the Polytechnic Institute of Viseu for their support. This work was prepared in the ambit of the multinational project EATMOT from CI&DETS Research Centre (Polytechnic Institute of Viseu, Portugal) with reference PROJ/CI&DETS/CGD/0012.

Conflicts of Interest: The authors declare no conflict of interest.

References

1. Köster, E.P. Diversity in the determinants of food choice: A psychological perspective. *Food Qual. Prefer.* **2009**, *20*, 70–82. [CrossRef]
2. Lent, R. *Cem Bilhões de Neurónios: Conceitos Fundamentais de Neurociencia*; Atheneu: São Paulo, Brasil, 2004.
3. Fonseca, V. Importância das emoções na aprendizagem: Uma abordagem neuropsicopedagógica. *Rev. Psicopedag.* **2016**, *33*, 365–384.
4. Ogden, J. *The Psychology of Eating: From Healthy to Disordered Behavior*; John Wiley & Sons: Malden, MA, USA, 2002; ISBN 978-0-631-23374-9.
5. GHDX. *Global Burden of Disease Study 2017*; Institute for Health Metrics and Evaluation: Washington, DC, USA, 2017.
6. Annunziata, A.; Vecchio, R. Organic farming and sustainability in food choices: An analysis of consumer preference in southern Italy. *Agric. Sci. Procedia* **2016**, *8*, 193–200. [CrossRef]
7. Danner, H.; Menapace, L. Using online comments to explore consumer beliefs regarding organic food in German-speaking countries and the United States. *Food Qual. Prefer.* **2020**, *83*, 103912. [CrossRef]
8. Rana, J.; Paul, J. Consumer behavior and purchase intention for organic food: A review and research agenda. *J. Retail. Consum. Serv.* **2017**, *38*, 157–165. [CrossRef]
9. Costa, C.; García-Lestón, J.; Costa, S.; Coelho, P.; Silva, S.; Pingarilho, M.; Valdiglesias, V.; Mattei, F.; Dall'Armi, V.; Bonassi, S.; et al. Is organic farming safer to farmers' health? A comparison between organic and traditional farming. *Toxicol. Lett.* **2014**, *230*, 166–176. [CrossRef]
10. Kamp, M.E.; Saridakis, I.; Verkaik-Kloosterman, J. Iodine content of semi-skimmed milk available in the Netherlands depending on farming (organic versus conventional) and heat treatment (pasteurized versus UHT) and implications for the consumer. *J. Trace Elem. Med. Biol.* **2019**, *56*, 178–183. [CrossRef]
11. Armesto, J.; Rocchetti, G.; Senizza, B.; Pateiro, M.; Barba, F.J.; Domínguez, R.; Lucini, L.; Lorenzo, J.M. Nutritional characterization of *Butternut squash* (*Cucurbita moschata* D.): Effect of variety (Ariel vs. Pluto) and farming type (conventional vs. organic). *Food Res. Int.* **2020**, *132*, 109052. [CrossRef]
12. Martí, R.; Leiva-Brondo, M.; Lahoz, I.; Campillo, C.; Cebolla-Cornejo, J.; Roselló, S. Polyphenol and l-ascorbic acid content in tomato as influenced by high lycopene genotypes and organic farming at different environments. *Food Chem.* **2018**, *239*, 148–156. [CrossRef]
13. Reeve, J.R.; Hoagland, L.A.; Villalba, J.J.; Carr, P.M.; Atucha, A.; Cambardella, C.; Davis, D.R.; Delate, K. Chapter six—Organic farming, soil health, and food quality: Considering possible links. In *Advances in Agronomy*; Sparks, D.L., Ed.; Academic Press: Cambridge, MA, USA, 2016; Volume 137, pp. 319–367.
14. Hyland, C.; Bradman, A.; Gerona, R.; Patton, S.; Zakharevich, I.; Gunier, R.B.; Klein, K. Organic diet intervention significantly reduces urinary pesticide levels in U.S. children and adults. *Environ. Res.* **2019**, *171*, 568–575. [CrossRef]
15. Melgarejo, M.; Mendiola, J.; Koch, H.M.; Moñino-García, M.; Noguera-Velasco, J.A.; Torres-Cantero, A.M. Associations between urinary organophosphate pesticide metabolite levels and reproductive parameters in men from an infertility clinic. *Environ. Res.* **2015**, *137*, 292–298. [CrossRef] [PubMed]
16. Kuang, L.; Hou, Y.; Huang, F.; Hong, H.; Sun, H.; Deng, W.; Lin, H. Pesticide residues in breast milk and the associated risk assessment: A review focused on China. *Sci. Total Environ.* **2020**, *727*, 138412. [CrossRef]
17. Sabarwal, A.; Kumar, K.; Singh, R.P. Hazardous effects of chemical pesticides on human health–Cancer and other associated disorders. *Environ. Toxicol. Pharmacol.* **2018**, *63*, 103–114. [CrossRef] [PubMed]
18. Martin, F.L.; Martinez, E.Z.; Stopper, H.; Garcia, S.B.; Uyemura, S.A.; Kannen, V. Increased exposure to pesticides and colon cancer: Early evidence in Brazil. *Chemosphere* **2018**, *209*, 623–631. [CrossRef] [PubMed]
19. Philippat, C.; Barkoski, J.; Tancredi, D.J.; Elms, B.; Barr, D.B.; Ozonoff, S.; Bennett, D.H.; Hertz-Picciotto, I. Prenatal exposure to organophosphate pesticides and risk of autism spectrum disorders and other non-typical development at 3 years in a high-risk cohort. *Int. J. Hyg. Environ. Health* **2018**, *221*, 548–555. [CrossRef] [PubMed]
20. Forman, J.; Silverstein, J. Organic foods: Health and environmental advantages and disadvantages. *Pediatrics* **2012**, *130*, e1406–e1415. [CrossRef]
21. USDA. *Pesticide Data Program*; United States Department of Agriculture: Washington, DC, USA, 2016.
22. Jackson, B.; Cooper, M.L.; Mintz, L.; Albino, A. Motivations to eat: Scale development and validation. *J. Res. Personal.* **2003**, *37*, 297–318. [CrossRef]

23. Gibson, E.L. Emotional influences on food choice: Sensory, physiological and psychological pathways. *Physiol. Behav.* **2006**, *89*, 53–61. [CrossRef] [PubMed]
24. Gold, P.W.; Chrousos, G.P. Organization of the stress system and its dysregulation in melancholic and atypical depression: High vs low CRH/NE states. *Mol. Psychiatry* **2002**, *7*, 254–275. [CrossRef]
25. Paans, N.P.G.; Gibson-Smith, D.; Bot, M.; van Strien, T.; Brouwer, I.A.; Visser, M.; Penninx, B.W.J.H. Depression and eating styles are independently associated with dietary intake. *Appetite* **2019**, *134*, 103–110. [CrossRef]
26. Love, H.; Bhullar, N.; Schutte, N.S. Psychological aspects of diet: Development and validation of three measures assessing dietary goal-desire incongruence, motivation, and satisfaction with dietary behavior. *Appetite* **2019**, *138*, 223–232. [CrossRef] [PubMed]
27. Lazarevich, I.; Camacho, M.E.I.; Velázquez-Alva, M.d.C.; Zepeda, M. Relationship among obesity, depression, and emotional eating in young adults. *Appetite* **2016**, *107*, 639–644. [CrossRef] [PubMed]
28. Ferrão, A.C.; Guine, R.P.F.; Correia, P.M.R.; Ferreira, M.; Lima, J.D. Development of a questionnaire to assess people's food choices determinants. *Curr. Nutr. Food Sci.* **2019**, *15*, 281–295. [CrossRef]
29. Ferrão, A.C.; Correia, P.; Ferreira, M.; Guiné, R.P.F. Perceptions towards healthy diet of the portuguese according to area of work or studies. *Zdr Varst* **2019**, *58*, 40–46. [CrossRef] [PubMed]
30. Ferrão, A.C.; Guiné, R.P.F.; Correia, P.; Ferreira, M.; Cardoso, A.P.; Duarte, J.; Lima, J. Perceptions towards a healthy diet among a sample of university people in Portugal. *Nutr. Food Sci.* **2018**, *48*, 669–688. [CrossRef]
31. Likert, R. A technique for the measurement of attitudes. *Arch. Psychol.* **1932**, *22*, 1–55.
32. Pestana, M.H.; Gageiro, J.N. *Análise de Dados para Ciências Sociais—A complementaridade do SPSS*; Edições Sílabo: Lisbon, Portugal, 2014.
33. Witten, R.; Witte, J. *Statistics*, 9th ed.; Wiley: Hoboken, NJ, USA, 2009.
34. Lê, J.; Dallongeville, J.; Wagner, A.; Arveiler, D.; Haas, B.; Cottel, D.; Simon, C.; Dauchet, L. Attitudes toward healthy eating: A mediator of the educational level-diet relationship. *Eur. J. Clin. Nutr.* **2013**, *67*, 808–814. [CrossRef]
35. Thow, A.M.; Verma, G.; Soni, D.; Soni, D.; Beri, D.K.; Kumar, P.; Siegel, K.R.; Shaikh, N.; Khandelwal, S. How can health, agriculture and economic policy actors work together to enhance the external food environment for fruit and vegetables? A qualitative policy analysis in India. *Food Policy* **2018**, *77*, 143–151. [CrossRef]
36. Sharps, M.; Robinson, E. Encouraging children to eat more fruit and vegetables: Health vs. descriptive social norm-based messages. *Appetite* **2016**, *100*, 18–25. [CrossRef]
37. Park, H.; Yu, S. Policy review: Implication of tax on sugar-sweetened beverages for reducing obesity and improving heart health. *Health Policy Technol.* **2019**, *8*, 92–95. [CrossRef]
38. Carbone, S.; Lavie, C.J.; Elagizi, A.; Arena, R.; Ventura, H.O. The impact of obesity in heart failure. *Heart Fail. Clin.* **2020**, *16*, 71–80. [CrossRef] [PubMed]
39. DiNicolantonio, J.J.; Lucan, S.C.; O'Keefe, J.H. The evidence for saturated fat and for sugar related to coronary heart disease. *Prog. Cardiovasc. Dis.* **2016**, *58*, 464–472. [CrossRef] [PubMed]
40. Teixeira, B.; Afonso, C.; Sousa, A.S.; Guerra, R.S.; Santos, A.; Borges, N.; Moreira, P.; Padrão, P.; Amaral, T.F. Adherence to a mediterranean dietary pattern status and associated factors among Portuguese older adults: Results from the nutrition up 65 cross-sectional study. *Nutrition* **2019**, *65*, 91–96. [CrossRef] [PubMed]
41. Dammann, K.W.; Smith, C. Food-related environmental, behavioral, and personal factors associated with body mass index among urban, low-income African-American, American Indian, and Caucasian women. *Am. J. Health Promot.* **2011**, *25*, e1–e10. [CrossRef]
42. Rustad, C.; Smith, C. Nutrition knowledge and associated behavior changes in a holistic, short-term nutrition education intervention with low-income women. *J. Nutr. Educ. Behav.* **2013**, *45*, 490–498. [CrossRef]
43. Strien, T. Causes of emotional eating and matched treatment of obesity. *Curr. Diab. Rep.* **2018**, *18*. [CrossRef]
44. Chambers, D.; Phan, U.T.X.; Chanadang, S.; Maughan, C.; Sanchez, K.; Di Donfrancesco, B.; Gomez, D.; Higa, F.; Li, H.; Chambers, E.; et al. Motivations for Food Consumption during specific eating occasions in Turkey. *Foods* **2016**, *5*, 39. [CrossRef]
45. Ashurst, J.; van Woerden, I.; Dunton, G.; Todd, M.; Ohri-Vachaspati, P.; Swan, P.; Bruening, M. The association among emotions and food choices in first-year college students using mobile-ecological momentary assessments. *BMC Public Health* **2018**, *18*, 573. [CrossRef]
46. Bennett, J.; Greene, G.; Schwartz-Barcott, D. Perceptions of emotional eating behavior. A qualitative study of college students. *Appetite* **2013**, *60*, 187–192. [CrossRef]

47. Boggiano, M.M. Palatable eating motives scale in a college population: Distribution of scores and scores associated with greater BMI and binge-eating. *Eat. Behav.* **2016**, *21*, 95–98. [CrossRef]
48. Bartkiene, E.; Steibliene, V.; Adomaitiene, V.; Juodeikiene, G.; Cernauskas, D.; Lele, V.; Klupsaite, D.; Zadeike, D.; Jarutiene, L.; Guiné, R.P.F. Factors affecting consumer food preferences: Food taste and depression-based evoked emotional expressions with the use of face reading technology. *Bio. Med. Res. Int.* **2019**, *2019*, 2097415. [CrossRef] [PubMed]
49. Guiné, R.; Ferrão, A.C.; Ferreira, M.; Correia, P.; Cardoso, A.P.; Duarte, J.; Rumbak, I.; Shehata, A.-M.; Vittadini, E.; Papageorgiou, M. The motivations that define eating patterns in some Mediterranean countries. *Nutr. Food Sci.* **2019**, *49*, 1126–1141. [CrossRef]
50. Hidalgo-Mora, J.J.; García-Vigara, A.; Sánchez-Sánchez, M.L.; García-Pérez, M.-Á.; Tarín, J.; Cano, A. The Mediterranean diet: A historical perspective on food for health. *Maturitas* **2020**, *132*, 65–69. [CrossRef] [PubMed]
51. Latha, S. Vuca in engineering education: Enhancement of faculty competency for capacity building. *Procedia Comput. Sci.* **2020**, *172*, 741–747. [CrossRef]
52. Bezanilla, M.J.; Fernández-Nogueira, D.; Poblete, M.; Galindo-Domínguez, H. Methodologies for teaching-learning critical thinking in higher education: The teacher's view. *Think. Ski. Creat.* **2019**, *33*, 100584. [CrossRef]
53. Castro, J.M.; Bellisle, F.; Feunekes, G.I.J.; Dalix, A.-M.; De Graaf, C. Culture and meal patterns: A comparison of the food intake of free-living American, Dutch, and French students. *Nutr. Res.* **1997**, *17*, 807–829. [CrossRef]

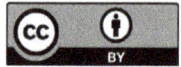

© 2020 by the authors. Licensee MDPI, Basel, Switzerland. This article is an open access article distributed under the terms and conditions of the Creative Commons Attribution (CC BY) license (http://creativecommons.org/licenses/by/4.0/).

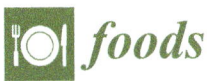

Article

Comparison of Supercritical CO_2-Drying, Freeze-Drying and Frying on Sensory Properties of Beetroot

Nikola Tomic [1,*], Ilija Djekic [1], Gerard Hofland [2], Nada Smigic [1], Bozidar Udovicki [1] and Andreja Rajkovic [1,3]

1 Department of Food Safety and Quality Management, Faculty of Agriculture, University of Belgrade, Nemanjina 6, 11080 Belgrade, Serbia; idjekic@agrif.bg.ac.rs (I.D.); nadasmigic@agrif.bg.ac.rs (N.S.); bozidar.udovicki@agrif.bg.ac.rs (B.U.); arajkovic@agrif.bg.ac.rs (A.R.)
2 FeyeCon Carbon Dioxide Technologies, Rijnkade 17A, 1382 GS Weesp, The Netherlands; gerard.hofland@feyecon.com
3 Department of Food Technology, Food Safety and Health, Faculty of Bioscience Engineering, Ghent University, Coupure Links 653, B-9000 Ghent, Belgium
* Correspondence: tsnikola@agrif.bg.ac.rs; Tel.: +381-64-1298623

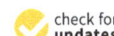

Received: 20 July 2020; Accepted: 26 August 2020; Published: 31 August 2020

Abstract: The aim of this study was to compare the sensory quality and acceptance of dried ready-to-eat beetroot snacks as a result of different drying methods applied: supercritical CO_2-drying (scCO_2-drying), frying, and freeze-drying. Descriptive sensory analysis, quality rating (10 assessors), and consumer acceptance testing ($n = 102$) were performed. Mean overall quality scores within the range of "very good" quality were found only in non-precooked scCO_2-dried samples which were characterized by typical magenta color, low level of shape and surface deformations, pronounced brittleness and crispiness, and good rehydration during mastication. The other samples were in the range of "good" quality. The pre-cooking step before scCO_2-drying negatively influenced the sensory quality parameters, particularly appearance. Around 60% of tested consumers showed a preference for the fried and non-precooked scCO_2-dried samples. The drivers of liking were mostly related to the characteristics of the product, which was salted, fried, and crispy, with an oily and overburnt flavor, i.e., the product most similar to commercial potato chips products. Freeze-drying had a negative effect primarily on appearance and flavor. According to the sensory evaluation conducted, direct scCO_2-drying without a pre-cooking step showed itself as a promising alternative drying technology in the production of dried beetroot snacks.

Keywords: supercritical CO_2-drying; beetroot snacks; preference mapping; mean drop analysis

1. Introduction

Drying of biological material is a controlled effort to preserve the structure or create a new one that serves for functional purposes [1]. The main technological objectives of food drying are [2]: preservation; reduction in weight and volume; transport and storage facilitation; and achieving a desirable sensory profile of different flavors, chewiness, crispiness, firmness, etc.

The food product's microstructure is often negatively affected by the movement and ultimate loss of water during the drying process which influences physical properties, nutritional availability, and also chemical and microbiological stability [3,4]. Consumers nowadays demand high-quality, nutritious, fresh, convenient, additive-free, safe food products with a natural flavor and taste, and an extended shelf-life [5–7]. To achieve dehydrated fruit or vegetable commodities of high quality at a reasonable cost, in the sense of minimizing the loss of volatiles, loss of flavors, changes in texture, changes in color, and also a decrease in nutritional value [5], dehydration must occur fairly rapidly [8]. Enhancing drying rates has been a major challenge for food engineers [1]. Air-drying, which is still the most commonly used drying operation in the food industry [3,5,9], can bring many reconstituted products, such as powdered milk or dry pasta, with sensory profiles very similar to the original material. Further, certain air-dried commodities such as grains and legumes show desirable textural characteristics after cooking due to high rehydration capability, but the structure of most fruits and vegetables is usually negatively affected during air-drying resulting in poor reconstitution properties when compared to their fresh state [1]. Structural changes are important since food texture, as a complex sensory attribute which can be perceived and described only by human beings, is directly influenced by the structure of food, i.e., it derives from the structure (molecular, microscopic, or macroscopic) of food [10]. A decrease in the sensory quality [5] influenced by application of higher temperatures during air-drying (typically 65–85 °C) is most often reflected in the small volume, great shrinkage, high density, low porosity, and increased hardness of the dried product [4,11]. Heat can also affect the color of the dried commodity. As a part of the cellular structure, betalains are the main red pigments in beetroot. These compounds are very sensitive to heat, light, and oxygen, and therefore air-drying triggers the oxidation of betalains in beetroot due to prolonged exposure to higher temperatures [12].

Although primarily considered as a thermal preservation technique, according to Oreopoulou et al. [13], frying can be defined as a process of cooking and drying through contact with hot oil. Its preservative effect is reflected through both thermal destruction of microorganisms and enzymes and a reduction in water activity at the surface or throughout the product. Food products that are fully dried during the frying process, such as potato chips or other extruded snacks, have a shelf-life up to several months, which is usually limited by quality deterioration of the absorbed oil and development of a rancid odor and flavor. During food frying, heat is transferred by convection from the surrounding oil to the surface of the food and by conduction within the solid food. Mass transfer is reflected through the vaporization of water from the surface of the product and on the other side through the penetration of oil into the food. Along with water removal, the surface of the product becomes more and more dry causing the formation of a crust. Considering the process temperature and time, in general, the lower the temperature and the longer the process time, the slower the cooking rate of the product, the firmer the crust and texture, and the higher the oil content absorbed by the product [13]. The unique texture–flavor combination of fried snack foods makes them highly appreciated within different categories of consumers.

Freeze-drying is considered as a superior drying method for many fruits and vegetables and the best solution for food drying in general, which can deliver dried products of high commercial value with good sensory quality and a high level of nutrients retention [8,14]. Since the process implies a direct transition from solid to gaseous state without melting and without exposing the product to high temperatures, the structure of the product remains porous which facilitates rapid product rehydration, structural changes and shrinkage are largely avoided, movement of the soluble solids is minimized, thermal damage is minimized, and flavor, color, and appearance are highly preserved [8,15]. On the other side, freeze-drying is a highly energy-consuming technology with high capital costs which limits its industrial application to high added value products such as baby foods, instant products (coffee, soups), exotic fruits and vegetables, or mushrooms [16].

Application of supercritical fluids (SCFs) as extraction solvents in the food industry dates back to the mid-20th century [9,17]. Being at a temperature and pressure above the critical point, SCFs have the special combination of liquid-like solvating properties and density, and gas-like diffusivity and viscosity which makes them excellent solvents [18], while the fluid can be recovered and reused. Carbon dioxide is the most intensively used agent in supercritical processes applied to food [19]. CO_2 is nontoxic, non-carcinogenic, non-flammable, odorless, colorless, and thermodynamically stable, with the possibility of adjusting its thermophysical properties, such as viscosity, diffusivity, density, or dielectric constant, by varying the temperature and/or pressure [18], and its usage in food industry is approved without declaration [19]. The removal of water during supercritical CO_2-drying is not based on sublimation or vaporization, but on dissolving water in the scCO$_2$ [9]. Due to these gas–liquid properties of scCO$_2$, the structure of the dried material remains preserved to a high extent. Problems that occur with conventional air-drying processes, in which the solid structure can collapse due to surface tension effects at the vapor–liquid interfaces, are absent in the case of scCO$_2$-drying [3,17]. Further on, due to the low critical parameters of CO$_2$ (304.1 K, 7.38 MPa) [20], the drying process can be conducted at relatively low temperatures (e.g., 40 °C). The main drawback is the relatively low solubility of water in scCO$_2$ (2.5 mg/g at 40 °C, 20 MPa) [3,21]. The drying conditions are most often reflected in the application of scCO$_2$ under pressure within the range of 10 to 14 MPa and temperature between 40 and 60 °C with the fluid flow rate of 80–220 kg/h [22–24]. The drying time that must be ensured, in order to achieve an appropriate level of dehydration of a plant material under these conditions, ranges from 6 to 16 h [24]. According to the findings of Zambon et al. [24], the most influential process variable in reaching an appropriate level of water activity is temperature, as it acts directly on the water solubility in scCO$_2$. The pressure significantly influences the drying efficiency only at lower temperatures and a longer drying time [24]. For the purpose of commercial drying, scCO$_2$ is widely used for the drying of gels [25] and also there are studies that reported its practical application for the preservation of decellularized esophageal scaffolds [26]. Application of scCO$_2$ in food drying is still limited to few products at the small pilot scale [22,24,27–29] and additional studies are still needed for scCO$_2$-drying technology to be developed at industrial scale. The pilot scale scCO$_2$-drying unit used in this study still has a low technology readiness level and requires further work in order to reach industrial application [30], first of all to validate its effectiveness in various working regimes [31].

Previous studies reported that the application of scCO$_2$ showed a potent antimicrobial effect against both bacteria and fungi [32–34] which allows scCO$_2$-drying to be used as a promising "green" technology than can combine drying and pasteurization in one single step. On the other side, recent studies showed that scCO$_2$-drying can bring and retain, for at least six months, dried apple slices with similar sensory quality and consumer acceptance levels as obtained by freeze-drying, in the case of using non-permeable materials and an inert atmosphere for packing the products [22,23].

The aim of this study was to investigate the effects of the supercritical CO$_2$ drying method, as compared to the freeze-drying and frying techniques, on the sensory quality and acceptance of dried beetroot cuts intended to be eaten as ready-to-eat snacks.

2. Materials and Methods

2.1. Dried Beetroot Samples

Fresh red beetroot (*Beta vulgaris*) was purchased at a local market in the Netherlands (Kruythof aardappelhandel, 3291 CN Strijen, The Netherlands). After thorough washing, beetroot was sliced without removing the skin into flat or "wavy" circular cuts of relatively similar size (around 3 mm in thickness). Three different drying methods were applied: supercritical drying using CO$_2$ (scCO$_2$-drying), freeze-drying, and frying. ScCO$_2$-drying was performed in a patented equipment [35] under a pressure of 10.0 MPa at 40 °C for 14 h. ScCO$_2$-drying was combined with a pre-cooking step, and also two types of cutting were applied to obtain flat and wavy beetroot discs, in which way three experimental scCO$_2$-dried samples were obtained: scCO$_2$-dried-Flat (not pre-cooked; raw sliced, flat cuts); scCO$_2$-dried-LT (not pre-cooked; raw sliced, wavy cuts); and scCO$_2$-dried-HT (pre-cooked in boiling water and sliced; wavy cuts). "Wavy" shape was introduced in order to examine the influence of this type of appearance on consumer acceptance. Freeze-drying of flat raw beetroot cuts was performed in a 20-L freeze-dryer SuperModulyo (Thermo Scientific, Waltham, MA, USA) within 48 h. The pressure during sublimation was kept at 20 Pa and during desorption at 5 Pa, while the temperature of −25 °C during sublimation was gradually increased up to 40 °C during desorption. Deep fat frying of flat beetroot cuts was done in boiling vegetable oil at 160 °C for 3.5 min (raw beetroot cuts were first salted with around 25 g of salt per 1 kg of beetroot and then fried). Water activity of the dried samples was 0.32 ± 0.02. Appearance of the beetroot samples used in the study is shown in Figure 1.

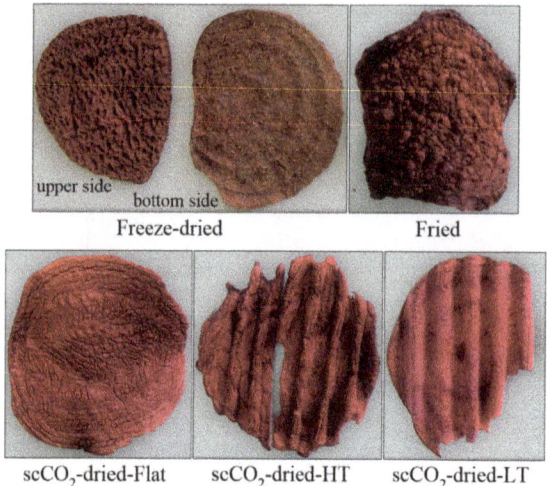

Figure 1. Images of the dried beetroot samples used in this study. Supercritical CO_2-dried-HT sample was cooked in boiling water before drying, the rest were subjected to the drying processes in a raw state. The upper and bottom sides of a beetroot chip substantially differed from each other in appearance only in the case of freeze-dried samples.

After drying, the samples (100–200 g) were packed under 100% N_2 in aluminum-polyethylene (Alu-PE) pouches (thickness: 98 µm, aluminum layer: 8 µm; Goglio S.p.A, Milan, Italy) and placed in the dark at ambient temperature (≈22 °C). All of the beetroot samples were produced within two separate batches (two replications). The samples were evaluated between the third and fourth week upon packing.

2.2. Sensory Analysis

The sensory tests were conducted in the sensory testing laboratory at the University of Belgrade. Testing conditions such as sample serving procedures, instructions to panelists, palate cleansing, and training sessions are described in Tomic et al. (2019) [22]. In short, random 3-digit numbers were used for the sample-coding, the panelists used low-sodium mineral water for palate cleansing, no strict instructions were given to the panelists regarding the swallowing/expectorating of individual bites, additional beetroot samples were kept in closed glass jars for the purpose of orthonasal olfaction during evaluation. Environmental conditions during testing were in accordance with ISO 8589:2007 (Sensory analysis—General guidance for the design of test rooms) and ISO 11136:2014 (Sensory analysis—Methodology—General guidance for conducting hedonic tests with consumers in a controlled area). The trained panelists who participated in descriptive analysis and quality judging were of good general health, of normal range for BMI of 18–25 kg/m^2, with no dental wearers and reported dental problems, which is in line with the recommendations of Forde et al. [36]. For this particular reason, the descriptive/objective quality sensory panel had six 2-h additional training sessions in total prior to the analyses. These calibration trainings were performed using different types of dried commodities (bell pepper, apple, and beetroot). Considering consumer sensory testing, all volunteers gave verbal consent that they were of good general health with no dental issues before conducting the test.

2.2.1. Descriptive Sensory Testing

Descriptive sensory testing was performed by a 10-university members sensory panel (4 men and 6 women) experienced in fruits and vegetables quality judging.

The testing was done in two replications by assessing the intensity of 20 sensory attributes using 15 cm line-scales with verbal anchors at both ends. Since there were no reference standards, the assessors were using the scales in their own way by comparing the samples to each other [37,38]. The list of the attributes with terminal verbal anchors is shown in Table 1. A Latin square design was used in the samples' presentation scheme.

Table 1. The list of sensory properties and descriptors used in the descriptive sensory evaluation of dried beetroot samples.

Attribute	Definition	Anchors
APPEARANCE		
Flesh color intensity	The intensity or color strength of the flesh.	light-dark
Surface deformation	Presence of furrows, cracks, or holes on the flesh surface.	none-lots of
Degree of shape deformation	Deformation of the shape in relation to the flat disc (distortion, bending).	none-much
ODOR (orthonasal olfaction)		
Overall odor intensity	The intensity of the overall odor of the product.	none-intensive
Beetroot odor	The intensity of the beetroot-like odor.	none-intensive
Hay-like odor	The intensity of the hay-like and dried vegetables-like odor.	none-intensive
Musty odor [1]	The intensity of odor associated with a damp cellar, or stale vegetables.	none-intensive
Oil odor	The intensity of the fried vegetable oil odor.	none-intensive
Nasal pungency	The intensity of nasal pungent and sourish feelings.	none-intensive
FLAVOR		
Overall flavor intensity	The intensity of the overall flavor of the product.	none-intensive
Beetroot flavor	The intensity of the beetroot-like flavor.	none-intensive
Sweetness	The taste stimulated by sugars.	none-intensive
Overburnt/Grime flavor	The intensity of the overburnt, grime-like flavor.	none-intensive
Bitterness	The taste stimulated by chemical substances such as caffeine or quinine.	none-intensive
TEXTURE		
Flesh surface roughness	Degree to which the surface is uneven, related to the amount of irregularity, bumps, grains, or protrusions present on the surface.	smooth-rough
Hardness	The force required to bite through the dried beetroot disc.	soft-hard
Cohesiveness	Amount of product that deforms rather than breaks during chewing.	breaks-deforms
Denseness [1]	Cross-section compactness.	airy-dense/compact
Crispiness	The force and noise with which the beetroot slice breaks during chewing.	not crispy-very crispy
Adhesiveness	Degree to which mass sticks to the teeth.	not sticky-very sticky

[1] These attributes were excluded from further multivariate statistical analysis because 3-way ANOVA showed they did not significantly discriminate ($p < 0.05$) among the tested samples.

2.2.2. Sensory Quality Rating

Sensory quality rating was also done in two replications by the same assessors used in the descriptive analysis.

The evaluation was conducted using a 5-level quality scoring system described in Djekic et al. (2018) [23] supported by the internal laboratory guidelines for fruits and vegetables quality judging. By dividing each of the five integer quality scores into quarters, the 0–5 score range was transformed into a 20-responses category scale. Four groups of sensory attributes were evaluated in order to assess overall sensory quality: appearance, flavor, texture, and odor. In order to distinguish the selected sensory attributes according to their impact on overall quality, each attribute was assigned an appropriate correction factor (CI—coefficient of importance): 2, 8, 6, and 2, respectively. Overall sensory quality score was calculated by multiplying individual scores with appropriate CIs and by dividing the sum of the obtained corrected scores by the sum of CIs.

2.2.3. Consumer Sensory Testing

Consumer acceptance tests were performed by 103 students from the university (102 responses in total were further processed: 43 males and 59 females). Students between the ages of 19 and 25 were randomly selected and were chosen if they were relatively frequent consumers (more than two times per month) of dried fruits/vegetables (regardless of direct consumption of the products as snacks or through other food products and meals such as cereal breakfasts/bars).

A 9-point hedonic scale [39,40] was used to evaluate overall acceptance, appearance acceptance, as well as flavor acceptance. Further on, just-about-right (JAR) scales of 9 points (1 = too little, 5 = JAR, 9 = too much) [41] were used to assess the samples for accepted intensities of "hardness", "chewiness", "crispiness", "color", "saltiness", and "bitterness" (only "too much" part of the scale).

2.3. Statistical Analysis

2.3.1. Descriptive Data and PREFMAP

The significance of the multivariate effect for samples was tested by multivariate analysis of variance (MANOVA) with "samples" as the fixed factor. After that, three-way ANOVA (followed by Tukey's HSD test) was conducted in order to identify those characteristics that significantly discriminate among the tested products ("samples" = fixed factor; "assessors" and "replications" = random factors). Original descriptive data were first standardized for each assessor before applying both MANOVA and ANOVA. As a result, two sensory characteristics ("musty odor" and "denseness") were excluded from subsequent dimensional reduction analysis (Table 1) since they did not significantly discriminate ($p < 0.05$) among the samples. Original descriptive data for the attributes that remained after removing the two, divided into personal data matrices, were subjected to generalized Procrustes analysis (GPA). Then, principal component analysis (PCA) was applied to the obtained consensus data. External preference mapping (PREFMAP) [42] was done by applying linear multiple regression analysis in which the extracted PC space was regressed against the overall hedonic data. K-means cluster analysis was used to segment the obtained regression coefficients.

2.3.2. Quality Data

Three-way ANOVA was applied on raw quality data ("samples" = fixed factor; "assessors" and "replications" = random factors) together with Tukey's HSD post hoc test.

2.3.3. Consumer Data

In order to examine the differences both between the consumer clusters obtained by K-means cluster analysis in PREFMAP (within the samples) and between the samples within the clusters, raw hedonic data were subjected to ANOVA ("samples" = fixed factor).

One-way ANOVA was also performed in order to test for gender differences in hedonic scores.

Mean drop analysis was done as described by Schraidt (2009) [43]. In brief, for each sensory attribute evaluated by using the appropriate JAR scale, the tested consumers were first grouped into three categories according to their JAR scores: 1, 2, and 3 = "below JAR (i.e., too little of an attribute)"; 4, 5, and 6 = "at JAR"; and 7, 8, and 9 = "above JAR (i.e., too much of an attribute)". The mean overall hedonic scores were calculated for each category and then the mean drops were obtained by subtracting the mean hedonic score of each non-JAR category from the mean of the JAR category. Statistical significance of the mean drops was tested by applying ANOVA and Tukey's HSD test. The cutoff was set at 20% of the total number of respondents.

2.3.4. Software

The statistical analyses were performed using both Idiogrid software version 2.4/2008 (Oklahoma State University, Stillwater, OK, USA) [44] (GPA, PCA) and SPSS Statistics 17.0 (IBM, Armonk, NY, USA) (MANOVA, ANOVA, PCA), at a 0.05 level of statistical significance.

3. Results and Discussion

3.1. PREFMAP

Generalized Procrustes analysis of the descriptive data showed strong agreement among the assessors and replications (consensus proportion = 0.94; $p < 0.05$) with relatively small differences in overall variability of the individual data matrices (isotropic scaling values ranged from 0.72 to 1.44 which are relatively close to 1) [45]. Upon PCA of the consensus data matrix, 18 original variables fit into the new four-dimensional PC space. The Kaiser criterion [46] was used for making a decision on the number of PCs that should be retained for the overall variability explanation (6.9, 4.0, 4.0, and 3.1, PC-1 to PC-4, respectively).

Figure 2 shows the PC space of the first four principal components extracted. The freeze-dried beetroot sample was characterized by the presence of various relatively large holes and cracks on the upper surface of the cuts (the side which was free during the drying), highly pronounced flesh surface roughness, pronounced beetroot and hay-like odor, pronounced cohesiveness, and lower level of crispiness. Surface deformation and flash surface roughness were the most pronounced in the freeze-dried sample when compared to the rest of the evaluated products ($p < 0.05$). The fried sample, on the far right side of both score plots (Figure 2), was characterized by a pronounced over-burnt/grime flavor, oil odor, nasal pungency, the highest degree of shape deformation ($p < 0.05$), bitterness, and lower levels of sweetness, beetroot flavor, and cohesiveness. This sample was also the darkest one in color, and with the highest levels of crispiness and bitterness ($p < 0.05$). The surface lumpiness observed in fried samples (Figure 1) originates from vapor bubbles entrapped under the formed crust on the very surface of the snack product during frying [13]. As it was expected, oil notes were noticed only in the fried sample. Certain characteristics that were typical for the fried sample, such as over-burnt flavor, nasal pungency, and shape deformation, were also noticed in the precooked scCO$_2$-dried-HT sample. According to sweetness, three homogenous ($\alpha = 0.05$) subsets of the samples without overlaps emerged (ANOVA data not shown) with increasing sweetness in the following order: (i) fried; (ii) scCO$_2$-dried-HT; (iii) freeze-dried, scCO$_2$-dried-Flat, and scCO$_2$-dried-LT. It seems that the application of high temperatures during or before the drying process influences the perception of sweetness in dried beetroot. In addition, hay-like odor and common dried vegetables-like odor were at the highest level in the freeze-dried and scCO$_2$-dried-HT samples as compared to the rest ($p < 0.05$), while totally absent in the fried beetroot cuts. The ScCO$_2$-dried-HT sample differed to a certain extent in sensory profile from the other scCO$_2$-dried samples which were not thermally treated before drying. Beside the mentioned flavor notes, the scCO$_2$-dried HT sample was less hard, less cohesive, less crispy, and more adhesive ($p < 0.05$) than the other two which were characterized by a pronounced beetroot flavor, sweetness, less surface deformations and flesh surface roughness, and also shape deformations to a lesser degree.

Individual consumer overall hedonic scores (N = 102) were regressed against the four PCs. Cluster analysis revealed three consumer clusters with individual proportions of tested consumers greater than 20% (Cluster 1 = 41.2%; Cluster 2 = 33.3%; and Cluster 3 = 25.5%). The clusters are mapped within the PC space (Figure 2) by averaging the regression coefficients across the clusters. The results of the hedonic acceptance testing with the scores averaged across the clusters are shown in Table 2. Cluster 3 (25.5%) showed a preference for the scCO$_2$-dried-Flat (7.5 ± 1.3) and fried (7.3 ± 2.1) beetroot samples, while Cluster 2 (33.3%) preferred the scCO$_2$-dried-LT (7.5 ± 1.5) and fried (6.5 ± 2.7) samples. This means that around 59% of the tested consumers showed a preference for the scCO$_2$-dried beetroot samples not subjected to the cooking step before the drying process.

Similar results related to consumer acceptance were reported for scCO$_2$-dried red bell pepper and apple fruits [22,24]. ScCO$_2$-dried red bell pepper was assessed as acceptable by more than 60% of the tested consumers [24]. Preference of the consumer within Cluster 1 cannot be explained in this four-dimensional PC space since the position of the cluster is mainly close to the origin in the plots (PC1 to PC4 score values were less than 0.35). According to the average overall and flavor hedonic scores (6.6 and 6.2, respectively), the consumers within Cluster 1 slightly preferred also the fried sample (the rest of the scores were less than 6). It appeared that, in general, tested consumers showed their preference for the beetroot product which was salted, fried, crispy, with an oily and overburnt flavor, in other words, most similar to commercial potato chips products. Freeze-dried and scCO$_2$-dried-HT samples did not gain the consumers' attention and were scored with relatively low (<6) overall and flavor hedonic scores (Table 2). It seems also that the "wavy" shape of the scCO$_2$-dried-LT and scCO$_2$-dried-HT samples did not have an influence on the shape acceptance scores of the scCO$_2$-dried beetroot products. Taking into account that descriptive analysis and quality judging showed that precooked scCO$_2$-dried-HT beetroot wavy discs suffered shape deformations, the mean shape acceptance scores for the scCO$_2$-dried-LT sample were not statistically higher within any consumer cluster when compared with the scCO$_2$-dried-Flat beetroot sample.

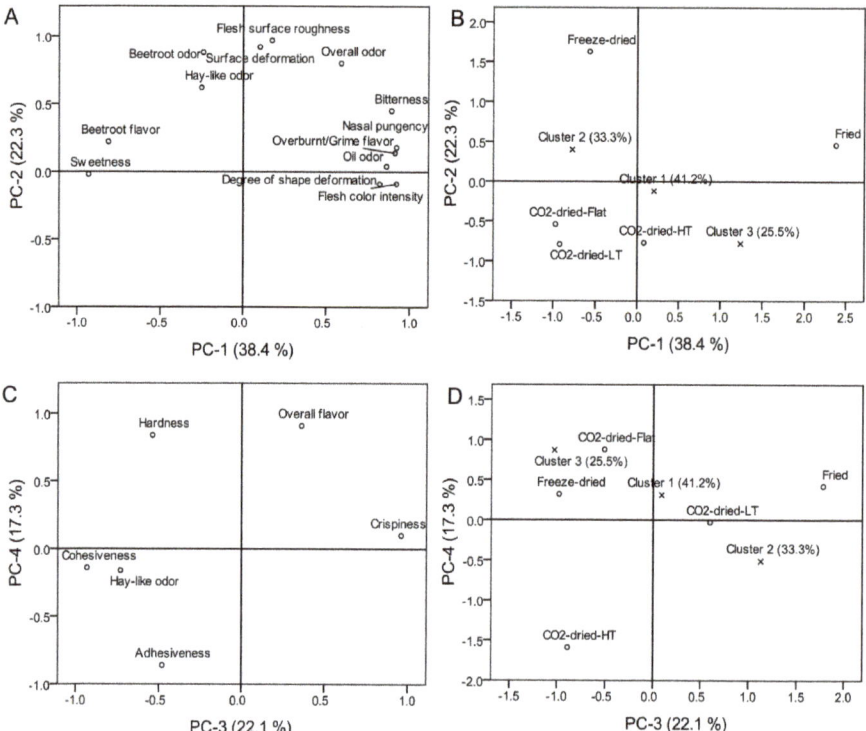

Figure 2. Four-dimensional principal component-space (PC-1 to PC-4) of the sensory descriptive data (10 assessors × 2 replications) of dried beetroot samples, previously subjected to generalized Procrustes analysis, regressed against the overall hedonic data (PREFMAP). (**A,C**): loading plots; (**B,D**): scores plots. Loadings cutoff was set at 0.60. Consumers (N = 102) are grouped within the three clusters. Samples abbreviations: "Flat" = not pre-cooked, flat cuts; "LT" = not pre-cooked, wavy cuts; and "HT" = pre-cooked, wavy cuts.

Table 2. Consumer hedonic acceptance [1] for dried beetroot samples.

Beetroot Samples	Consumers [2] (N = 102)		
	Cluster 1 (41.2%)	Cluster 2 (33.3%)	Cluster 3 (25.5%)
Overall Liking			
CO_2-dried Flat	5.9 ± 2.8 [b,B,C]	4.3 ± 2.1 [a,A]	7.5 ± 1.3 [c,C]
CO_2-dried LT	5.2 ± 2.5 [a,A,B,C]	7.5 ± 1.5 [b,C]	4.0 ± 2.0 [a,A]
CO_2-dried HT	4.0 ± 2.2 [a,A]	5.0 ± 2.2 [a,b,A,B]	5.7 ± 1.8 [b,B]
Fried	6.6 ± 2.7 [C]	6.5 ± 2.7 [B,C]	7.3 ± 2.1 [C]
Freeze-dried	4.9 ± 2.6 [A,B]	5.2 ± 2.6 [A,B]	4.6 ± 2.0 [A,B]
Appearance Liking			
CO_2-dried Flat	7.3 ± 2.1 [a,b,C]	6.7 ± 1.9 [a,B,C]	8.2 ± 1.1 [b,B]
CO_2-dried LT	6.6 ± 2.4 [a,B,C]	7.4 ± 1.5 [b,C]	5.5 ± 2.3 [a,b,A]
CO_2-dried HT	5.8 ± 2.8 [A,B]	5.9 ± 2.3 [A,B]	6.5 ± 2.1 [A]
Fried	5.9 ± 2.7 [A,B,C]	5.7 ± 2.6 [A,B]	5.9 ± 2.5 [A]
Freeze-dried	5.0 ± 2.5 [A]	4.7 ± 2.6 [A]	4.9 ± 2.4 [A]
Flavor Liking			
CO_2-dried Flat	5.5 ± 2.7 [a,b,B]	4.8 ± 2.2 [a,A]	6.6 ± 2.1 [b,B]
CO_2-dried LT	5.1 ± 2.4 [a,B]	7.1 ± 1.8 [b,C]	4.5 ± 2.4 [a,A]
CO_2-dried HT	3.1 ± 2.4 [a,A]	4.8 ± 2.3 [b,A]	5.0 ± 2.2 [b,A,B]
Fried	6.2 ± 3.1 [B]	6.5 ± 2.9 [B,C]	6.7 ± 2.7 [B]
Freeze-dried	5.1 ± 2.8 [B]	5.1 ± 2.8 [A,B]	4.4 ± 2.9 [A]

[1] Arithmetic mean ± standard deviation. The same lowercase letter within a row and the same uppercase letter within a column indicate values that are not statistically different (α = 0.05). [2] K-means cluster analysis of the consumer PCA scores.

Acceptance ratings of the total number of tested consumers, measured by using the hedonic scales, were also compared in order to assess the gender effect. The gender of the tested consumers did not influence liking for the examined dried beetroot snacks. Analysis of variance showed that there were no statistically significant differences ($p > 0.05$) between females and males within any of the examined modalities: overall, appearance, and flavor liking (data not shown).

Beside acceptable appearance and palatability, it is also expected of dried ready-to-eat agricultural commodities such as fruits and vegetables to preserve their nutritional content [47]. Since beetroot is rich in valuable active compounds such as carotenoids, betalains, polyphenols, and flavonoids, and also saponins, it has attracted significant scientific and consumer attention in recent years as a health-promoting functional food product [12]. As being mostly strong antioxidants, these compounds are sensitive to the promoters of oxidation such as oxygen, light, and heat. Due to prolonged exposure to elevated temperatures typical for hot air-drying (65–85 °C), in the presence of oxygen, oxidation and degradation of these compounds are inevitable, which causes the loss of their nutritional and health values [48,49]. Within the optimal pH range, temperature is the most influential factor for betalains degradation [50], betalains being the main red pigments in beetroot with intense antibacterial and antiviral activity that comes from their strong antioxidant potential [51]. Relatively low temperatures (e.g., 40 °C) observed in the case of using $scCO_2$ for drying purposes are recognized as a nutritionally friendly preservation technology meeting these consumers' demands [52]. In addition, reduced water activity, inactivation of enzymes, and increased light impermeability of dried plant tissue can decrease the sensitivity of these phytochemicals as compared to the raw state [12], as it was shown in the case of betalains in beetroot [50]. Stability of these kinds of products during storage can be increased by using protective packaging materials and an inert gas atmosphere for packing. According to the findings of Tomic et al. [22], $scCO_2$-drying can bring and retain the same acceptance level of dried apples for at least 6–12 months as it can be obtained by the freeze-drying process provided the products were packed in the packaging material with low gas permeability (such as aluminum-polyethylene pouches used in their study) under an inert atmosphere (N_2).

3.2. Mean Drop Analysis

The results of the mean drop analysis are shown in Figure 3 only for the scCO$_2$-dried beetroot samples.

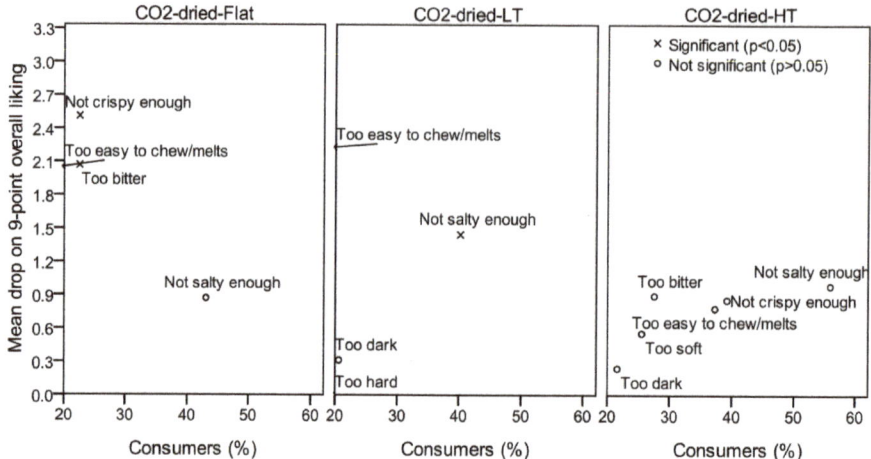

Figure 3. Mean drop analysis for supercritical CO$_2$-dried beetroot samples (N = 102 respondents).

Points in the mean drop plot represent the drops of the averaged hedonic scores linked to the consumer groups who felt a particular attribute "too little" or "too much" in regard to the "just about right" level. The direction of potential product modification is sought among those points with a large proportion of consumers and a statistically significant mean drop [39]. There were two large consumer groups (≥20%) with statistically significant ($p < 0.05$) mean drops (Figure 3), one of which felt the scCO$_2$-dried-Flat sample was "not crispy enough" (22.5%), and one who felt the dried product was "too bitter" (22.5%). The scCO$_2$-dried-LT sample was felt by the consumers as "not salty enough" (40.2% of the consumers, $p < 0.05$). As for the scCO$_2$-dried-HT sample, there were no points in the plot with large consumer groups and significant mean drops, but it is worth mentioning that all of the mean acceptance scores for the "just right" consumer groups were less than 5.4 (data not shown), i.e., not in the range of acceptable products. The freeze-dried sample was rated as "too light/pale" in color, "not crispy enough" and "too bitter", while the fried sample appeared to be felt as "too hard" and "too bitter" according to the tested consumers.

3.3. Sensory Quality Rating

Table 3 shows the results of the sensory quality rating of the dried products. Mean overall quality scores in the range of "very good" quality (i.e., above 3.5) were found only in the scCO$_2$-dried-Flat and scCO$_2$-dried-LT samples (3.7 both). Overall sensory quality levels of the other samples were in the range of "good" quality with the scores significantly lower as compared to the former two ($p < 0.05$). The non-pre-cooked scCO$_2$-dried samples (Flat and LT) were characterized by the typical beetroot magenta color evenly distributed over the surface to a large extent, low level of shape and surface deformations, non-intensive beetroot odor and flavor, pronounced brittleness and crispiness, and good rehydration during mastication. The pre-cooking step before drying negatively influenced the sensory quality parameters, at first appearance. The scCO$_2$-dried-HT sample appeared shrunken and distorted, the waves obtained after initial slicing with the curved knife were mostly damaged after drying, the surface was darker in color with the occurrence of dark discolorations as compared with the other two scCO$_2$-dried products, flavor was empty and hay-like with the beetroot flavor totally lost, and it was harder, more cohesive, and less airy than the Flat and LT scCO$_2$-dried samples.

Similar negative effects of scCO$_2$-drying on sensory quality were observed also in red bell pepper and apple fruits. In the case of red bell pepper, the main defects were related to the loss of color and flavor intensities, with the simultaneous occurrence of a hay-like odor [24], while the apples suffered partial shape deformation, the appearance of cracks on the flesh surface, and the appearance of reddish/pinkish discoloration in flesh originating from the skin color [22,23]. Satisfied textural characteristics such as crispiness, airy denseness, good chewiness, and good rehydration during mastication were observed in both pepper and apple cases. Frying of beetroot slices led to the product being characterized by pronounced shape deformation (mostly bended in the shape of a saddle), very dark in magenta color with the grime-black areas on the surface, the presence of airborne blisters on the surface indicating that the product was oil-fried, pronounced oil-like odor and over-burnt/grime flavor, bitterness, and mild sourness. On the other hand, the fried product was very crispy, firm, but not too hard or brittle, with a relatively good rehydration rate during chewing (with residual small solid particles in the mass), and accordingly the texture was assessed as "very good" (4.1 ± 0.8, Table 3). Contrary to expectations based on the experience with red bell pepper and apple in the previous studies [23,24], freeze-dried beetroot got relatively low quality scores in general. The score-lowering factors in the case of the freeze-dried sample were primarily related to the appearance attributes such as the presence of numbers of relatively large holes and cracks on the upper surface of the beetroot slices, uneven distribution of magenta color on the upper surface with the presence of discolorations and ash-gray color notes which are not characteristic of beetroot, absence of magenta color on the bottom surface of the cuts with dominating dark brownish-ash-gray color, but also to less intensive beetroot flavor with the presence of the common root vegetables-like flavor notes. Despite the freeze-dried sample was brittle and crispy, firm but not too hard, airy, and easy-to-chew, the texture quality score was below 3.5 (in the range of "good" quality) compared with the scCO$_2$-dried samples not pre-cooked (Flat and LT) whose texture scores were within the range of "very good" quality. These findings indicate the different behavior of red beetroot in comparison with red bell pepper and apple when exposed to freeze-drying. In both latter cases, freeze-drying resulted in the highest sensory quality scores of the dried commodities among the applied drying techniques [23,24]. As reported by the same authors, air-drying was not indicated as a good solution for the production of this kind of dried ready-to-eat fruit/vegetable snacks as it delivers products with very pronounced hardness which negatively influences chewiness, presence of off-flavors, and distinct shape deformation, which all together result in a reduction of both consumer acceptance and objective sensory quality score [22–24].

Table 3. Sensory quality scores [1] for dried beetroot samples.

Beetroot Samples	Overall Quality	Appearance	Odor	Texture	Flavor
CO$_2$-dried Flat	3.7 ± 0.6 [b]	4.3 ± 0.6 [c]	2.6 ± 1.2 [a,b]	3.9 ± 0.7 [a,b]	4.0 ± 0.7 [b]
CO$_2$-dried LT (Curvy)	3.7 ± 0.6 [b]	3.9 ± 0.7 [c]	2.5 ± 1.3 [a]	4.2 ± 0.8 [b]	3.9 ± 0.8 [b]
CO$_2$-dried HT (Curvy)	2.9 ± 0.6 [a]	3.8 ± 0.8 [c]	2.3 ± 0.8 [a]	3.4 ± 0.8 [a]	2.4 ± 1.0 [a]
Fried	3.0 ± 0.9 [a]	2.8 ± 0.7 [b]	2.3 ± 1.2 [a]	4.1 ± 0.8 [b]	2.6 ± 1.4 [a]
Freeze-dried	3.0 ± 1.0 [a]	1.8 ± 1.1 [a]	3.2 ± 1.1 [b]	3.4 ± 0.9 [a]	2.9 ± 1.4 [a]

[1] Arithmetic mean ± standard deviation (10 assessors × 2 replications). The same letter within a column indicates values that are not statistically different ($\alpha = 0.05$).

4. Conclusions

According to the sensory evaluation conducted, direct scCO$_2$-drying, without a pre-cooking step and application of high temperatures, showed promising potential to be used as an alternative drying technology in the production of dried beetroot snacks, but an economic justification is required for the industrial application at a large scale. The trials with beetroot revealed that scCO$_2$-drying can bring the dried product with significantly higher levels of sensory quality and consumer acceptance than can be obtained by freeze-drying which is considered today as the best drying method for many fruits and vegetables. Among the tested beetroot samples, a "very good" level of overall sensory quality was found only in those two samples dried using scCO$_2$ without applying the thermal treatment before drying. Mean overall sensory quality score for freeze-dried beetroot was in the range of "good" quality. Further, almost 59% of tested consumers showed a preference for the two scCO$_2$-dried beetroot samples not subjected to the cooking step before drying, which were characterized by typical beetroot magenta color, low level of shape and surface deformations, pronounced brittleness and crispiness, and good rehydration during mastication. Freeze-drying had negative effects primarily on appearance attributes, but also on the flavor of dried beetroot, resulting in partial loss of the typical beetroot flavor. The main defect in the fried beetroot was related to overburnt/grime flavor notes and appearance. Nevertheless, according to the acceptance testing, the consumers from all of the obtained clusters scored the fried beetroot product as acceptable. This could be explained by the fact that the product was salted and relatively similar to commercial potato chips or extruded corn snacks—the products that are ready-to-eat and that are commonly consumed as a fast food within the population tested in this study (university students).

Author Contributions: Conceptualization, G.H., A.R., N.T. and I.D.; methodology, N.T.; validation, N.T. and I.D.; formal Analysis, N.T.; investigation, N.T., I.D., N.S. and B.U.; resources, G.H. and N.T.; data Curation, N.T. and I.D.; writing—original draft preparation, N.T.; writing—review and editing, I.D., N.S., B.U. and A.R.; visualization, N.T.; supervision, I.D. and A.R.; project administration, I.D.; funding acquisition, G.H. All authors have read and agreed to the published version of the manuscript.

Funding: This research has received funding from the European Union's Horizon 2020 research and innovation programme under grant agreement No 635759: Faster Upcoming Technology Uptake Relevant for the Environment in FOOds Drying ("FUTURE-FOOD").

Conflicts of Interest: The authors declare no conflict of interest.

References

1. Aguilera, J.M.; Chiralt, A.; Fito, P. Food dehydration and product structure. *Trends Food Sci. Technol.* **2003**, *14*, 432–437. [CrossRef]
2. Berk, Z. Chapter 22—Dehydration. In *Food Process Engineering and Technology*, 2nd ed.; Berk, Z., Ed.; Academic Press: San Diego, CA, USA, 2013; pp. 511–566.
3. Brown, Z.K.; Fryer, P.J.; Norton, I.T.; Bakalis, S.; Bridson, R.H. Drying of foods using supercritical carbon dioxide—Investigations with carrot. *Innov. Food Sci. Emerg. Technol.* **2008**, *9*, 280–289. [CrossRef]
4. Witrowa-Rajchert, D.; Rząca, M. Effect of Drying Method on the Microstructure and Physical Properties of Dried Apples. *Dry. Technol.* **2009**, *27*, 903–909. [CrossRef]
5. Nijhuis, H.H.; Torringa, H.M.; Muresan, S.; Yuksel, D.; Leguijt, C.; Kloek, W. Approaches to improving the quality of dried fruit and vegetables. *Trends Food Sci. Technol.* **1998**, *9*, 13–20. [CrossRef]
6. Rizzolo, A.; Vanoli, M.; Cortellino, G.; Spinelli, L.; Contini, D.; Herremans, E.; Bongaers, E.; Nemeth, A.; Leitner, M.; Verboven, P.; et al. Characterizing the tissue of apple air-dried and osmo-air-dried rings by X-CT and OCT and relationship with ring crispness and fruit maturity at harvest measured by TRS. *Innov. Food Sci. Emerg. Technol.* **2014**, *24*, 121–130. [CrossRef]
7. Mayor, L.; Sereno, A.M. Modelling shrinkage during convective drying of food materials: A review. *J. Food Eng.* **2004**, *61*, 373–386. [CrossRef]
8. Jayaraman, K.S.; Das Gupta, D.K. Drying of Fruits and Vegetables. In *Handbook of Industrial Drying*, 4th ed.; Mujumdar, A.S., Ed.; CRC Press, Taylor & Francis Group: Boca Raton, FL, USA, 2015; pp. 611–635.
9. Bourdoux, S.; Li, D.; Rajkovic, A.; Devlieghere, F.; Uyttendaele, M. Performance of Drying Technologies to Ensure Microbial Safety of Dried Fruits and Vegetables. *Compr. Rev. Food Sci. Food Saf.* **2016**, *15*, 1056–1066. [CrossRef]
10. Szczesniak, A.S. Texture is a sensory property. *Food Qual. Prefer.* **2002**, *13*, 215–225. [CrossRef]
11. Krokida, M.K.; Maroulis, Z.B. Effect of drying method on shrinkage and porosity. *Dry. Technol.* **1997**, *15*, 2441–2458. [CrossRef]
12. Nistor, O.-V.; Seremet, L.; Andronoiu, D.G.; Rudi, L.; Botez, E. Influence of different drying methods on the physicochemical properties of red beetroot (*Beta vulgaris* L. var. *Cylindra*). *Food Chem.* **2017**, *236*, 59–67. [CrossRef]

13. Oreopoulou, V.; Krokida, M.; Marinos-Kouris, D. Frying of Foods. In *Handbook of Industrial Drying*, 4th ed.; Mujumdar, A.S., Ed.; CRC Press, Taylor & Francis Group: Boca Raton, FL, USA, 2015; pp. 1189–1207.
14. Pei, F.; Shi, Y.; Mariga, A.M.; Yang, W.-J.; Tang, X.-Z.; Zhao, L.-Y.; An, X.-X.; Hu, Q.-H. Comparison of Freeze-Drying and Freeze-Drying Combined with Microwave Vacuum Drying Methods on Drying Kinetics and Rehydration Characteristics of Button Mushroom (*Agaricus bisporus*) Slices. *Food Bioprocess Technol.* **2014**, *7*, 1629–1639. [CrossRef]
15. Berk, Z. Chapter 23—Freeze Drying (Lyophilization) and Freeze Concentration. In *Food Process Engineering and Technology*, 2nd ed.; Berk, Z., Ed.; Academic Press: San Diego, CA, USA, 2013; pp. 567–581.
16. Donsì, G.; Ferrari, G.; Matteo, D.I. Utilization of Combined Processes in Freeze-Drying of Shrimps. *Food Bioprod. Process.* **2001**, *79*, 152–159. [CrossRef]
17. Benali, M.; Boumghar, Y. Supercritical Fluid-Assisted Drying. In *Handbook of Industrial Drying*, 4th ed.; Mujumdar, A.S., Ed.; CRC Press, Taylor & Francis Group: Boca Raton, FL, USA, 2015; pp. 1261–1270.
18. Knez, Ž.; Markočič, E.; Leitgeb, M.; Primožič, M.; Knez Hrnčič, M.; Škerget, M. Industrial applications of supercritical fluids: A review. *Energy* **2014**, *77*, 235–243. [CrossRef]
19. Brunner, G. Supercritical fluids: Technology and application to food processing. *J. Food Eng.* **2005**, *67*, 21–33. [CrossRef]
20. Djas, M.; Henczka, M. Reactive extraction of carboxylic acids using organic solvents and supercritical fluids: A review. *Sep. Purif. Technol.* **2018**, *201*, 106–119. [CrossRef]
21. Sabirzyanov, A.N.; Il'in, A.P.; Akhunov, A.R.; Gumerov, F.M. Solubility of Water in Supercritical Carbon Dioxide. *High Temp.* **2002**, *40*, 203–206. [CrossRef]
22. Tomic, N.; Djekic, I.; Zambon, A.; Spilimbergo, S.; Bourdoux, S.; Holtze, E.; Hofland, G.; Sut, S.; Dall'Acqua, S.; Smigic, N.; et al. Challenging chemical and quality changes of supercritical CO_2 dried apple during long-term storage. *LWT* **2019**, *110*, 132–141. [CrossRef]
23. Djekic, I.; Tomic, N.; Bourdoux, S.; Spilimbergo, S.; Smigic, N.; Udovicki, B.; Hofland, G.; Devlieghere, F.; Rajkovic, A. Comparison of three types of drying (supercritical CO_2, air and freeze) on the quality of dried apple—Quality index approach. *LWT Food Sci. Technol.* **2018**, *94*, 64–72. [CrossRef]
24. Zambon, A.; Tomic, N.; Djekic, I.; Hofland, G.; Rajkovic, A.; Spilimbergo, S. Supercritical CO_2 Drying of Red Bell Pepper. *Food Bioprocess Technol.* **2020**, *13*, 753–763. [CrossRef]
25. Şahin, İ.; Özbakır, Y.; İnönü, Z.; Ulker, Z.; Erkey, C. Kinetics of Supercritical Drying of Gels. *Gels* **2018**, *4*, 3. [CrossRef]
26. Giobbe, G.G.; Zambon, A.; Vetralla, M.; Urbani, L.; Deguchi, K.; Pantano, M.F.; Pugno, N.M.; Elvassore, N.; De Coppi, P.; Spilimbergo, S. Preservation over time of dried acellular esophageal matrix. *Biomed. Phys. Eng. Express* **2018**, *4*, 65021. [CrossRef]
27. Braeuer, A.; Schuster, J.; Gebrekidan, M.; Bahr, L.; Michelino, F.; Zambon, A.; Spilimbergo, S. In Situ Raman Analysis of CO_2—Assisted Drying of Fruit-Slices. *Foods* **2017**, *6*, 37. [CrossRef] [PubMed]
28. Michelino, F.; Zambon, A.; Vizzotto, M.T.; Cozzi, S.; Spilimbergo, S. High power ultrasound combined with supercritical carbon dioxide for the drying and microbial inactivation of coriander. *J. CO_2 Util.* **2018**, *24*, 516–521. [CrossRef]
29. Vetralla, M.; Ferrentino, G.; Zambon, A.; Spilimbergo, S. A study about the effects of supercritical carbon dioxide drying on apple pieces. *Int. J. Food Eng.* **2018**, *4*, 186–190. [CrossRef]
30. Djekic, I.; Tomic, N.; Smigic, N.; Udovicki, B.; Hofland, G.; Rajkovic, A. Hygienic design of a unit for supercritical fluid drying—Case study. *Br. Food J.* **2018**, *120*, 2155–2165. [CrossRef]
31. Režek Jambrak, A.; Vukušić, T.; Donsi, F.; Paniwnyk, L.; Djekic, I. Three Pillars of Novel Nonthermal Food Technologies: Food Safety, Quality, and Environment. *J. Food Qual.* **2018**, *2018*, 18. [CrossRef]
32. Ferrentino, G.; Spilimbergo, S. High pressure carbon dioxide pasteurization of solid foods: Current knowledge and future outlooks. *Trends Food Sci. Technol.* **2011**, *22*, 427–441. [CrossRef]
33. Bourdoux, S.; Rajkovic, A.; De Sutter, S.; Vermeulen, A.; Spilimbergo, S.; Zambon, A.; Hofland, G.; Uyttendaele, M.; Devlieghere, F. Inactivation of Salmonella, Listeria monocytogenes and Escherichia coli O157:H7 inoculated on coriander by freeze-drying and supercritical CO_2 drying. *Innov. Food Sci. Emerg. Technol.* **2018**, *47*, 180–186. [CrossRef]
34. Zambon, A.; Michelino, F.; Bourdoux, S.; Devlieghere, F.; Sut, S.; Dall'Acqua, S.; Rajkovic, A.; Spilimbergo, S. Microbial inactivation efficiency of supercritical CO_2 drying process. *Dry. Technol.* **2018**, *36*, 2016–2021. [CrossRef]

35. Agterof, W.G.M.; Bhatia, R.; Hofland, G.W. Dehydration Method. European Patent Bulletin 2009/42 EP 1,771,074 B1, 14 October 2009.
36. Forde, C.G.; van Kuijk, N.; Thaler, T.; de Graaf, C.; Martin, N. Oral processing characteristics of solid savoury meal components, and relationship with food composition, sensory attributes and expected satiation. *Appetite* **2013**, *60*, 208–219. [CrossRef]
37. ASTM. Manual on Descriptive Analysis Testing for Sensory Evaluation. In *ASTM Manual Series: MNL 13*; Hootman, R.C., Ed.; ASTM—American Society for Testing and Materials: Philadelpfia, PA, USA, 1992.
38. Romano, R.; Brockhoff, P.B.; Hersleth, M.; Tomic, O.; Næs, T. Correcting for different use of the scale and the need for further analysis of individual differences in sensory analysis. *Food Qual. Prefer.* **2008**, *19*, 197–209. [CrossRef]
39. Lawless, H.T.; Heymann, H. *Sensory Evaluation of Food: Principles and Practices*, 2nd ed.; Springer Science+Business Media, LLC: New York, NY, USA, 2010.
40. Meilgaard, M.; Civille, G.V.; Carr, T.B. *Sensory Evaluation Techniques*, 3rd ed.; CRC Press LLC: Boca Raton, FL, USA, 1999.
41. Rothman, L.; Parker, M.J. Structure and Use of Just-About-Right Scales. In *ASTM Manual Series: MNL 63—Just-About-Right (JAR) Scales: Design, Usage, Benefits and Risks*; Rothman, L., Parker, M.J., Eds.; ASTM International—American Society for Testing and Materials: Bridgeport, NJ, USA, 2009; pp. 1–13.
42. McEwan, J.A. Preference mapping for product optimization. In *Multivariate Analysis of Data in Sensory Science*; Naes, T., Risvik, E., Eds.; Elsevier Science B.V.: Amsterdam, The Netherlands, 1996; pp. 71–102.
43. Schraidt, M. Appendix L: Penalty analysis or mean drop analysis. In *ASTM Manual Series: MNL 63—Just-About-Right (JAR) Scales: Design, Usage, Benefits and Risks*; Rothman, L., Parker, M.J., Eds.; ASTM International—American Society for Testing and Materials: Bridgeport, NJ, USA, 2009; pp. 50–53.
44. Grice, J.W. Idiogrid: Software for the management and analysis of repertory grids. *Behav. Res. Methods Instrum. Comput.* **2002**, *34*, 338–341. [CrossRef] [PubMed]
45. Grice, J.W.; Assad, K.K. Generalized Procrustes Analysis: A tool for exploring aggregates and persons. *Appl. Multivar. Res.* **2009**, *13*, 93–112. [CrossRef]
46. Stevens, J.P. *Applied Multivariate Statistics for the Social Sciences*, 5th ed.; Taylor & Francis Group, LLC: New York, NY, USA, 2009.
47. Rahman, M.S. Dried Food Properties: Challenges Ahead. *Dry. Technol.* **2005**, *23*, 695–715. [CrossRef]
48. Figiel, A. Drying kinetics and quality of beetroots dehydrated by combination of convective and vacuum-microwave methods. *J. Food Eng.* **2010**, *98*, 461–470. [CrossRef]
49. Kaur, K.; Singh, A.K. Drying kinetics and quality characteristics of beetroot slices under hot air followed by microwave finish drying. *Afr. J. Agric. Res.* **2014**, *9*, 1036–1044.
50. Ravichandran, K.; Saw, N.M.M.T.; Mohdaly, A.A.A.; Gabr, A.M.M.; Kastell, A.; Riedel, H.; Cai, Z.; Knorr, D.; Smetanska, I. Impact of processing of red beet on betalain content and antioxidant activity. *Food Res. Int.* **2013**, *50*, 670–675. [CrossRef]
51. Kowalski, S.J.; Szadzińska, J. Kinetics and Quality Aspects of Beetroots Dried in Non-Stationary Conditions. *Dry. Technol.* **2014**, *32*, 1310–1318. [CrossRef]
52. Ferrentino, G.; Balzan, S.; Spilimbergo, S. Supercritical Carbon Dioxide Processing of Dry Cured Ham Spiked with Listeria monocytogenes: Inactivation Kinetics, Color, and Sensory Evaluations. *Food Bioprocess Technol.* **2013**, *6*, 1164–1174. [CrossRef]

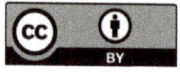

© 2020 by the authors. Licensee MDPI, Basel, Switzerland. This article is an open access article distributed under the terms and conditions of the Creative Commons Attribution (CC BY) license (http://creativecommons.org/licenses/by/4.0/).

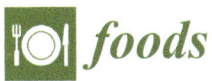

Article

Edible Flowers, Old Tradition or New Gastronomic Trend: A First Look at Consumption in Portugal versus Costa Rica

Raquel P. F. Guiné [1], Sofia G. Florença [2], Keylor Villalobos Moya [3] and Ofélia Anjos [4,5,*]

1. CERNAS Research Centre, Polytechnic Institute of Viseu, 3504-510 Viseu, Portugal; raquelguine@esav.ipv.pt
2. Faculty of Food and Nutrition Sciences, University of Porto, 4200-465 Portugal; sofiaguine@gmail.com
3. School of Agrarian Sciences, National University of Costa Rica, Heredia, Costa Rica; keylorvm87@gmail.com
4. Polytechnic Institute of Castelo Branco, 6001-909 Castelo Branco, Portugal
5. Forest Research Centre, School of Agriculture, University of Lisbon, 1349-017 Lisbon, Portugal
* Correspondence: ofelia@ipcb.pt; Tel.: +351-272-339-900

Received: 21 June 2020; Accepted: 20 July 2020; Published: 23 July 2020

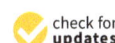

Abstract: This study investigated the knowledge and use of edible flowers (EF) in two countries, Portugal, in Europe, and Costa Rica, in Latin America, and aimed to evaluate the similarities and/or differences regarding the utilization of EF in gastronomy. This work consisted of a questionnaire survey, undertaken on a sample of 290 participants. The results indicate that most people surveyed (87%) have heard about EF but believe there is not enough information about them (96%). Only one third of participants consider there are risks associated with the consumption of EF, being those related to toxicity and pesticides. Significant differences ($p < 0.05$) were found between participants from the two countries but not with different professional areas. About half (48%) of the participants had already consumed EF, mostly for decoration or confection of dishes (77% positive answers) and in salads (75%). The flowers consumed most frequently were chamomile and rose, respectively, in Costa Rica and Portugal. Reasons pointed out to consume EF include decoration, taste, novelty and aroma, while aspects such as nutritional value or antioxidant capacity are prized by fewer consumers. EF were mostly acquired in supermarkets, cultivated at home or collected in the wild. In general, most participants (85%) consider the use of EF in gastronomy interesting, but less than one third (27%) believe we should eat EF more often. Finally, discriminant function analysis revealed that country was the variable for which the differences in the consumption of EF was more pronounced, while education level and age group showed the lowest variability between groups.

Keywords: edible flowers; food security; gourmet kitchen; knowledge; questionnaire survey

1. Introduction

The consumption of flowers in ancient time is known, on one hand, for being a part of traditional culinary practices, while being also used in the field of alternative medicines. In civilizations in ancient Rome and Greece, as well as in China, the tradition of using edible flowers (EF) is linked to a historic concept, being their use in food preparation, as aroma enhancers, to add flavor and aesthetic value. For example, roses (*Rosa* spp. L.) were used in ancient Rome to provide flavor and sweetness to dishes, in drinks, salads, purees, omelets, and desserts. In France, during the Middle Ages, flowers of calendula (*Calendula officinalis*) were consumed in a wide variety of salads. Documented use of violets (*Viola odorata* L.) in the 17th century related to their ability to confer sweetness and color to syrups [1–3].

Although EF have been consumed over the ages, their use is not as widespread as other foods and their inclusion in gastronomic preparations is more often linked to special occasions, gourmet cuisine and certain chefs' recipes or suggestions. The health and aesthetic properties of EF represent a niche market nowadays; however, from a strategic point of view, the food industry and food service operators might greatly benefit from a wider inclusion of EF in food products, pre-prepared meals, drinks, freshly prepared dishes and desserts, as a way of positive differentiation and service enhancement [4,5].

According to a review by Fernandes et al. [6] about the benefits of EF for human health, they possess nutritional value—being rich in moisture, carbohydrates and protein, and being low in lipids. They also contain interesting amounts of ash, including dietary minerals such as calcium, iron, potassium, magnesium, phosphorous or zinc. Furthermore, they contain bioactive components, such as phenolic compounds, which contribute to their high antioxidant activity, while also conferring color and aroma. Other biological effects include antimicrobial and anti-inflammatory activities which are also reported to inhibit cell proliferation, turning them into a potential ally for cancer treatment and prevention [7–10]. Still, it is important to bear in mind what amounts need to be ingested for these health effects to be effective on the human body. From this point of view, many of these possible health claims are not yet established through recommended intake dosages.

As with other food categories, the consumption of edible flowers involves a complex decision process, when making food choices. These food choices are related to the products' characteristics but also to the individual's history and context, including integration of personal ideas, resources and social influences with the social, cultural and physical environments [11–16]. With regard to EF, some people consider the unique combination of their pleasant visual aspect, color, aroma, taste, shape and nutrition, consequently invoking these reasons when deciding to consume EF. On the other hand, some people value their nutritional composition more and them being fresh, unprocessed or minimally processed food products, making these the reasons for eating them [4,17].

This study was carried out to assess the knowledge and use of EF in two countries situated in different parts of the globe, Portugal in Europe and Costa Rica in Latin America, possibly representing different realities regarding the utilization of EF in gastronomy.

2. Materials and Methods

2.1. Data Collection and Sample Characterization

This survey was based on a questionnaire that was applied to a convenience sample in two countries, Portugal and Costa Rica. The convenience sample was chosen according to the facility to recruit and place of residence, and it was intended to have a minimum of approximately 150 responses in each of the countries. Therefore, the questionnaire was sent to a high number of people in each of the countries, but the responses obtained were limited in number, a little higher in Portugal than in Costa Rica (151 and 139, respectively). Convenience samples have both the advantages of easy recruitment and not allowing generalization according to estimates of sociodemographic differences. In addition, they can be a good tool for exploratory research [18–21]. All data collected were treated with confidentiality and met all ethical issues, so that it was impossible to link the answers to a particular individual. The survey was conducted with adult participants only, who answered the questionnaire voluntarily. The data collection was approved by the Ethical Committee at Polytechnic Institute of Viseu and all participants gave explicit consent prior to the data collection.

This survey included 290 participants, of which 47.9% were from Costa Rica and 52.1% were from Portugal, leading to an even distribution between countries (Table 1). The average age of the participants was 40 ± 13 years, slightly higher in Portugal (41 ± 13 years) than in Costa Rica (38 ± 12 years). Most of the participants were aged between 31 and 50 years (52.7%), and the elderly were those least represented (2.1%). Regarding the highest level of education, most of the participants had completed a university degree (83.1%), however, fewer had just completed basic education (3.1%). As for the living environment, the great majority lived in urban (67.2%), followed by rural (22.8%) and then suburban (10.0%) environment. For the combined results of both countries, for all sociodemographic variables considered, a relative homogeneity between the samples from Portugal and Costa Rica was observed—the sex variable was an exception, for which the percentage of men was considerably higher in Costa Rica (37.4%) than Portugal (19.2%).

Table 1. Sociodemographic characterization of the study sample.

	Variable	Costa Rica	Portugal	Total [1]
	Dimension: N (%)	139 (47.9)	151 (52.1)	290 (100)
	Age [2] (MV ± SD years)	38 ± 12	41 ± 13	40 ± 13
Age group	Young adults (18–30 years) (%)	30.2	23.8	26.9
	Middle aged adults (31–50 years) (%)	52.6	53.0	52.7
	Senior adults (51–65 years) (%)	15.8	20.5	18.3
	Elderly (≥66 years) (%)	1.4	2.6	2.1
Sex	Women (%)	62.6	80.8	72.1
	Men (%)	37.4	19.2	27.9
Education level	Basic (%)	2.9	3.3	3.1
	Secondary (%)	12.2	15.2	13.8
	University (%)	84.9	81.5	83.1
Living environment	Urban (%)	66.2	68.0	67.2
	Suburban (%)	12.9	7.3	10.0
	Rural (%)	20.9	24.7	22.8

[1] Combined results of Portugal and Costa Rica. [2] Age expressed as mean value (MV) ± standard deviation (SD).

The professional area of the participants (either regarding work or studies) was also assessed considering its possible influence on the level of information and consumptions habits towards EF. The results in Table 2 indicate that, while in Portugal a high percentage of participants had professional areas related with food and nutrition (58.0%), in Costa Rica the percentage for these areas was much smaller (only 17.3%). Additionally, the professionals linked with restaurants and hotels were more frequent in Portugal (12.1%) than in Costa Rica (5.0%). Regarding professions or studies in the domain of agriculture or agricultural sciences, both countries had a similar representation (31.2% in Costa Rica and 29.3% in Portugal).

Table 2. Professional area of the participants.

Professional Area	Costa Rica		Portugal		Total [1]	
	Yes (%)	No (%)	Yes (%)	No (%)	Yes (%)	No (%)
Nutrition/Food	17.3	82.7	58.0	42.0	38.4	61.6
Agriculture	31.2	68.8	29.3	70.7	30.2	69.8
Hotels/Restaurants	5.0	95.0	12.1	87.9	8.7	91.3
Not related to any of the above	43.5	56.5	38.3	61.7	47.0	53.0

[1] Combined results of Portugal and Costa Rica.

2.2. Data Analysis

Exploratory analysis was done using SPSS software V25 (IBM, United States Inc.). The crosstabs and chi-square test were used to evaluate possible relations between some of the categorical variables studied at a level of significance of 5%. The coefficient Cramer's V was used to express the strength of the significant relations found between variables. This coefficient varies, ranging from 0 (no association) to 1 (perfect association), and for V ≈ 0.1 the association is considered weak, V ≈ 0.3 the association is moderate and V ≈ 0.5 or higher, the association is strong [22]. When the conditions did not allow the use of the chi-square test, the Fisher's exact test was used.

Discriminant function analysis (DFA) was performed using statistic software from StatSoft (Vs 7.09). This is a statistical procedure that classifies unknown individuals and estimates the probability of their classification into a certain group (for example sex or country). DFA assumes a normal distribution for the sample, and the subsequent probability and typicality probability are applied to calculate the classification probabilities [23].

3. Results and Discussion

3.1. Information about Edible Flowers

Flowers have traditionally been used in gastronomy in various cultures, such as European, Asian, East Indian, Victorian English, and Middle Eastern [24]. Up to the present, EF have been greatly used as garnish in high-end foodservice establishments. However, their potential is considerably greater. EF can be used fresh as a garnish or as an integral part of a dish, for example in salads, but some other applications include stuffing or use in stir-fry dishes. Flowers can also be used to add color and flavor to foods, for example soups, entrées, desserts or drinks. Finally, EF have also been introduced into processed foods to add diversity and innovation to the food market, besides the nutritional and health benefits for consumers [2,24,25].

This led us to investigate the knowledge and habits relating to EF in Portugal and Costa Rica, which have different social and cultural backgrounds. Table 3 shows the results obtained for the whole sample, separated by country, as well as the results of the chi-square tests made to evaluate if there were statistically significant differences between countries in relation to various aspects of information linked with EF. The first aspect investigated was whether the participants knew what EF were. The results of this survey showed that the great majority of the participants had already heard about EF (86.9%), particularly in Portugal where almost everyone knew about EF (96.7%), while in Costa Rica that percentage was lower, but still high (76.3%). The differences between both countries were statistically significant ($p < 0.0005$) and there was a moderate association between these two variables, country and having heard about EF ($V = 0.302$).

Table 3. Information about edible flowers (EF), according to country.

Question		Total [1]	Costa Rica	Portugal	CST [2]		CC [3]
					x^2	p	V
Have you heard about EF?	Yes (%)	86.9	76.3	96.7	26.530	<0.0005 [5]	0.302
	No (%)	13.1	23.7	3.3			
Do you think there is enough information about EF?	Yes (%)	3.8	3.6	4.0	0.028	0.557 [5]	-
	No (%)	96.2	96.4	96.0			
Do you think there are risks associated with consumption of EF?	Yes (%)	35.2	27.4	42.4	7.342	0.025	0.159
	No (%)	31.0	33.8	28.5			
	M [4] (%)	33.8	38.8	29.1			
Do you think toxicity is a risk?	Yes (%)	83.8	71.2	93.5	12.237	0.001 [5]	0.300
	No (%)	16.2	28.8	6.5			
Do you think pesticides are a risk?	Yes (%)	80.9	68.3	91.8	12.105	<0.0005 [5]	0.298
	No (%)	19.1	31.7	8.2			
Do you think there are other risks?	Yes (%)	50.5	39.6	58.7	3.995	0.035	0.190
	No (%)	49.5	60.4	41.3			

[1] Combined results of Portugal and Costa Rica. [2] CST: chi-square test (level of significance of 5%: $p < 0.05$) for country differences. [3] CC: Cramer's coefficient, only indicated if there were significant differences. [4] This option accounts for Maybe/I do not know. [5] Fisher's exact test.

A good level of information is fundamental to help make food decisions in general, and this is even more true when it comes to EF. Hence, some of the aspects investigated aimed to evaluate the degree of knowledge that the participants had about different aspects related with EF. In appearance, EF are similar to ornamental flowers, since many of the species are used in both contexts. They are beautiful but also interesting from the organoleptic and nutritional point of view while at the same time being safe for human consumption. Nevertheless, if it is true that all edible species can be used for decorative purposes, the contrary is not true, and it is crucial to distinguish them for their edibility by using chemical and biological parameters [1,26]. The results obtained showed differences between

Portugal and Costa Rica in relation to some aspects that measure the level of knowledge about EF. This has been reported previously by Rodrigues et al. in [25]. Despite the attention that EF have been gaining in the past years, it appears that they are not popular for consumption in Latin America, being considered unfamiliar to some cultures in the American continent. Information and knowledge about EF are fundamental to help consumers understand whether they can be used and how, as well as what benefits they provide from the organoleptic, nutritional or even medicinal points of view [4,27,28].

As for the question regarding the availability of information about EF, very similar results were found in both countries, with practically all participants stating that they considered the information about EF as not enough (about 96%) (Table 3). For this question, no significant differences were found between countries.

Aspects linked to safety and possible risks involved in the consumption of EF were also investigated. The obtained results indicated that only about one third of the participants (35.1%) considered that there were risks associated with the consumption of EF; specifically, the Portuguese participants were more aware of this possibility (42.4%) than Costa Rican participants (27.4%) (Table 3). Furthermore, a very important percentage of participants (33.8%) could not express an opinion about this fact, replying maybe or I do not know. The differences found between countries were statistically significant ($p = 0.025$) but the association was weak ($V = 0.159$).

In the 21st century, the agro-food industry faces many challenges, including food security (the need to provide enough food to be consumed) and food safety (products that are safe to eat). EF meet these challenges and additionally they allow for introducing innovative products with nutraceutical properties and health benefits to the market [26,29]. Regarding the food safety domain, EF pose some additional concerns. While purely decorative flowers sometimes have toxic components that can lead to intoxication or even death, the flowers used for human consumption have to be absolutely safe. Additionally, in many cases, the cultivation of decorative flowers involves the use of harmful chemicals, whereas EF, aimed for gastronomic purposes or other consumption options, such as medicinal preparations, for example, are usually obtained through organic production [6]. Seeing as two main aspects linked to the safety of EF are important, specific questions were formulated to evaluate if the participants considered toxicity and/or pesticides as risks associated with EF consumption. In fact, regarding these questions the great majority of participants assumed they believed toxicity (83.8%) and pesticides (80.9%) to be effective risks when consuming EF (Table 3). Again, very marked differences were encountered between participants from Portugal and Costa Rica, with the percentages for those who consider these as risks being much higher in the Portuguese sample (93.5% and 91.8%, respectively, for toxicity and pesticides) as compared with Costa Rica (71.2% and 68.3%, respectively). These differences were significant ($p = 0.001$ and $p < 0.0005$, respectively, for Portugal and Costa Rica) and the associations between variables were moderate in both cases ($V = 0.300$ and $V = 0.298$, respectively). One last question investigated if the participants considered that other risks could be associated with EF, and in this case the percentage of agreement was lower. Here, 50.5% of participants believed other risks could be involved in the consumption of EF, again, the higher percentage being Portugal, with significant differences between both countries ($p = 0.035$) but a relatively weak association ($V = 0.190$).

As well as hypothesizing that some professionals working in some specific areas could possibly have a different pattern of answers when compared with the common participants, it was also investigated if there were differences between participants not related and those related with the following areas: Agriculture, Food and Nutrition, Hotels and Restaurants. These results are presented in Table 4 where Portugal and Costa Rica are considered together.

The results in Table 4 show significant differences ($p < 0.0005$) between the participants related within the professional areas previously specified and those who were not related for the question about having already heard about EF, with a significantly higher percentage of yes for the participants related (94.7% against 22.2%, respectively, for related and not related). Furthermore, the association between being or not being related with the specified professional areas and having heard about EF was moderate ($V = 0.250$). Regarding the question of whether the participants considered if there is enough information about EF, no significant differences were found, and in both groups the percentage of participants that considered the information to be scarce was very high.

Table 4. Information about edible flowers (EF), according to professional areas in Portugal and Costa Rica (considered together).

Question		Related [1]	Not Related [1]	CST [2]		CC [3]
				χ^2	p	V
Have you heard about EF?	Yes (%)	94.7	22.2	17.901	<0.0005 [5]	0.250
	No (%)	5.3	77.8			
Do you think there is enough information about EF?	Yes (%)	5.3	2.2	1.794	0.151 [5]	-
	No (%)	94.7	97.8			
Do you think there are risks associated with consumption of EF?	Yes (%)	46.7	22.2	19.234	0.442	-
	No (%)	27.0	35.6			
	M [4] (%)	26.3	42.2			
Do you think toxicity is a risk?	Yes (%)	86.7	77.8	1.738	0.142 [5]	-
	No (%)	16.3	22.2			
Do you think pesticides are a risk?	Yes (%)	80.5	81.3	0.012	0.552 [5]	-
	No (%)	19.5	18.7			
Do you think there are other risks?	Yes (%)	50.0	50.0	0.000	0.579 [5]	-
	No (%)	50.0	50.0			

[1] Related or not related with the following areas: Nutrition/Food, Agriculture, Hotels/Restaurants. [2] CST: chi-square test (level of significance of 5%: $p < 0.05$) for country differences. [3] CC: Cramer's coefficient, only indicated if there were significant differences. [4] This option accounts for Maybe/I do not know. [5] Fisher's exact test.

In the question regarding the risk associations of EF, participants with professional links with Food and Nutrition, Agriculture or Hotels and Restaurants are more aware of the risks in general (46.7% against 22.2% for those not related), more alert to the risk of toxicity (86.7% against 77.8%) but not to the risk of pesticides (80.5% against 81.3%) or other risks (50% for both). Nevertheless, these differences were not statistically significant.

EF bring interesting elements to culinary and dietary habits; therefore, chefs find in EF valuable allies to their gastronomic preparations due to their aromas and bouquet, their color, shapes and the sensations they evoke [30]. Because of their nutritive and bioactive compounds, such as polyphenols and their antioxidant properties, they also contain important dietary elements with nutritional and health benefits, recognized by the professionals linked with nutrition and health [31,32]. The cultivation of EF has to obey special requirements, usually in organic mode, and farmers are expected to be aware of the effects of the utilization of chemical products in their farms [6,30]. Nevertheless, despite these aspects, it was found that the professional area did not significantly impact the level of knowledge about EF.

3.2. Use of Edible Flowers

About half of the participants in this survey (47.6%) had already consumed EF, and this percentage was very similar for both countries (47.7% and 47.5% for Costa Rica and Portugal, respectively). For those who had already consumed EF, it was asked in what ways and/or for what purposes they consumed EF. The results showed that 77% had consumed EF for decoration and confection of dishes, 75% had consumed EF in salads, 49% in starters, 43% as aroma intensifiers, 26% in jellies and 33% in other non-specified possibilities. Figure 1 shows the ways consumption differentiated by country and similar results were found for the use of EF as decoration and confection of dishes (70% for Costa Rica and 83% for Portugal) as well as in salads (71% for Costa Rica and 78% for Portugal), these being the most frequent forms of consumption in both countries. The use in jellies showed the lowest incidence in both countries (less than 30%) but the use in starters and as aroma intensifiers was more pronounced among Portuguese participants (64% and 50%, respectively) than among those from Costa Rica (32% and 35%, respectively). Although traditionally EF have been mainly used due to their smell and visual appeal, new and innovative value has been attributed to flowers as part of the food market and chefs' resources. Apart from being consumed fresh or cooked, they can be used in savory dishes containing meat and fish, in soups and drinks (such as wine, beer, vinegar or spirits), in desserts, sweets, jellies, as well as spices, and dyes. Furthermore, they can also be used in a dried form, ground into powder, crystallized or used as foams in molecular gastronomy [2,4].

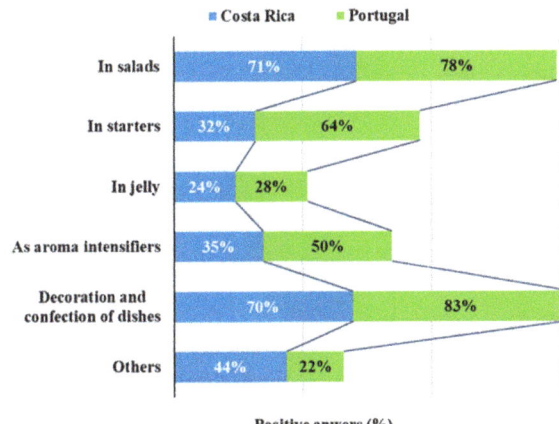

Figure 1. Possible ways in which the participants consumed edible flowers.

One other question of the survey investigated which flowers the participants had already consumed. There are many flowers that are safe for human consumption and their usage can be varied according to availability and the chef's discretion. Some of the most frequently reported EF include violet, pansy, marigold, rose, daisy, chicory, gardenia, hibiscus or jasmine, to name a few [6,32], and those most consumed by the participants in this study are included in this list. In this study, the most consumed flowers were chamomile and rose (by 62% of the participants in both cases). Then came the pumpkin flower (49%), pansy (38%), sunflower (32%), calendula (26%), orchid (10%), and others not specified were consumed by 53% of the participants. The results shown in Figure 2, which separates the consumption by country, indicate that most of the flowers which are popular in Costa Rica are also popular in Portugal and vice-versa: chamomile (64% and 61%, respectively, for Costa Rica and Portugal) and rose (55% and 69%, respectively) as the most popular, and orchid (15% and 6%, respectively) as the least. The usage of EF is very much dependent on tradition on one side, but also on innovation and new gastronomic trends on the other. While in Europe and Asia there is an old tradition linked with the usage of flowers for human consumption which is well documented, in some other parts of the world this habit is not so present among the population. Additionally, European chefs are among those who use creativity to explore the application of EF into their recipes [5,25], and this helps to explain some differences found when comparing the usage of EF in Portugal and in Costa Rica.

Regarding the frequency of consumption, 94% consumed EF sporadically (100% of the participants from Costa Rica and 88% of the participants from Portugal) and only 6% consumed them regularly. Some differences could be observed between the two countries, while in Portugal 12% already consume EF on a regular basis, in Costa Rica no one does.

Decoration, novelty, taste and aroma were cited as the most relevant reasons to use EF, while nutrition and antioxidant activity have the lowest importance. Nevertheless, the nutritional importance of many different EF has been established, as well as the value associated with some of the bioactive compounds that they contain that bear biological activities beneficial for human health—for example, the high antioxidant activity provided by phenolic compounds [6,33,34]. The reasons why participants consumed EF were varied and included their ability to decorate dishes or other food preparations (66%), their exquisite taste (62%), the perception of novelty associated with their utilization

(62%), their aroma and bouquet (57%), their bioactive compounds that bear antioxidant activity (37%), their nutritional value, most especially regarding micronutrients lime vitamins and minerals (26%), among others (21%). Figure 3 represents the reasons indicated by the participants, separated by country, and some differences could be identified. While Portuguese consumers value more decoration (74%) and novelty (69%) those from Costa Rica value more taste (70%) followed by decoration (58%). In addition, differences were found for the value of nutrition and antioxidant properties, which were much more prized by the consumers in Costa Rica (33% and 44%, respectively) than in Portugal (19% and 31%, respectively).

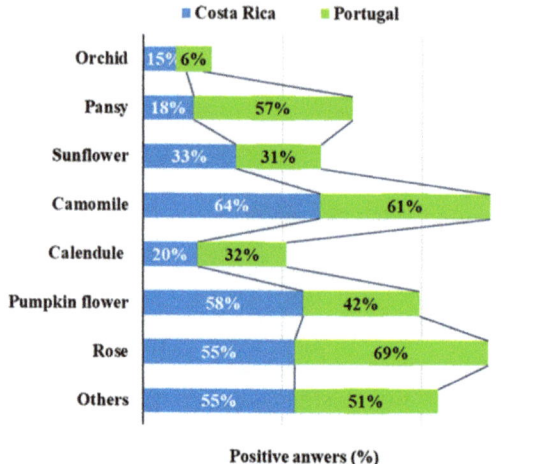

Figure 2. Types of flowers consumed by the participants.

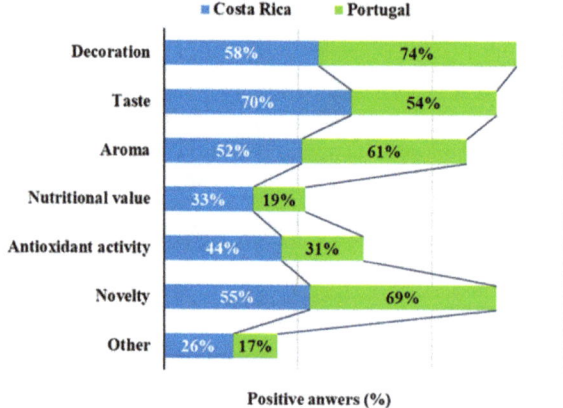

Figure 3. Reasons pointed out by the participants for consumption of EF.

The places where the participants ate EF for the first time were in restaurants (for 46%), followed by the participants' own homes (30%) and only a small percentage ate them for the first time in cafés or pastry shops (4%). According to Figure 4, the first consumption for the Portuguese occurred mostly at restaurants (57%) and with a lower expression at home (25%), while in Costa Rica both places were even (35% and 36%, respectively, for homes and restaurants). As chefs know already that some aspects linked with culinary pleasure captured through our senses are closely connected to emotions, they explore this by using ingredients and raw materials which are able to awaken these sensations. Hence, flowers, due to their varied colors, intense aromas and exquisite taste, are among those ingredients, and restaurants are, therefore, places where EF can be found in gastronomic preparations [35,36].

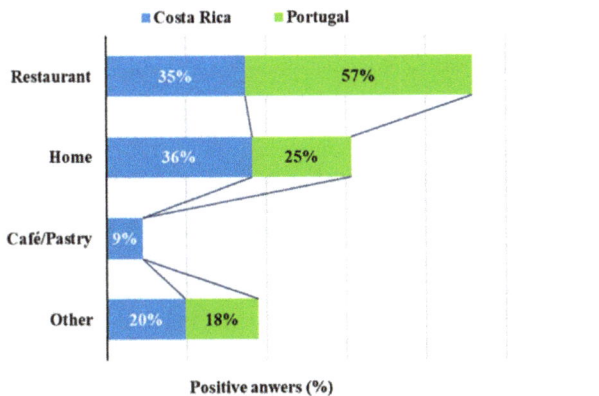

Figure 4. Places where participants consumed EF for the first time.

It was observed that 29% of the participants used EF for gastronomic preparations, this percentage being equal in both countries. Additionally, it was observed that the fresh state was the preferred form of consumption, by 75% of participants, while 43% used them cooked. Some differences were found between countries for the utilization of EF in the cooked form, being more expressive among consumers in Costa Rica (58%) than in Portugal (29%) (Figure 5).

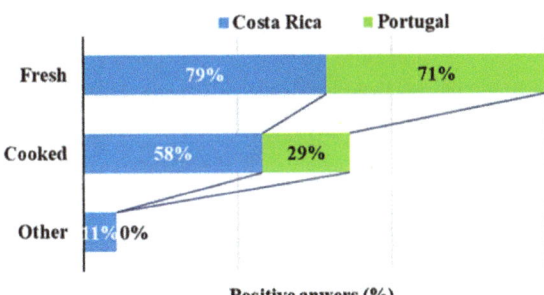

Figure 5. Forms of consumption of EF.

The marketing of fresh EF poses some challenges as both dehydration and oxidation make them highly perishable, diminishing their nutritional and bioactive characteristics. On the other hand, they are easily contaminated by insects, thus compromising their safety while also decreasing their attractiveness. For these reasons, fresh edible flowers are sold packed in rigid plastic containers [4]. Regarding the places where consumers obtain EF, most participants buy them in supermarkets (43%) or collect them in the wild (58%) or grow them at home (53%). Still a worrying fraction admit buying EF in flower shops (13%), which is highly critical, since ornamental flowers may not, and many times do not, comply with the necessary quality criteria to be ingested as foods [1]. Flowers can carry traces of pesticides and insects, and therefore, flowers grown for ornamental purposes may be among the edible species but should not be used for human consumption because they may be contaminated with pesticides or special fertilizers for better blooming. The flowers used in gastronomy should be cultivated purposely by the cook who will use them or bought from organic vegetable producers, as safe foods [5].

Some differences were found also for this question among participants from different countries (Figure 6), since in Costa Rica home cultivation is the most frequent way to obtain EF (58%), followed by the supermarket (53%) and then collection in the wild (47%), while in Portugal the most expressive way to obtain EF is to collect them from the wild (67%), then home cultivation (48%) and the supermarket comes in third (33%). The buying of EF in flower shops is more pronounced in Costa Rica (16%) compared to Portugal (10%).

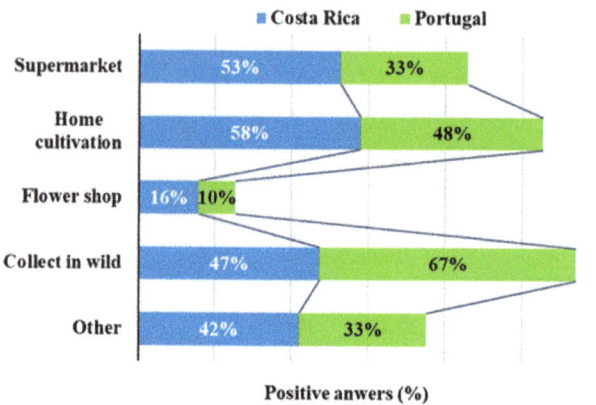

Figure 6. Places where the participants buy EF.

Another aspect investigated in this study, related to the ease of obtaining EF, is only 15% consider it is easy to obtain EF, while 36% think not, but almost half of the participants (49%) think maybe or do not know. These results were very similar for both countries, as indicated in Figure 7. As EF are still a niche in the food market, it is natural that their availability is lower when compared with other food categories such as fruits and vegetables [5].

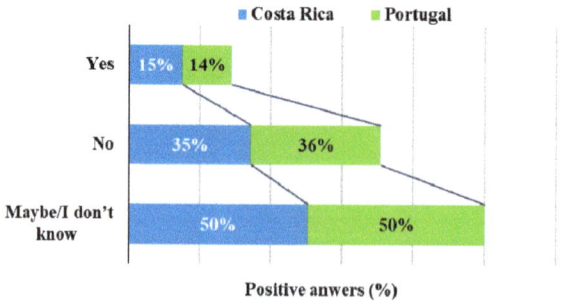

Figure 7. Availability of EF.

Finally, two questions were dedicated to gathering the participants' opinions about the usage of EF in gastronomy. The results obtained showed that most participants (85%) consider the use of EF for gastronomic purposes interesting, particularly those from Costa Rica (89%) with a higher expression than Portugal (80%) (Figure 8). Regarding the second question, only 27% believe that we should eat EF more often, being a higher percentage for participants from Costa Rica (35%) than Portugal (20%).

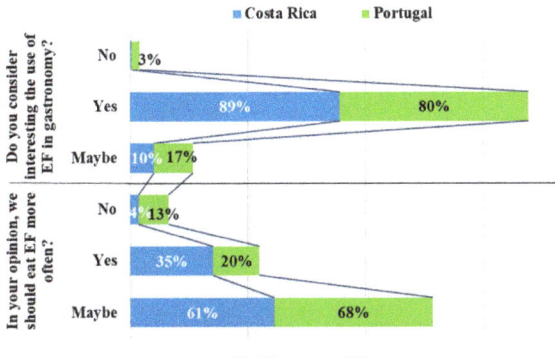

Figure 8. Opinions about the use of EF for culinary purposes.

3.3. Effect of Sociodemographic Variables in Edible Flowers' Consumption

DFA is used to determine which variables discriminate between two or more naturally occurring groups. In this study, DFA was used to determine which variable(s) are the best predictors for the consumers' subsequent choice. The discriminant function is a linear function of the predictor variables such that it can discriminate between groups of respondents, i.e., differentiate low probability or high probability for a specific consumption attitude group. This is estimated by including all the predictors simultaneously and using the direct method of discriminant analysis.

For the question "How did you eat the flowers?" it was observed that education level, living environment and age group do not influence the consumers' attitudes (Table 5). Nevertheless, statistical differences were found between sex groups for the use of EF in decoration and confection of dishes (female participants eat the flowers more in decoration and confection of dishes than male participants do). The differences observed between the two countries were assigned by the different uses of EF in starters.

Concerning the question "Which flowers have you already eaten?" for both age group and education level, no significate differences were observed (Table 5). However, significant differences were found in the pansy and pumpkin flower consumption in both countries. Additionally, it was further observed that the pansy flowers were consumed differently according to gender. It was observed also that the living environment influences the consumption of pumpkin flowers and roses.

For the frequency of the consumption of EF, only in the country and education level groups were significant differences found. For almost all sociodemographic groups studied, the motives for the consumption of EF did not present statistical differences. Conversely, the age group presented statistical differences concerning the use as decoration and for nutritional purposes (Table 5). The way the participants in each country consume flowers is significantly different when it comes to the consumption in the fresh form or cooked. This result is in accordance with the aforementioned statistic discussed in Figure 5, which shows that participants from Costa Rica eat cooked EF in much higher percentages than those from Portugal.

For the question "If you use EF, where do you buy them?" significant differences were found only for the living environment variable and regarding the option "others", which accounts for other ways to buy EF not specified in the answering possibilities (Table 5). Furthermore, no significant differences were found in the question "Is there enough information about EF?" for country, age group, sex and education level variables. In this case only the different sex groups showed different opinions about the availability of information on EF. Regarding the risks associated with the consumption of EF, only for the risks associated with pesticides were there differences found in the participants from both countries and for both sexes (Table 5).

Table 5. Discriminant function analysis summary (p-value).

Questions		Country	Age Group	Sex	Living Environment	Education Level
How did you eat the flowers?	In salads	ns	ns	ns	ns	ns
	In starters	0.0019 **	ns	ns	ns	ns
	In jelly	ns	ns	ns	ns	ns
	As aroma intensifiers	ns	ns	ns	ns	ns
	Decoration and confection of dishes	ns	ns	0.0307 *	ns	ns
	Others	0.0232 *	ns	ns	ns	ns
Which flowers have you already eaten?	Orchid	ns	ns	ns	ns	ns
	Pansy	0.0001 ***	ns	0.0125 *	ns	ns
	Sunflower	ns	ns	ns	ns	ns
	Chamomile	ns	ns	ns	ns	ns
	Calendula	ns	ns	ns	ns	ns
	Pumpkin flower	0.0405 *	ns	ns	0.0007 ***	ns
	Rose	ns	ns	ns	0.0209 *	ns
	Others	ns	ns	ns	ns	ns
Frequency of consumption of EF?		0.0021 **	ns	ns	ns	0.0199 *
What motivates you to consume them?	Decoration	ns	0.0287 *	ns	ns	ns
	Taste	ns	ns	ns	ns	ns
	Aroma	ns	ns	ns	ns	ns
	Nutrition	ns	0.0346 *	ns	ns	ns
	Antioxidant activity	ns	ns	ns	ns	ns
	Novelty	ns	ns	ns	ns	ns
	Other	ns	ns	ns	ns	ns
If you consume EF, in what form?	Fresh	0.0251 *	ns	ns	ns	ns
	Cooked	0.0053 **	Δ	ns	ns	Δ
	Other	ns	ns	ns	ns	ns
If you use EF, where do you buy them?	Supermarket	ns	ns	ns	ns	ns
	Home cultivation	ns	ns	ns	ns	ns
	Flower shop	ns	Δ	ns	ns	Δ
	Collect in wild	ns	ns	ns	ns	ns
	Other	ns	ns	ns	0.0051 **	ns
Is there enough information about EF?		ns	ns	0.0396 *	ns	ns
Risks associated with consumption of EF	Toxicity	ns	ns	ns	ns	ns
	Pesticides	0.0055 **	ns	0.0032 **	ns	Δ
EF are easy to obtain?	Other	ns	ns	ns	ns	ns
		ns	ns	ns	ns	ns
In your opinion we should eat EF more often?		ns	ns	ns	ns	ns

EF: edible flowers. ns: $p > 0.05$; * $0.01 < p < 0.05$; ** $0.001 < p < 0.01$; *** $p < 0.001$. Δ—some groups contain only a valid case.

For the questions "EF are easy to obtain?" and "In your opinion we should eat EF more often?" no significant differences were found for all sociodemographic groups.

4. Conclusions

The present work concluded that the level of information about EF is significantly different between participants form the two countries evaluated, namely Costa Rica and Portugal. The highest differences were found in the knowledge about EF, or the risks associated with their consumption, particularly concerning toxicity and pesticides, for which the associations were moderate. As for the differences in information considering different professional groups, no significant differences were found except for having heard about EF, for which the association was moderate.

Regarding the use of EF, they are used mainly for decoration and confection of dishes and in salads, and those most consumed are rose and chamomile, which are consumed sporadically. Reasons for the consumption of EF include decoration, novelty, taste and aroma. Most participants ate EF for the first time in restaurants, and they consume them mostly fresh. In regard to obtaining EF, it consists mainly in collecting them in the wild, followed by home cultivation and then supermarkets, but consumers believe it is quite difficult to acquire. A great majority of the participants believe that the use of EF for gastronomic purposes is interesting, but a much smaller fraction believe that we should eat EF more often.

Finally, DFA revealed that country was the variable for which the differences in the consumption of EF between groups was more pronounced, while education level and age group showed the lowest variability between groups.

As our sample was recruited by convenience, more women and more people with university degrees volunteered to participate in the survey, and this constitutes one limitation of the study, also considering the limited number of responses obtained. However, this study is a first approach to understanding the habits of EF consumption in these two countries, highlighting which aspects are more relevant for the consumption of this type of product, from the point of view of the consumer. Additionally, this study allows for some complementing future lines of work, namely the importance of safety assurance, quality control and marketing issues, including labelling as a way to protect and inform consumers.

Author Contributions: Conceptualization, R.P.F.G. and O.A.; methodology, R.P.F.G. and O.A.; software, R.P.F.G. and O.A.; validation, R.P.F.G. and O.A.; formal analysis, R.P.F.G. and O.A.; investigation, all authors; resources, R.P.F.G.; data curation, R.P.F.G.; writing—original draft preparation, R.P.F.G., S.G.F. and O.A.; writing—review and editing, all authors; visualization, R.P.F.G.; supervision, R.P.F.G.; project administration, R.P.F.G.; funding acquisition, R.P.F.G. and O.A. All authors have read and agreed to the published version of the manuscript.

Funding: This research was funded by CI&DETS Research Centre (Polytechnic Institute of Viseu, Portugal) grant number PROJ/CI&DETS/2017/0028. The APC was funded by FCT—Foundation for Science and Technology (Portugal) project Reference UIDB/00681/2020 and project Reference UIDB/00239/2020.

Acknowledgments: This work was supported by National Funds through the FCT—Foundation for Science and Technology, I.P., within the scope of the project Reference UIDB/00681/2020. Furthermore, we would like to thank the CERNAS Research Centre and the Polytechnic Institute of Viseu for their support. This work was prepared in the ambit of the project from CI&DETS Research Centre (Polytechnic Institute of Viseu, Portugal) with reference PROJ/CI&DETS/2017/0028. Thanks to project reference POCI-01-0145-FEDER-029305, co-financed by the Foundation for Science and Technology (FCT) and the European Regional Development Fund (ERDF), through Portugal 2020—Competitiveness and Internationalization Operational Program (POCI). Thanks to Forest Research Centre, a research unit funded by FCT (UIDB/00239/2020).

Conflicts of Interest: The authors declare no conflict of interest.

References

1. Mlcek, J.; Rop, O. Fresh edible flowers of ornamental plants—A new source of nutraceutical foods. *Trends Food Sci. Technol.* **2011**, *22*, 561–569. [CrossRef]
2. Takahashi, J.A.; Rezende, F.A.G.G.; Moura, M.A.F.; Dominguete, L.C.B.; Sande, D. Edible flowers: Bioactive profile and its potential to be used in food development. *Food Res. Int.* **2020**, *129*, 108868. [CrossRef]

3. Vinokur, Y.; Rodov, V.; Reznick, N.; Goldman, G.; Horev, B.; Umiel, N.; Friedman, H. Rose Petal Tea as an Antioxidant-rich Beverage: Cultivar Effects. *J. Food Sci.* **2006**, *71*, S42–S47. [CrossRef]
4. Chen, N.-H.; Wei, S. Factors influencing consumers' attitudes towards the consumption of edible flowers. *Food Qual. Prefer.* **2017**, *56*, 93–100. [CrossRef]
5. Guiné, R.; Florença, S.G.; Ferrão, A.C.; Correia, P.M. Investigation about the consumption of edible flowers in Portugal. *Indian J. Tradit. Knowl. (IJTK)* **2019**, *18*, 579–588.
6. Fernandes, L.; Casal, S.; Pereira, J.A.; Saraiva, J.A.; Ramalhosa, E. Edible flowers: A review of the nutritional, antioxidant, antimicrobial properties and effects on human health. *J. Food Compos. Anal.* **2017**, *60*, 38–50. [CrossRef]
7. Guiné, R.P.F.; Pedro, A.; Matos, J.; Barracosa, P.; Nunes, C.; Gonçalves, F.J. Evaluation of phenolic compounds composition, antioxidant activity and bioavailability of phenols in dried thistle flower. *Food Meas.* **2017**, *11*, 192–203. [CrossRef]
8. Kucekova, Z.; Mlcek, J.; Humpolicek, P.; Rop, O.; Valasek, P.; Saha, P. Phenolic compounds from *Allium schoenoprasum*, *Tragopogon pratensis* and *Rumex acetosa* and their antiproliferative effects. *Molecules* **2011**, *16*, 9207–9217. [CrossRef]
9. Nowak, R.; Olech, M.; Pecio, L.; Oleszek, W.; Los, R.; Malm, A.; Rzymowska, J. Cytotoxic, antioxidant, antimicrobial properties and chemical composition of rose petals. *J. Sci. Food Agric.* **2014**, *94*, 560–567. [CrossRef]
10. Skowyra, M.; Calvo, M.; Gallego, M.; Azman, N.; Almajano, M. Characterization of Phytochemicals in Petals of Different Colours from Viola × wittrockiana Gams and Their Correlation with Antioxidant Activity. *J. Agric. Sci.* **2014**, *6*, 93–105. [CrossRef]
11. Biondi, B.; Van der Lans, I.A.; Mazzocchi, M.; Fischer, A.R.H.; Van Trijp, H.C.M.; Camanzi, L. Modelling consumer choice through the random regret minimization model: An application in the food domain. *Food Qual. Prefer.* **2019**, *73*, 97–109. [CrossRef]
12. O'Connor, E.L.; Sims, L.; White, K. Ethical food choices: Examining people's Fair Trade purchasing decisions. *Food Qual. Prefer.* **2017**, *60*, 105–112. [CrossRef]
13. Reddy, G.; van Dam, R.M. Food, culture, and identity in multicultural societies: Insights from Singapore. *Appetite* **2020**, *149*, 104633. [CrossRef] [PubMed]
14. Risso, D.S.; Giuliani, C.; Antinucci, M.; Morini, G.; Garagnani, P.; Tofanelli, S.; Luiselli, D. A bio-cultural approach to the study of food choice: The contribution of taste genetics, population and culture. *Appetite* **2017**, *114*, 240–247. [CrossRef] [PubMed]
15. Sirasa, F.; Mitchell, L.; Silva, R.; Harris, N. Factors influencing the food choices of urban Sri Lankan preschool children: Focus groups with parents and caregivers. *Appetite* **2020**, *150*, 104649. [CrossRef]
16. Zoltak, M.J.; Veling, H.; Chen, Z.; Holland, R.W. Attention! Can choices for low value food over high value food be trained? *Appetite* **2018**, *124*, 124–132. [CrossRef]
17. Rop, O.; Mlcek, J.; Jurikova, T.; Neugebauerova, J.; Vabkova, J. Edible flowers—A new promising source of mineral elements in human nutrition. *Molecules* **2012**, *17*, 6672–6683. [CrossRef]
18. Hill, M.M.; Hill, A. *Investigação por Questionário*, 2nd ed.; Sílabo: Lisboa, Portugal, 2008.
19. Marôco, J. *Análise Estatística com o SPSS Statistics*, 7th ed.; Report Number: Lisboa, Portugal, 2018.
20. Robinson, O.C. Sampling in Interview-Based Qualitative Research: A Theoretical and Practical Guide. *Qual. Res. Psychol.* **2014**, *11*, 25–41. [CrossRef]
21. Bornstein, M.H.; Jager, J.; Putnick, D.L. Sampling in developmental science: Situations, shortcomings, solutions, and standards. *Dev. Rev.* **2013**, *33*, 357–370. [CrossRef]
22. Witten, R.; Witte, J. *Statistics*, 9th ed.; Wiley: Hoboken, NJ, USA, 2009.
23. Moore, M.K. Chapter 4—Sex Estimation and Assessment. In *Research Methods in Human Skeletal Biology*; DiGangi, E.A., Moore, M.K., Eds.; Academic Press: New York, NY, USA, 2013; pp. 91–116. ISBN 978-0-12-385189-5.
24. Kaisoon, O.; Siriamornpun, S.; Weerapreeyakul, N.; Meeso, N. Phenolic compounds and antioxidant activities of edible flowers from Thailand. *J. Funct. Foods* **2011**, *3*, 88–99. [CrossRef]
25. Rodrigues, H.; Cielo, D.P.; Goméz-Corona, C.; Silveira, A.A.S.; Marchesan, T.A.; Galmarini, M.V.; Richards, N.S.P.S. Eating flowers? Exploring attitudes and consumers' representation of edible flowers. *Food Res. Int.* **2017**, *100*, 227–234. [CrossRef] [PubMed]
26. Pires, T.C.S.P.; Barros, L.; Santos-Buelga, C.; Ferreira, I.C.F.R. Edible flowers: Emerging components in the diet. *Trends Food Sci. Technol.* **2019**, *93*, 244–258. [CrossRef]

27. Cunningham, E. What Nutritional Contribution Do Edible Flowers Make? *J. Acad. Nutr. Diet.* **2015**, *115*, 856. [CrossRef]
28. Shi, J.; Gong, J.; Liu, J.; Wu, X.; Zhang, Y. Antioxidant capacity of extract from edible flowers of *Prunus mume* in China and its active components. *LWT Food Sci. Technol.* **2009**, *42*, 477–482. [CrossRef]
29. Scotter, M.J. 6—Methods of analysis for food colour additive quality and safety assessment. In *Colour Additives for Foods and Beverages*; Scotter, M.J., Ed.; Woodhead Publishing Series in Food Science, Technology and Nutrition; Woodhead Publishing: Oxford, UK, 2015; pp. 131–188. ISBN 978-1-78242-011-8.
30. Matyjaszczyk, E.; Śmiechowska, M. Edible flowers. Benefits and risks pertaining to their consumption. *Trends Food Sci. Technol.* **2019**, *91*, 670–674. [CrossRef]
31. Chen, G.-L.; Chen, S.-G.; Xie, Y.-Q.; Chen, F.; Zhao, Y.-Y.; Luo, C.-X.; Gao, Y.-Q. Total phenolic, flavonoid and antioxidant activity of 23 edible flowers subjected to in vitro digestion. *J. Funct. Foods* **2015**, *17*, 243–259. [CrossRef]
32. Pires, T.C.S.P.; Dias, M.I.; Barros, L.; Calhelha, R.C.; Alves, M.J.; Oliveira, M.B.P.P.; Santos-Buelga, C.; Ferreira, I.C.F.R. Edible flowers as sources of phenolic compounds with bioactive potential. *Food Res. Int.* **2018**, *105*, 580–588. [CrossRef]
33. Benvenuti, S.; Bortolotti, E.; Maggini, R. Antioxidant power, anthocyanin content and organoleptic performance of edible flowers. *Sci. Hortic.* **2016**, *199*, 170–177. [CrossRef]
34. Villavicencio, A.L.C.H.; Heleno, S.A.; Calhelha, R.C.; Santos-Buelga, C.; Barros, L.; Ferreira, I.C.F.R. The influence of electron beam radiation in the nutritional value, chemical composition and bioactivities of edible flowers of *Bauhinia variegata* L. var. candida alba Buch.-Ham from Brazil. *Food Chem.* **2018**, *241*, 163–170. [CrossRef]
35. Egebjerg, M.M.; Olesen, P.T.; Eriksen, F.D.; Ravn-Haren, G.; Bredsdorff, L.; Pilegaard, K. Are wild and cultivated flowers served in restaurants or sold by local producers in Denmark safe for the consumer? *Food Chem. Toxicol.* **2018**, *120*, 129–142. [CrossRef]
36. Lightner, M.; Rand, S. The enhancement of natural colors to provoke seasonality. *Int. J. Gastron. Food Sci.* **2014**, *2*, 55–59. [CrossRef]

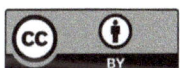

© 2020 by the authors. Licensee MDPI, Basel, Switzerland. This article is an open access article distributed under the terms and conditions of the Creative Commons Attribution (CC BY) license (http://creativecommons.org/licenses/by/4.0/).

MDPI
St. Alban-Anlage 66
4052 Basel
Switzerland
Tel. +41 61 683 77 34
Fax +41 61 302 89 18
www.mdpi.com

Foods Editorial Office
E-mail: foods@mdpi.com
www.mdpi.com/journal/foods

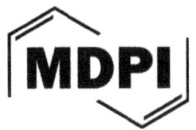

www.ingramcontent.com/pod-product-compliance
Lightning Source LLC
LaVergne TN
LVHW070500100526
838202LV00014B/1760